Handbook ✐ W9-DJB-323 and the Kidney

Sixth Edition

William E. Mitch, MD
Gordon A. Cain Chair in Nephrology
Director, Division of Nephrology
Professor of Medicine
Baylor College of Medicine
Houston, Texas

T. Alp Ikizler, MD
Catherine McLaughlin-Hakim Professor of Medicine
Department of Medicine
Division of Nephrology
Vanderbilt University School of Medicine
Nashville, Tennessee

◉. Wolters Kluwer | Lippincott Williams & Wilkins
Health
Philadelphia · Baltimore · New York · London
Buenos Aires · Hong Kong · Sydney · Tokyo

Acquisitions Editor: Lisa McAllister
Product Manager: Michelle LaPlante
Vendor Manager: Alicia Jackson
Senior Manufacturing Manager: Benjamin Rivera
Marketing Manager: Kimberly Schonberger
Design Coordinator: Teresa Mallon
Production Service: Maryland Composition Inc.

©2010 by **LIPPINCOTT WILLIAMS & WILKINS, a WOLTERS KLUWER business**

530 Walnut Street
Philadelphia, PA 19106 USA
LWW.com

Printed in The People's Republic of China

Library of Congress Cataloging-in-Publication Data
9780781795173
0781795176

Handbook of nutrition and the kidney / [edited by] William E. Mitch, T. Alp Ikizler. — 6th ed.
    p.; cm.
Includes bibliographical references and index.
  ISBN 978-0-7817-9517-3
  1. Kidneys—Diseases—Diet therapy—Handbooks, manuals, etc.
  2. Kidneys—Diseases—Nutritional aspects—Handbooks, manuals, etc. I. Mitch, William E. II. Ikizler, T. Alp.
  [DNLM: 1. Kidney Diseases—diet therapy—Handbooks.
2. Kidney Diseases—metabolism—Handbooks. 3. Nutritional Requirements—Handbooks. WJ 39 H2357 2009]
  RC903.N87 2009
  616.6'10654—dc22

                              2009005096

Care has been taken to confirm the accuracy of the information presented and to describe generally accepted practices. However, the authors, editors, and publisher are not responsible for errors or omissions or for any consequences from application of the information in this book and make no warranty, expressed or implied, with respect to the currency, completeness, or accuracy of the contents of the publication. Application of the information in a particular situation remains the professional responsibility of the practitioner.

The authors, editors, and publisher have exerted every effort to ensure that drug selection and dosage set forth in this text are in accordance with current recommendations and practice at the time of publication. However, in view of ongoing research, changes in government regulations, and the constant flow of information relating to drug therapy and drug reactions, the reader is urged to check the package insert for each drug for any change in indications and dosage and for added warnings and precautions. This is particularly important when the recommended agent is a new or infrequently employed drug.

Some drugs and medical devices presented in the publication have Food and Drug Administration (FDA) clearance for limited use in restricted research settings. It is the responsibility of the health care provider to ascertain the FDA status of each drug or device planned for use in their clinical practice.

To purchase additional copies of this book, call our customer service department at (800) 638-3030 or fax orders to (301) 223-2320. International customers should call (301) 223-2300.

Visit Lippincott Williams & Wilkins on the Internet: at LWW.com. Lippincott Williams & Wilkins customer service representatives are available from 8:30 am to 6 pm, EST.

10 9 8 7 6

Dedication

We dedicate this book to two outstanding investigators: Saulo Klahr and the late Mackenzie Walser. Each made many contributions to the investigation of mechanisms underlying kidney diseases and to the designs of treatments for patients with kidney disease. Besides his many studies of mechanism causing kidney damage, Saulo Klahr was a co-editor of the first five editions of this book, the editor of Kidney International, and served as President of the American Society of Nephrology. Mackenzie Walser was a pioneer in devising nutritionally-based methods to treat patients with chronic kidney disease. His landmark studies introduced a new level of sophistication to the study of the metabolism of kidney disease. We are honored to dedicate this book to these giants in our field.

Contents

Contributing Authors

Naji N. Abumrad, MD
Chairman, Department of Surgery
Vanderbilt University School of Medicine
Nashville, Tennessee

Joanne M. Bargman, MD, FRCPC
Professor of Medicine
University Health Network at the University of Toronto
Toronto General Hospital
Toronto, Ontario, Canada

Ishir Bhan, MD, MPH
Instructor
Department of Medicine
Division of Nephrology
Harvard Medical School
Massachusetts General Hospital
Boston, Massachusetts

Melissa B. Bleicher, MD
Fellow, Renal, Electrolyte, and Hypertension Division
Department of Medicine
University of Pennsylvania
Philadelphia, Pennsylvania

Lilian Cuppari, PhD
Affiliate Professor
Division of Nephrology
Department of Medicine
Federal University of São Paulo
São Paulo, Brazil

Gary C. Curhan, MD, ScD
Associate Professor of Medicine
Channing Laboratory and Renal Division
Department of Medicine
Brigham and Women's Hospital and Harvard Medical School
Associate Professor of Epidemiology
Harvard School of Public Health
Boston, Massachusetts

Ian H. de Boer, MD, MS
Assistant Professor of Medicine
Department of Medicine, Division of Nephrology
University of Washington
Seattle, Washington

Wilfred Druml, MD
Professor of Medicine and Nephrology
Medical University of Vienna
Department of Nephrology
Vienna General Hospital
Vienna, Austria

Denis Fouque, MD, PhD
Professor of Renal Medicine
Chief, Department of Nephrology, Dialysis, and Renal Nutrition
University Claude Bernard Lyon 1
INSERM U870
Hôpital Edouard Herriot
Lyon, France

Simin Goral, MD
Associate Professor of Medicine
Renal, Electrolyte, and Hypertension Division
University of Pennsylvania
Philadelphia, Pennsylvania

Jane H. Greene, RD, CSR
Clinical Instructor
Vanderbilt School of Nursing
Nephrology Dietitian
Vanderbilt Medical Center
Nashville, Tennessee

Fitsum Guebre-Egziabher, MD
Senior Nephrologist
Department of Nephrology, Dialysis, and Renal Nutrition
University Claude Bernard Lyon 1
INSERM U870
Hôpital Edouard Herriot
Lyon, France

Olof Heimbürger, MD, PhD
Associate Professor of Nephrology
Division of Renal Medicine
Baxter Novum Department of Clinical Science, Intervention
  and Technology
Karolinska Institutet
Department of Renal Medicine
Karolinska University Hospital
Stockholm, Sweden

Jonathan Himmelfarb, MD
Professor of Medicine
Joseph W. Eschbach Endowed Chair for Kidney Research
Division of Nephrology
Department of Medicine
University of Washington
Seattle, Washington

T. Alp Ikizler, MD
Catherine McLaughlin-Hakim Professor of Medicine
Department of Medicine
Division of Nephrology
Vanderbilt University School of Medicine
Nashville, Tennessee

Kirsten L. Johansen, MD
Associate Professor of Medicine
Department of Medicine, Epidemiology, and Biostatistics
University of California, San Francisco
San Francisco, California

George A. Kaysen, MD, PhD
Professor of Medicine
Chief, Division of Nephrology
Professor and Acting Chair, Division of Biochemistry and
*   Molecular Medicine*
University of California Davis School of Medicine
Davis, California;
Department of Veterans Affairs Health Care System
Mather, California

Bryan Kestenbaum, MD, MS
Assistant Professor of Medicine
Department of Medicine/Nephrology
University of Washington
Seattle, Washington

Joel D. Kopple, MD
Professor of Medicine and Public Health
Division of Nephrology and Hypertension
Department of Medicine
Harbor-UCLA Medical Center
Torrance, California

Maarit Korkeila, MD, PhD
Nephrologist, Department of Renal Medicine
Karolinska University Hospital at Huddinge
Stockholm, Sweden

Vera Krane, MD
Assistant Professor of Medicine
Department of Medicine
Division of Nephrology
University Hospital
University of Würzburg
Würzburg, Germany

Bengt Lindholm, MD, PhD
Adjunct Professor/Director
Division of Baxter Novum
Department of Clinical Science, Intervention, and Technology
Karolinska Institutet
Karolinska University Hospital Huddinge
Stockholm, Sweden

Tahsin Masud, MD
Associate Professor of Medicine
Renal Division, Department of Medicine
Emory University School of Medicine
Atlanta, Georgia

William E. Mitch, MD
Gordon A. Cain Chair in Nephrology
Director, Division of Nephrology
Professor of Medicine
Baylor College of Medicine
Houston, Texas

Sharon J. Nessim, MD
Lecturer
University of Toronto
Department of Medicine
Division of Nephrology
St. Michael's Hospital
Toronto, Ontario, Canada

Eberhard Ritz, MD
Professor of Medicine
Department of Nephrology
University Heidelberg
Heidelberg, Germany

Jabbar Saliba, MD
Surgical Research Fellow
Vanderbilt University School of Medicine
Nashville, Tennessee

Peter Stenvinkel, MD, PhD
Professor of Nephrology
Department of Renal Medicine
Karolinska University Hospital at Huddinge
Stockholm, Sweden

Ravi Thadhani, MD, MPH
Associate Professor of Medicine
Renal Unit and Department of Medicine
Massachusetts General Hospital
Harvard Medical School
Boston, Massachusetts

Christoph Wanner, MD
Professor of Medicine
Chief, Division of Nephrology
University Hospital
University of Würzburg
Würzburg, Germany

Christopher S. Wilcox, MD, PhD
George E. Schreiner Chair of Nephrology
Chief, Division of Nephrology and Hypertension
Department of Medicine
Georgetown University
Washington, District of Columbia

Jane Y. Yeun, MD
Professor of Clinical Medicine
Director, Nephrology Fellowship Program
University of California Davis School of Medicine
Davis, California;
Sacramento Veterans Administration Medical Center
Mather, California

Michel Zakari, MD
Division of Nephrology
University of California Davis School of Medicine
Davis, California

Preface

In the sixth edition of the *Handbook of Nutrition and the Kidney*, there are important changes and additions. First, there are 13 new authors, including experts from Germany, Canada, Sweden, and Brazil. These authors bring additional new perspectives to the international flavor of the book. Second, we have added new topics to broaden the scope of how changing the diet can influence the course of kidney disease. The new topics include the influence of dietary salt, how diets affect kidney stones, and strategies for obese patients plus the influence of exercise on dietary recommendations. Third, we continue to emphasize practical and clinically relevant aspects of manipulating the diet while making the Handbook more accessible and useful for physicians, dietitians, nurses, and other professionals who provide care to patients with kidney disease. We continue to emphasize the use of figures and tables to demonstrate nutritional principles.

Our goal is to integrate scientific lessons with clinical wisdom to provide readers with clinically useful information that contains a rational approach to supplying the nutritional needs of patients with acute and chronic kidney disease, for patients undergoing maintenance dialysis (both hemodialysis and peritoneal dialysis) or kidney transplantation, for patients with kidney stones, hypertension, diabetic nephropathy, or with the nephrotic syndrome. We have made these changes because we believe the role of nutritional principals in the treatment of patients with kidney disease cannot be overestimated. Specifically, the requirements for protein, energy, minerals, and other elements change substantially with advancing kidney disease, and ignoring these changes can contribute to complications. Besides the new topics, each chapter has been revised and updated by experts in nephrology and clinical nutrition.

We are grateful to the chapter authors for their timely and thoughtful contributions to the Handbook. We especially thank Ms. Carmelita Mitra and Ms. Rebeca Barroso for their expert editorial help, and we thank Ms. Michelle LaPlante, Senior Product Manager, at Lippincott Williams & Wilkins for her patience and advice.

William E. Mitch, MD
T. Alp Ikizler, MD

Nutrition and Energy for Healthy Adults

Naji N. Abumrad and Jabbar Saliba

INTRODUCTION

Nutrition refers to the provision of cells and organisms with the necessary material to support life's growth and maintenance. While in prehistoric time food availability for humans was scarce, eating was a must to provide energy and maintain life. Nowadays food is plentiful, occasionally overabundant, and present in many tasty forms and restriction is sometimes needed to maintain health. Disequilibrium in nutrition will favor a malnutritious state. Currently, the number of obese far exceeds the number of hungry. Knowledge of the basics of food biology and the interactions among its different components are crucial to combat such "epidemics." Sugars, proteins, and lipids are different but work in concert to provide energy and nutrition. Appropriate knowledge of the interactions among these nutrients would likely promote health and prevent disease. The current chapter will examine the basic structures and digestive processes of these nutrients. Food functionality and outcome will be assessed in an interactive context with our metabolic needs and possible effects on human health.

CARBOHYDRATES AND FIBERS

Historical Highlights and Definitions

Carbohydrates are the most widely distributed naturally occurring organic compounds on earth. Sites of primitive sugarcane cultivation plants were found in New Guinea and in northeast India dating as early as 10,000 and 6,000 years BC, respectively. Papyrus, composed mainly of cellulose and wheat starch, was used for writing around the years 4,000 BC especially by the Egyptians. In August 1492, Christopher Columbus stopped at the Canary Islands where he stayed for a month after he became romantically involved with the governor of the island. When leaving, she gave him cuttings of sugarcane which became the first to reach the New World.

The name carbohydrate, or hydrate of carbon, actually makes the chemical definition. An alternative term used for carbohydrate is saccharide, from the Greek language meaning sugar. The general stoichiometric formula of an unmodified simple carbohydrate molecule or monosaccharide is $(C \cdot H_2O)_n$ or $(CHOH)_n$. The number of carbon atoms per molecule can be as few as three or triose(s) ($C_3H_6O_3$: i.e., glyceraldehyde and dihydroxyacetone, which are important in mitochondrial respiration), to as many as nine or nonose(s) ($C_9H_{18}O_9$: like neuraminic acid also called sialic acid, widely found in glycoproteins and gangliosides). Although all these monosaccharides are found in nature, by far the most abundant and the most commonly used in cellular metabo-

1

lism are the hexoses ($C_6H_{12}O_6$), mainly glucose, galactose, fructose, and mannose. Another important class of monosaccharides is the pentoses ($C_5H_{10}O_5$) like the ribose sugar, a main constituent of the cellular deoxyribonucleic acid (DNA) and ribonucleic acid (RNA).

Carbohydrates are classified according to the number of saccharide molecules forming the sugar. They are subdivided into mono-, di-, oligo-, and polysaccharides. Monosaccharides have one molecule like glyceraldehyde, ribose, glucose, galactose, fructose, etc., as described in the previous paragraph. Disaccharides have two molecules; examples include maltose (glucose-glucose), lactose (glucose-galactose), and sucrose (glucose-fructose) or table sugar which is also called saccharose, from the Greek language meaning sweet sugar. Oligosaccharides contain between 3 and 10 monosaccharides, they are often found as components of glycolipids and glycoproteins. An important oligosaccharide is the glycoprotein of the ABO blood type specificity. Finally, polysaccharides have more than 10 molecules although usually the number is much higher between 200 and 2500. The sugar moieties are linked together in a multi-branched structure. Starch is the main plant's polysaccharide whereas glycogen makes its counterpart as the animal's prototype. Both of them are polymers of glucose but glycogen has more extensive branching than starch.

The description of fibers was originally coined in 1953, when Hipsley et al. reported a possible association between dietary fibers and the lower occurrence of pregnancy toxemia. Dietary fibers were analytically defined for the first time in 1972 by Trowell et al. as "the skeletal remains of plant cells resistant to digestion by human enzymes." This definition was subsequently modified by the same group in 1976 into "all plant polysaccharides and lignins which are resistant to hydrolysis by digestive enzymes of the man." Dietary fibers contain mainly complex polysaccharides within their structures, thus their inclusion in the carbohydrate section. It is well known that dietary fibers have many beneficial, though sometimes debatable, effects on human health. In view of the variety of physiological effects and the methodology used to identify and quantify them, various definitions for "dietary fiber" have been proposed and adopted. Substances of animal origins were also described as having similar characteristics as the plants' dietary fibers (e.g., chitosan). In 2005, the Institute of Medicine of the National Academics defined the "fiber concept" as the following:

- Dietary fiber: nondigestible carbohydrates and lignins, those are intrinsic and intact in plants.
- Functional fiber: isolated, nondigestible carbohydrates that have physiological effects in humans.
- Total fiber: the sum of dietary and functional fiber.

Structures

The structure and/or the chemical configuration of the sugar confer its availability for utilization by the metabolic processes in humans. Glucose ($C_6H_{12}O_6$), the most common monosaccharide, exists in ring (cyclic) and open chain (noncyclic) forms. The cyclic form is predominant in nature. Depending on the atomic arrange

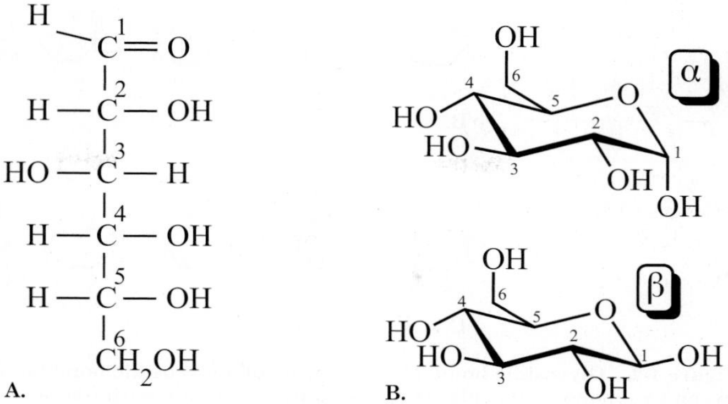

Figure 1-1.   D-glucose. (A) Representation of Dextro-glucose (D-glucose) stereoisomer through Fisher linear projection.
(B) Cyclic representation of D-glucose in a three dimensional perspective or chair conformation, also called Haworth projection.
When the hydroxyl (OH) group on C-1 is on the opposite side of the methyl (CH$_2$OH) group on C-6 the anomer is called (α) and when both chemical groups are on the same side the anomer is called (β).

ment of the spatial structure, or isomeric configuration, glucose (or any hexose) has two stereoisomers named dextro- (D) and levo- (L) isomers (Fig. 1-1A). D and L sugars are nonsuperimposable mirror images of each other; D sugars are the most naturally occurring. While both forms can diffuse into the cell, D-glucose absorption being much higher than L-glucose, only D-glucose contributes to energy production.

In the cyclic form, two spatial structures exist: designated alpha- (α) and beta- (β) anomers. The difference between α-glucose and β-glucose depends on the relative placements of the hydroxyl group (—OH) attached to the first carbon (C-1) and the —CH$_2$OH group attached to the fifth carbon (C-5). In the α anomer the —OH group and the CH$_2$OH group are on different sides of the ring, while in the β anomer both groups are on the same side (Fig. 1-1B). Under physiologic conditions and at equilibrium, the ratio of α-D-glucose to β-D-glucose in a solution is approximately 2:1. The differential uptake and metabolism by the cells of either α or β-D-glucose, also called anomeric specificity, is dependent on the type and function of different cells. Human studies show that β-D-glucose is more readily used for cellular transport and glycolysis in the erythrocyte at physiologic conditions. On the other hand, insulin release by the islets of Langerhans is more specific for the α-D-glucose; this occurs whether the sugar is injected intravenously or given by mouth. A change in the anomeric preference from the α-D-glucose toward the β-D-glucose in the pancreas has been proven in humans with noninsulin–dependent mellitus. Also, human subjects cannot differentiate by taste α- from β-D-glucose.

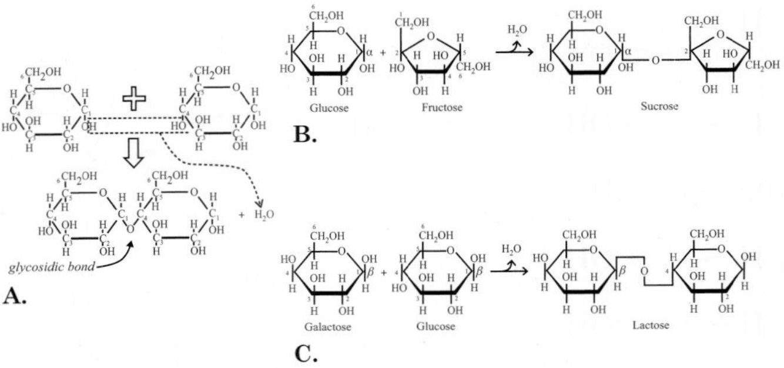

Figure 1-2. Glycosidic bond. (A) Formation of a glycosidic bond between two monosaccharides is a dehydration reaction with liberation of H₂O. (B) α-glycosidic bond: when the bond is on the opposite side of the substituent group (not H) connected to the carbon (C) flanking the oxygen (O). The O ring is considered as the reference plane (in the case of sucrose the substituent group is CH₂OH C-6 that is connected to C-5 of the glucose ring). (C) β-glycosidic bond: the substituent group and the bond are on the same side of the ring.

The structure of a di-, oligo-, or polysaccharide sugar is based on the bonding of two monosaccharides, called glycosidic bond. It is defined as a dehydration reaction between a sugar and another organic molecule. In the case of a disaccharide, two monosaccharides are joined with the loss of one molecule of water. This joining occurs between two —OH groups, one on each monosaccharide (Fig. 1-2A). The chemical formula will be the following:

$$(CHOH)_n + (CHOH)_{n'} \rightarrow (CHO)_nH_{n-1} - (CH)_{n'}(OH)_{n'-1} + H2O$$

Two important features of the glycosidic bond give the sugar its characteristic and also its name. First, the location of the carbon atom, meaning its number on the carbohydrate; second, the configuration α or β assumed by the glycosidic bond. In the cyclic form, carbon atoms are numbered according to their distance from the oxygen atom, which holds the center position, thus the name ring oxygen. One distinguishes between α and β forms depending on the spatial relation between the glycosidic bond and the substituent group, other than hydrogen, connected to the carbon flanking the ring oxygen. In a D sugar, α configuration is when the bond and the substituent group are on opposite sides of the ring (Fig. 1-2B), the β configuration is when both groups are on the same side of the ring (Fig. 1-2C), just like α- and β-D-glucose, respectively. These specifications are important for the sugar's availability for absorption and thus its utilization for energy production and/or storage.

A typical polysaccharide that is by far the most consumed by the human diet is starch. The main source of dietary starch is traditional staple foods such as cereals, roots, and tubers like potatoes. Starch is a polymer of glucose or homopolymer that has

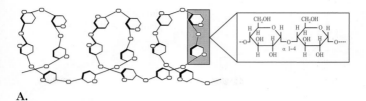

A.

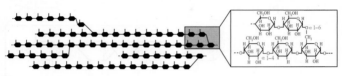

B.

Figure 1-3.   Starch structure. (A) Amylose portion of starch
showing helical formation because of the bend introduced by
the α-glycosidic bonds. The coiling is not interrupted because
all the attachments between the glucose moieties are bent in one
direction; they are all α (1-4) bonds. This configuration is useful
for storage because it relatively occupies less space. At the same
time it gives more resistance to enzymatic access and digestion.
(B) Amylopectin fraction of starch shows a branching structure
with less coiling because the bending introduced by α (1-4) bonds
is interrupted with the α (1-6) bonds that have different directions.

two components. The first is amylose, composed of linear chains
of α (1→4) D-glucose. Amylose is a long chain of glucose subunits,
the number usually ranging between 300 and 3000. The α (1-4)
bonds promote the formation of a helix structure that is important
for storage (Fig. 1-3A). The second macromolecule is amylopectin,
a branched homopolymer composed of linear chains of α (1-4)
D-glucose interconnected with α (1-6) bonding at the branching
points which take place every 20 to 30 molecules of glucose (Fig.
1-3B).

Cellulose, a typical fiber, is the most abundant natural organic
compound on earth. About 33% of all plant matter is cellulose.
It is the structural component of the primary cell wall of green
plants. Cellulose is a condensation of D-glucose moieties connected through β (1-4) glycosidic bonds. In contrast to α (1-4)
present in starch, the β bondings make the linear chain of cellulose less flexible than the amylose chain; accordingly, no coiling
occurs and the molecule adopts an extended and stiff, rod-like
conformation. The open chain configuration exposes multiple
—OH groups and promotes the formation of hydrogen bonds between the glucose residues. These connections stabilize further
the cellulose structure, which becomes organized in the form of
microfibrils with high tensile strength. This alignment provides
resistance to physical disruption of the cellulose molecule (Fig.
1-4). The digestion, thus the absorption, of nutrients containing
cellulose is harder to achieve if this architectural structure is
maintained.

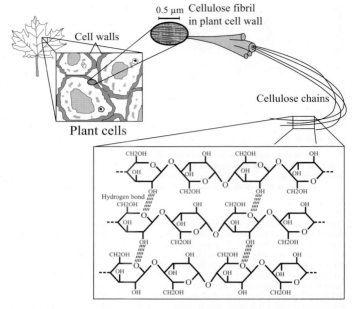

Figure 1-4. Physical and chemical structures of cellulose.
Macroscopic location of cellulose fibers in the cellular wall
gives the plant cells their shape and resilience to physical destruction. The alignment of the cellulose fibrils is enforced by hydrogen bonds that occur between different cellulose chains. The
β (1-4) glycosidic bonds will resist enzymatic digestion in humans.

Digestion

Intracellular metabolic pathways for carbohydrates use monosaccharides as their substrates. A sugar is absorbed by the enterocyte when it is in the monosaccharide form. The digestion of various sugars occurs at different levels in the gastrointestinal
system and by a multitude of enzymes. The end product is the
release of simple sugars or monosaccharides that will be used for
many metabolic functions, mainly energy storage or production.

The digestive process begins in the mouth with the salivary
amylase that is similar in function with the pancreatic amylase
secreted in the duodenum. They are both specific for α (1-4) glycosidic bonds present inside the polysaccharide chain but spare
other α linkages; that is, α (1-6), terminal α (1-4), and α (1-4)
adjacent to a branching point. The amylase digestion of a polysaccharide will yield shorter chain polysaccharides, oligosaccharides, and disaccharides. For example, the digestion of starch by
amylase will result in a group of different lengths' sugars containing maltose (a disaccharide: α-1,4 glucose-glucose), maltotriose
(an oligosaccharide: α-1,4 glucose-glucose-glucose), and α-dex-
trins (α-dextrin = shorter chain polysaccharide: α-1,6 glucose-

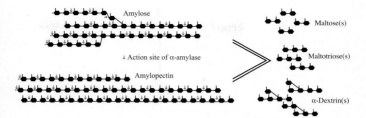

Figure 1-5.   Amylase hydrolysis of amylose and amylopectin, the two components of starch. The enzymatic effect of amylase on α (1-4) glycosidic bond will result in different types of oligo-saccharides. Maltose and maltotriose can originate from both amy-lose and amylopectin but α-dextrin is derived only from amylopectin.

glucose-(α-1,4(glucose-glucose)$_n$)) (Fig. 1-5). When the mixture of carbohydrates and amylase reach the stomach, the acidic pH in-hibits the hydrolytic activity of the enzyme. This activity is re-stored in the duodenum by the pancreatic secretions rich in bicar-bonate and amylase. Further digestion into monosaccharides occurs just outside the enterocyte in the intestinal lumen by an-other group of enzymes called oligosaccharidases. These en-zymes, secreted locally, break the glycosidic bonds present in the di- and oligosaccharides. The different human oligosacchari-dases, the site of their action, their substrates, and the products of their digestive processes are summarized in Table 1-1. As an overall result, this brush border digestion will transform a mix-ture of different sugars ingested into glucose, galactose, and fruc-tose. These three monosaccharides will constitute the carbohy-drate reservoir that will be absorbed, and accordingly utilized, in majority before the remains of a meal reaches the terminal part of the ileum.

Bioavailability

As one can concur from the preceding paragraph, the range of action for the digestive enzymes is restricted to few types of sugar connections. Likewise, the structural complexity of the carbohy-drate is a limiting factor for the enzyme's access to its site of action. Consequently, not all sugars are digestible and absorb-able. Also, incomplete absorption might occur for others even after digestion. The bioavailability of a sugar is the production of this digestive and absorptive process.

By definition, fibers are mainly polysaccharides resistant to digestion and absorption. Cellulose (polysaccharide of β (1-4) lin-ear glucose) is undigestible by humans. The main reason being that amylase, the only polysaccharidase in the intestinal tract, is specific for α (1-4) sugars. On the other hand, the table sugar sucrose (disaccharide: α (1-2) glucose-fructose) is completely hy-drolyzed by sucrase (Table 1-1) and totally absorbed. Starches from different sources have different contents and complexities of their macromolecules. Hence, each undergoes a different rate of digestion. A higher ratio of amylose:amylpectin, that is, longer

Table 1-1. Principle oligosaccharidases of the intestinal lumen

Enzyme	Maltase	Lactase	Sucrase	α-Dextrinase	Trehalase
Action site	α-1,4	β-1,4	α-1,2	α-1,6	α-1,1
Substrate (s)	Maltose	Lactose	Sucrose	α-Dextrins	Trehalose
	α-1,4 Glu*-glu	β-1,4 Glu-galactose	α-1,2 Glu-fructose		α-1,1 Glu-glu
	Maltotriose		Maltose		
	α-1,4 Glu-glu-glu		Maltotriose		
	α-Dextrins				
	α-1,6 Glu-glu-(α-1,4 glu-glu)$_n$				
Product (s)	Glu	Glu	Glu	Glu	Glu
	α-1,6 Glu-glu	Galactose	Fructose	(α-1,4 Glu-glu)$_n$	
Overall result	**Glu, galactose, and fructose**				

*, Glucose.

chain length of the amylose, slows the in vitro digestive rate of starch. Likewise, a higher content of α (1-6) bonding in the amylopectin molecule, meaning more branching points, has a similar effect. These characteristics will actually influence the physiologic changes that follow meal consumption. Rice varieties with similar fiber content were tested in healthy human volunteers; brands with higher amylose fractions induced lower postprandial glucose and insulin responses. Amylose content of starch was more beneficial than amylopectin in generating lower post-meal glucose peak and total quantity of insulin secretion while maintaining a comparable summed glucose measured postprandially. Although the impact of amylose/amylopectin ratio on the human metabolic responses was sometimes reported as marginal, diets high in amylose stimulated a lower glucose peak and more satiety than low amylose:amylopectin ratio diets. According to the rate and extent of in vitro digestion, starch is classified into three major fractions: (1) rapidly digestible starch, the portion of starch digested within the first 20 min of incubation; (2) slowly digestible starch, the portion of starch digested from 20 to 120 min; and (3) resistant starch, the remaining portion that cannot be further digested. Resistant starch is further subdivided into three categories according to the reason for resistance to digestion. Resistant starch corresponds to the sum of starch and degradation products not absorbed in the small intestine of healthy individuals.

In addition to lowering blood glucose levels, the undigested carbohydrates from dietary fibers and resistant starch reaching the colon undergo fermentation into short chain fatty acids by the resident bacteria of the colonic mucosa. Colonic carbohydrate fermentation enhances the suppression of postprandial hepatic glucose production and free fatty acids rise induced by oral glucose in humans. Food containing complete fibers induces a higher level of satiety and a lower spike of postprandial insulin than disrupted fibers diet, which may decrease overnutrition. Higher fiber meals consumed the night before have even a delayed favorable effect on reducing postprandial glycemia and free fatty acids the next morning, called second meal effect.

Glycemic Index and Glycemic Load

It becomes evident, from a nutritional concept, that the chemical classification of sugars (as simple vs. complex, digestible vs. nondigestible) does not permit sufficient insight into the sugar content and the physiologic outcome. In this regard, the same amounts of carbohydrates in various foods produce quite different blood glucose curves after ingestion. The "glycemic index" represents the quantification of the glycemic response to carbohydrates in different foods. The concept was defined in 1981 by Jenkins et al. The glycemic index for a specific food is calculated as the area under the 2-h blood glucose response curve expressed as a percentage of the area after taking the same amount of carbohydrate content as pure glucose. White bread can be used as the reference food instead of pure glucose and the postprandial blood sampling can be extended to 3 hours. The "glycemic load," defined as the mathematical product of the glycemic index of a food by its carbohydrate content, gives a global indication about the glucose response and insulin demand induced by a food serving. High glycemic index values are above 70, medium readings are from 55 to 70, and low values fall below 55, the reference food value is set to be 100. A glycemic load of 20 or more is high, between 11 and 19 is medium, and 10 or less is low. The classification of food according to the glycemic index places many variables in interaction. The type and quantity of the sugar measured in a serving, as reported on food labeling, are not enough to project the caloric outcome in vivo. Digestion, absorption, and usage differ between individuals and among the same individual at various metabolic states. Tailoring food intake according to the glycemic index could mean a better feedback, adaptable to physiologic response, than just looking at caloric content. In fact, healthy adolescents fed either a low glycemic index meal replacement (consisting of a shake and a nutrition bar) or a low glycemic index whole food and tested prospectively showed significantly decreased glucose and insulin response when compared to high glycemic index meal replacement. Also, beside a similar caloric intake between all groups, satiety was prolonged in the low glycemic index group. In a similar study, rapid absorption of glucose in the case of high glycemic index food promoted excessive food intake in obese adolescents. In another prospective study, obese subjects were given two types of energy restricted diets. The diets differed in the glycemic index content but matched in the level of energy limitation (−30% in relation to energy expenditure). At the end of the 8 weeks' dietary intervention, the lower glycemic index group significantly lost more weight. Besides, at 1 year follow-up, weight regain was statistically significant only in the high glycemic index group.

Glycemic Response and Health Outcome

Since its introduction in 1981, the practice of the novel food sorting according to the glycemic index/load gained huge momentum. Reports and studies examined the various associations between glycemic responses and diseases' risks. Most of these projects were designed to look at the direct and indirect results of food stratification according to the glycemic index or load in terms of weight change, diabetes, lipid profile, cardiovascular risk, and cancer. Possible mechanistic pathways are linked to hyperinsulinemia with other hormonal changes, lipid metabolism, and local inflammatory changes taking place in the intestines.

Many studies have reported that overweight and obese adults lose more weight if they consume a low glycemic index/load diet. In that group of the population, weight loss may be favored in overweight persons with higher insulin secretion or females with sedentary lifestyle. As for the prevention of obesity in healthy adults, positive association between low glycemic index/load diets and decreased risk of obesity did not result in strong evidence. The risk of type 2 diabetes was found to be associated with high glycemic index diets in various prospectively performed studies. At the same time, other reports denoted a higher protective role for the fiber content against the development of diabetes and not the glycemic response per se. Beneficial changes in the cardiovascular risk factors, high density lipoprotein, and triglyceride levels were observed to be positively correlated to low glycemic index or load diets in numerous epidemiological studies. Even though, few have reported a weak or no association between glycemic index/load and cardiovascular risks.

The controversy between different reports is even more important when it comes to linking the glycemic index and glycemic load on one side, to the risk of various cancers on the other side. Some studies reported significant association of high glycemic index or load diets with colorectal cancer, many others did not. While all of the aforementioned reports that found a lack of association with colorectal cancer studied female subjects, few reported a possible beneficial outcome for low glycemic index or load diets in males. Breast carcinogenesis was not tied to glycemic index/ load according to many authors. For others the association was significant among subpopulations of studied women in relation to their menopausal state or body weight. In a similar manner, for some studies, endometrial cancer was positively linked to glycemic index or load in women depending on their body mass index and/or hormonal replacement therapy. Many studies did not find a substantial increase in the risk of pancreatic cancer with higher glycemic diets. A possible beneficial effect was described among obese females.

It becomes obvious that outlining a straight forward conclusion regarding the health outcomes of the glycemic response food classification is still early at this stage. As much as the classification of food according to the inherent glycemic response appears more physiologically adaptable, scrutiny regarding the methodology and the variability of the testing used are also to be accounted for. Metabolic changes that occur in each individual will induce various blood sugar responses after a similar meal on different occasions. As a matter of fact, the coefficient of variation for the glycemic index is actually higher intra-individually than interindividually at 42.8% and 17.8%, respectively. These measures were done in healthy subjects who consumed white bread as the test meal and glucose as the reference meal on three occasions. Hätönen et al. tested the accuracy of capillary versus venous blood sampling and pure glucose versus white bread usage as the reference food. White bread as a reference produced glycemic index values 1.3 times higher than glucose as a reference food. The reference test, whether it is glucose or white bread, should be performed at least twice. The coefficients of variations based on capillary samples were significantly lower than those based on venous samples. The better accuracy of capillary testing was also described by other reports. Adding to this, the glycemic response would change for a single food type depending on various interaction(s); for example, the presence of fibers, the cooking methods, and the origins of the crops. A practical example is outlined in Table 1-2 that summarizes the glycemic indexes and the glycemic loads of certain common foods measured in normal subjects. Clinical measurements of the glycemic index are very difficult in large samples. Thus, all of the prospectively performed analyses for large cohorts categorize diets according to food questionnaires answered by the enrolled subjects. This is done at baseline and at different time points during the follow-up evaluations

Table 1-2. Glycemic index and glycemic load of various food products

Food	GI*	GL
White flour bread	70 ± 17.2	10
English muffin bread	77 ± 22.1	11
White bread + 15 g psyllium fiber	65	11
White bread eaten with powdered dried seaweed	48	7
White bread eaten with vinegar	45	7
Soy and linseed bread	50 ± 19	5
Whole wheat bread	75 ± 33.9	9
Whole wheat (80%) barley (20%) white flour bread	67	13
Coarse barley bread (80% kernels–20% wheat flour)	37	7.5
Cornflakes	76 ± 38.9	19
Whole wheat oat flour porridge	74	24
All bran breakfast cereal	40 ± 10.6	6.5
White rice, waxy (low amylose: 0%–2%), boiled	88 ± 11	38
Brown rice, steamed	55 ± 5	18
Spaghetti, white, boiled	49.6 ± 16.3	23.6
Spaghetti, whole wheat, boiled	42 ± 4	17
Beans, dried, boiled	36	11
Chickpeas, dried, boiled	23 ± 12.2	7
Lentils, dried, boiled	28 ± 7.9	4
Apple, raw	39 ± 3	6
Apple juice, unsweetened, reconstituted	39 ± 5	10
Apple, dried	29 ± 5	10
Banana, raw	66 ± 26.2	16
Orange, raw	36.5 ± 16.4	3.5
Orange juice, reconstituted from frozen concentrate	49.5 ± 22.4	10.5

*Numbers represent mean ± SD (if provided otherwise calculated from multiple studies' SDs).
GI, glycemic index, GL, glycemic load.

for some studies. Taking into account the high variability of the glycemic response, the analysis of the results can be largely biased by methodological inaccuracies of the dietary assessment tool.

In a review attempt, low glycemic index food and/or load provide more weight loss for overweight persons, better glycemic control for diabetics, and higher cardiovascular risk prevention for people with dyslipidemia. For chronic disease and cancer prevention in healthy population, a straight line of association between glycemic response and outcome cannot be drawn. Taking into account that lower glycemic index food does not harm, recommending its usage might not be a bad choice in the face of conflicting reports.

LIPIDS

Historical Landmarks and Definitions

The relationship between lipid and energy can be better appreciated by knowing that a car with a diesel engine was wholly run on vegetable oil (peanut oil) in 1900. The first appearance of the word "lipid" in a paper was in 1926. Cholesterol, derived from the Greek language as *Chole-* (bile), *stereos-* (solid), and the chemical suffix *ol* (alcohol), was first discovered in bile and in gallstones by Poulletier de la Salle in 1769. In 1818, Chevreul, a surgeon, described "cholesterol" but gave it the original name of cholesterine. Five years later he published a pioneering chemical description of several fatty acids. Claude Bernard had his share too; he demonstrated a lipase activity in the pancreas as early as 1846, then he proved the importance of the pancreatic juice and of bile for the digestion and absorption of fat in the duodenum in 1855. The term "essential fatty acids" was coined by Burr in 1930 when he discovered the importance of the long chain polyunsaturated fatty acids, linoleic, and linolenic acids not synthesized in mammals and for which deficiencies could be cured by dietary supplementation.

Lipids are broadly defined as any fat-soluble (lipophilic), naturally occurring molecule such as fats, oils, waxes, sterols (including cholesterol), fat-soluble vitamins, fatty acids, monoglycerides, diglycerides, phospholipids, and others. The word fats should not be confused with lipids, because fats or triglycerides are a subgroup of lipids. Beside acting as a structural component of cell membranes and participating in signaling systems, lipids exert another main biological function in the human body that is energy storage.

Chemistry and Structure

The largest portion of dietary lipids consumed by humans is made of triglycerides. A triglyceride, also known as triacylglycerol, is formed from a single molecule of glycerol, combined through ester bonds on each of the three -OH groups of glycerol with a fatty acid. A monoglyceride (monoacylglycerol) or diglyceride (diacylglycerol) has one glycerol connected to 1 or 2 fatty acids, respectively (Fig. 1-6).

A fatty acid is a carboxylic acid with often a long generally unbranched hydrocarbon tail (chain) which is either saturated or unsaturated (the chain has at least 2 carbons joined by a double bond). The chain's length and the number and arrangement of double bonds will determine the fatty acid's name and structure. The number of carbons in a fatty acid is even, usually ranging from 4 (such as butyric acid found in rancid butter, parmesan cheese, and body odor) to 26. Small quantities of longer chain length (32 carbons) can be found normally in most mammalian tissues and thus may exist in human diet. Ultra long chain length (36 carbons) were described in human and rat brain tissues. During biosynthesis the formation of fatty acids involves acetyl-CoA, a coenzyme which carries two-carbon-atom group, thus the even number of carbon atoms.

The double bond, characteristic of the unsaturated type, induces two conformations of the linear chain, *cis* and *trans*. The

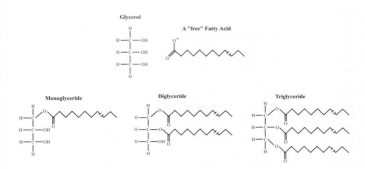

Figure 1-6.   Structures of mono-, di-, and triglycerides. Glyce-
rides whether mono-, di-, or triglycerides are formed through
esterification of the carboxyl group (COOH) on a fatty acid
to the hydroxyl group (OH) on the glycerol molecule with the release of a molecule of water (H_2O) for every esterification reaction.

"*cis*" form, with adjacent hydrogen atoms are on the same side,
causes the chain to bend and restricts the conformational freedom
of the fatty acid. This decreased flexibility of the *cis* conformation
hinders the ability of the fatty acids to be closely packed, for example, in lipid droplets. It favors a lower melting temperature than
the *trans* conformation. In contrast, in "*trans*" fatty acids (or trans
fats) adjacent hydrogen atoms are bound to opposite sides of the
double bond. This does not cause much bending and the chain
will look similar to straight saturated fatty acids (Fig. 1-7A). The
higher melting point and the higher conformational flexibility of
the trans fatty acids have major biological effects. Consumption
of trans fatty acids by humans has been positively associated with
harmful changes in serum lipids, systemic inflammation, and risk
of heart disease. All naturally occurring unsaturated fatty acids
are cis. Most trans fatty acids are the result of human processing.
In polyunsaturated fatty acids, subsequent double bond(s) almost
invariably occurs 3 carbon atoms farther along the chain from
the preceding one. Different systems of nomenclature for unsaturated fatty acids are described. The more commonly used in popular literature is "*n-x*" (n minus x; also "*w-x*" or omega minus x)
nomenclature. It starts by designating the total number of carbon
atoms and double bonds in a fatty acid by C:D called the code (C
is the number of carbon atoms and D is the number of double
bonds). Then, it identifies the placement of the double bond "x"
relative to the methyl end (CH3) of the carbon chain and the
conformation cis/trans. For example, linoleic acid is described as
"C18:2, n-6,9 all cis" or "C18:2, w-6,9 all cis." It indicates that
the chain has 18 carbons and 2 double bonds where the first one
is located between the sixth and seventh carbon atoms from the
methyl end. The second double bond is definitely located at the
ninth carbon. All double bonds are cis (Fig. 1-7B).

During de novo formation, the human enzymatic system is ca-

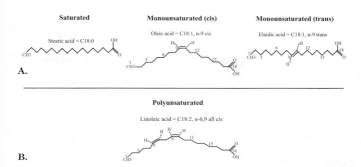

Figure 1-7.   Chemical structure of saturated and unsaturated fatty acids. (A) The presence of a double bond in a fatty acid chain charac-terizes the unsaturated state. In a *"cis"* configuration both hydrogen (H) atoms are present on one side of the double bond giving the chain a bent shape. In the *"trans"* configuration each H is on one side of the double bond and this keeps the chain in nearly a linear form. Metabolic consequences of these two forms are explained in the text. (B) Example of a polyunsaturated fatty acid structure illus-trating the *"n-x"* (or *"w-x"*) nomenclature style. Linoleic acid is an example for polyunsaturated fatty acid; in the *n-x* nomenclature it is written as C18:2, n-6-9 all cis, meaning that this is an 18 carbon (C) chain length with 2 double bonds, one located at C-6 (between C-6 and C-7) and the second one at C-9 (between C-9 and C-10), all in the *cis* configuration. Numbering of C atoms starts from the methyl end (CH$_3$).

pable of inserting double bonds at n-9 or higher. Meanwhile, mammalian tissues contain four families of polyunsaturated fatty acids (n-3, n-6, n-7, and n-9). Thus polyunsaturated fatty acids that have their first double bond below n-9 should be provided in the human diet and are therefore called essential fatty acids. The linoleic acid just mentioned is then an essential polyunsatu-rated fatty acid.

As much as the name cholesterol reflects disease in social mem-ory, it is a basic constituent and requirement for normal cell func-tion in the membrane of all mammalian cells; this is why it is only found in foods of animal origin. The molecular structure is made of a steroid nucleus (involves 17 carbons) and branched hydrocarbon tail (contains 10 carbons) (Fig. 1-8A). All of the 27 carbon atoms of cholesterol are derived from acetyl CoA, a com-mon metabolite of carbohydrate, fat, and protein metabolism. In the diet, cholesterol exists in both free form and esterified to fatty acids (called cholesteryl esters). Most of the dietary cholesterol is esterified. Plant material contains trace amounts of cholesterol but it contains another major constituent called phytosterol in-stead. Phytosterols are chemically related to cholesterol and also act as structural components of plant cell membranes. They have the same basic structure as cholesterol but differ mostly in the side chains attached to carbon 17 (Fig. 1-8B). Most phytosterols are found as stigmasterol, sitosterol (β-sitosterol), campesterol, and ergosterol.

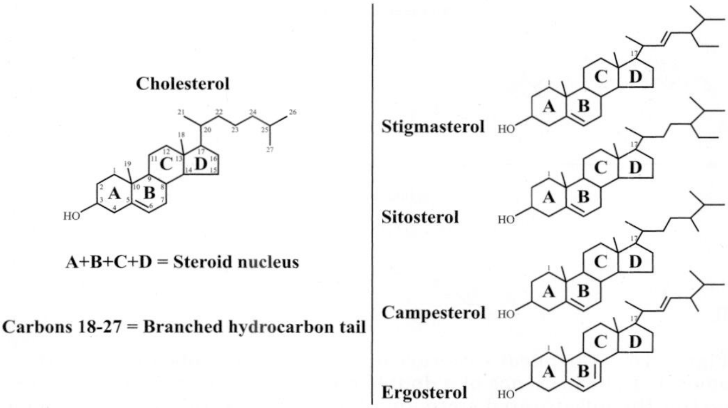

Cholesterol

A+B+C+D = Steroid nucleus

Carbons 18-27 = Branched hydrocarbon tail

Stigmasterol

Sitosterol

Campesterol

Ergosterol

A.   B.

Figure 1-8.   Chemical structure of different sterols. (A) Structure of the prototype of mammalian sterols. Cholesterol is composed of a steroid nucleus (17 carbons -C) and a linear chain (10 C) attached to it. Numbering of the C atoms is also shown. (B) Plant sterols have very similar structures to cholesterol (especially in the steroid nucleus) with differences mainly in the linear part (C-18 and above) of the chain.

Digestion and Absorption

As for the carbohydrates, instead of amylase, the digestive process of dietary lipids begins with the lingual lipase enzyme secreted in the oral cavity. A gastric lipase has a similar function in the stomach. A unique characteristic of these two enzymes is their ability to catalyze in a pH optimum of 4.5 to 5.4 for the lingual lipase and a pH of 3 to 6 for the gastric lipase. In contrast to the amylase enzymes that are nonfunctional in an acidic pH, the lingual lipases are active in the stomach; their substrates are triglycerides. These act on ester bonds present on the third carbon of the glycerol, releasing diacylglycerol and free fatty acids. Further digestion by the gastric lipase produces free fatty acids and glycerols. The contribution of both lingual and gastric lipases in fat hydrolysis is relatively minor, reaching in maximum 30% of the total dietary triglyceride load.

Most of the lipids' digestion starts in the duodenum. Pancreatic lipases hold a major role. In fact, two types of enzymes exist. The first type of pancreatic lipase acts mainly on the ester bonds of carbons 1 and 3 of the triglycerides with minimal action on the second carbon and the final products are free fatty acids and monoglycerides. This hydrolysis is greatly facilitated by co-lipase (a protein secreted by the exocrine pancreas and activated by trypsin in the intestinal lumen) and inhibited by bile salts. A second type of pancreatic lipases has been also described. The enzyme is called bile salt-activated lipase. In addition to its similar effect on triglycerides as the previous type, it also catalyzes the hydrolysis of cholesterol esters into cholesterol and fatty acids and it acts on the fat soluble vitamins and phospholipids. Cholesteryl esters are also digested by a cholesteryl ester hydrolase secreted by the exocrine pancreas. In addition, phospholipase A_2, an inactive enzyme (proenzyme) secreted by the pancreas, is activated by trypsin and releases free fatty acids from phospholipids.

The overall impact of the digestive process on ingested lipids is the formation of a mixture of substances made in majority by monoglycerides, free fatty acids, and cholesterol. Monoglycerides are relatively water soluble while free fatty acids and cholesterol are more hydrophobic molecules. The transport of the water insoluble products into the mucosal cells requires passage through an unstirred hydrophilic water layer at the mucosal brush border. This is accomplished by the formation of micelles formed mainly by bile salts and phospholipids. Through an amphipathic interaction between the bile salts and the phospholipids, free fatty acids and cholesterol are incorporated in a spherical shape. Thus, the polar (water soluble) extremities of the bile salts are exposed to the water milieu, while the nonpolar groups (i.e., hydrocarbon tails of the free fatty acids and cholesterol) are imbedded inside the sphere. Incorporation of monoglycerides in a micelle increases its ability to solubilize free fatty acids and cholesterol. On contact with the mucosal cell membrane the polar heads in the micelles and the hydrophilic side (external) of the cell membrane interact and open the way for the more lipophilic substances to pass through the lipid part of the membrane and into the cell.

Lipids: Function, Metabolism, and Energy

Lipids exert a wide array of biological functions in humans. To state some, structurally the lipids constitute approximately 30% of the plasma membrane. Their high caloric content (9 kcal/g) and their wide distribution in the body make lipids the energy reservoir by excellence. Lipids serve a variety of roles in cell signaling in parallel to the role played by the proteins. Other functions relating to immunology, endocrinology, inflammation, and cancer are also to be accounted for. Though in accordance to the scope of energy and nutrition of this chapter, the dietary intake of lipids will only be studied in terms of energy storage and disposal and the related impact on various metabolic outcomes.

Lipid intake is constituted mostly of triglycerides (>95%), the rest being made of cholesterol, free fatty acids, phospholipids, and plant sterols. In the cell, energy production involves the breaking down of fatty acids from triglycerides and/or other sources into acetyl-CoA by β-oxidation. On its turn acetyl-CoA enters the citric cycle producing ATP, H_2O, and CO_2 in cases of energy demand. And, as mentioned previously, the building blocks of fatty acids are made of acetyl-CoA condensations during biosynthesis. Also, during glucose metabolism acetyl-CoA is formed from pyruvate (a 3 carbon molecule). So, glucose can be converted to fatty acids through acetyl-CoA. In times of energy availability and excess (as happens postprandially), glucose and fatty acids metabolisms are shifted toward storing fat through the formation of fatty acids from acetyl-CoA. But when glucose is needed as a fuel (especially for cells that depend wholly on it as a source of energy, i.e., red blood cells), fast access to it from the lipid pool is limited. Why? The fatty acids cannot be transformed into glucose. The reason

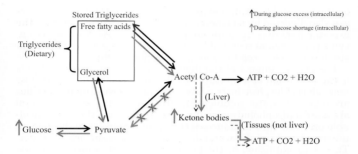

Figure 1-9.   Diagram showing energy pathways during different metabolic states. In postprandial periods the supply of glucose and free fatty acids provides enough ATP for energy consumption and the excess is driven toward storing this energy in the form of triglycerides with very little formation of ketone bodies. During fasting, especially prolonged ones, mobilization of triglycerides toward glucose is limited (no backward reaction forming glucose from acetyl Co-A, only glycerol can be transformed into glucose), with accumulation of more ketone bodies to be used as a source of alternative energy.

is the irreversible reaction that forms acetyl-CoA from pyruvate during glycogenolysis prohibits any backward reactions that would induce the formation of pyruvate from acetyl-CoA and thus the reproduction of glucose (Fig. 1-9). Usually glucose is supplemented either by intake or by glycogen degradation from the liver (which is not an enough supplier for periods more than 8–12 hours). Escape routes for longer glucose shortage are present through a reversible reaction called neo-glucogenesis changing glycerol into pyruvate and then into glucose, but this reaction is quantitatively unimportant. In lay terms, the human body is able to store fat easily in period of excess energy, while the production of glucose as a fast fuel in periods of energy needs is relatively a long and difficult process if a supply of intracellular glucose is not provided. In that case, alternatively, the liver induces the formation of ketone bodies, from acetyl Co-A, that are delivered in the bloodstream (the liver is incapable of metabolizing ketones). Other tissues have the capacity to metabolize a limited amount of these ketone bodies into ATP, CO_2, and H_2O as a source of energy. If glucose deprivation continues, the human body has a limited capacity to buffer the decline in blood pH secondary to the increase in ketone bodies. Accordingly, metabolic acidosis can ensue; examples include starvation, uncontrolled diabetes mellitus, and a high-fat low-carbohydrate diet.

Dietary Lipids, Body Weight, and Disease

Since the 1970s, dietary lipids, serum lipids, the associated lipoproteins (in particular, low density lipoprotein, high density lipoprotein, and very low density lipoprotein), and atherosclerosis have been linked together in different countries and various cohorts. The development of hyperlipidemia is known to rest on both genetic and environmental factor. Though the effect of dietary cholesterol on plasma cholesterol level and cardiovascular risk has been reported as not significant in some studies (reviewed in McNamara DJ, 1997), increases in dietary fats have been found by many others to promote a positive energy balance and body fat gain.

In recent years, interest in high-fat low-carbohydrate diets has been suggested as a recipe for weight loss. Such diets will deliver more lipids at the expense of carbohydrates (mainly glucose). Metabolically, as explained in the previous paragraph, more lipids will be mobilized to replenish glucose demands with the price of an increase in ketone bodies, thus the name "ketogenic diets." Ketogenic diets are well known in the United States and are used by many institutional weight loss programs. Popular names such as Atkins and Zone diets are some of the examples, with Atkins having the lower carbohydrate content. As early as 1973, Kasper et al. reported weight reduction in obese subjects given high-fat low-carbohydrate diets. Since then, many trials and manuscripts have described conflicting results. Even in the early 1970s, discrepancies of weight loss between ketogenic and nonketogenic diets (high-carbohydrate low-fat) were questioned as be differences in water instead of fat loss. In general, ketogenic diets have been found to generate weight loss as equal as or more than high-carbohydrate low-fat diets. While some argue against it, weight loss for overweight or obese persons is a common denominator for ketogenic diets in many studies.

The interest in this type of diet has grown very popular. At the same time, the scientific basis for its success is still unclear. While the theory of ketone bodies formation from stored lipids seems plausible, many have postulated the weight loss as being more related to decreased energy content as just to the change in the dietary lipid/carbohydrate ratio. Under isocaloric conditions Tay et al. found that obese subjects lost similar amounts of weight whether on high fat or high carbohydrate diets. Similar conclusions have been historically and recently described. To this regard, long-term controlled trials are few but most of them denote a similar benefit for the two types of diets, stressing the theory of restricted energy, not carbohydrate intake, in the case of high-fat low-carbohydrate diets. This being said, Dr. Atkins' books for weight loss have sold more than 45 million copies. Whether the ketogenic diet's theory is a hoax or not a clear cut border is hard to establish at this point. But, what is of evidence is that usage of such diets for the general population or for weight maintenance has not been recommended. The 2005 U.S. Department of Agriculture dietary guidelines recommend the total intake of lipids to be between 20% to 35% of the energy requirements. Meanwhile the percentage of calories derived from lipids in the high fat low carbohydrate diets is more than 50%.

Also, the increase in the lipid content of a diet is not without negative side effects. Particular attention should be made in patients with cardiovascular risk related to abnormal lipid profiles, of whom the overweight population makes the majority. Serum triglycerides decreased in overweight subjects on high fat diets. Even though the results in normal weight subjects are conflicting, some reported a decrease while others have found an increase in the triglyceride levels. High density lipoprotein cholesterol increased favorably in the obese subjects in two controlled trials, but positive changes in low density lipoprotein cholesterol were not of strong evidence in both of these trials. The significant changes in body weight that occur early for overweight persons on high fat diets might be offsetting unwanted shifts in the lipid profiles. So, as a general perception, in the absence of significant weight loss, ketogenic diets could have potential toxicities. The cardiovascular safety for these diets is to be closely monitored especially on the long-term when the rate of weight loss decreases. Low calorie diets instead of high fat diets might be a risk free choice especially if weight maintenance is contemplated (i.e., in the general population) or a bad baseline lipid profile is present in overweight subjects whose aim for the amount of weight loss is not drastic.

AMINO ACIDS AND PROTEINS

Historical Introduction

The word "protein" (*prota*) means "of primary importance" in the Greek language. Proteins were first described and named in 1838 by the Swedish chemist J.J. Berzelius. At that time, the organic material (protein) seemed to be the primitive substance of animal nutrition that plants prepare for the herbivores.

While the interaction between all carbohydrates, lipids, and proteins is mandatory for energy management, proteins hold a different type of importance. By now the central role of the double helix structure residing in the nucleus of every cell is very well appreciated. In 1957, Francis Crick laid out an influential presentation linking DNA-RNA-protein together and explained the coding processes involved. From a nutritional perspective, proteins are the only organic compounds that contain nitrogen. On average, protein is 16% by weight nitrogen while carbohydrates and lipids do not have any. Nitrogen, on the other hand, is the main atom involved in the chemical structure of the two types of nucleic acids, DNA and RNA. Putting all these together Berzelius' definition of "protein" as "of primary importance" holds very true today. In this chapter we limit our discussion of proteins and amino acids to their role in energy and nutrition. To that end, insulin was the first protein to be sequenced by F. Sanger, for which he won the Nobel Prize in chemistry in 1958.

Definition, Structure, and Synthesis

Amino acids form the building blocks of proteins. As the name implies, an amino acid is an organic acid with a carbon atom (C) in the center called α-carbon that is connected to a carboxylic acid (COOH) on one side and an amino group (NH_2) on the other side. The remaining two bonds of the α-carbon are linked to a hydrogen atom (H) and a side organic substituent chain designated (R). R is the only variant; it differs between various amino acids and it is called the functional group. The general formula of an amino acid molecule is NH_2-CHR-COOH (Fig. 1-10A). One exception to this definition is proline in which the amino group is cyclized in a five-edged ring with the side chain. Proline is actually called an imino acid or a cyclic amino acid and not amino acid (Fig.

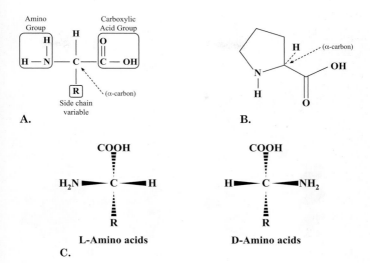

Figure 1-10.   Structure and configuration of the amino acids.
(A) General formula for an amino acid showing the specificity of
each group. The carboxylic acid (COOH) and the amino group
(NH₂) are constant while the side chain (R) attached to the main
carbon atom (called α-carbon) is variable and it defines the name
and structure of each amino acid. (B) Proline is the only amino
acid that does not follow the general rule. Its α-carbon is cyclized
within the side chain. (C) The α-carbon represents a rotational
center along which two different configurations can exist; they
are called optical Levo- (L) and Dextro- (D) isomers. L and D isomers are mirror images of each other and are not superimposable.

1-10B). The physical and chemical properties of an amino acid
are mainly dependent on the size, the structure, and the configuration of its functional group (R). R can vary from a single hydrogen atom to a linear or aromatic hydrocarbon chain. Nitrogen,
sulfur, and oxygen atoms can all take part in its chemical structure. The α-carbon of the amino acid represents a rotation center
around which the different substituents align in two possible configurations. These stereoisomers called "L" or "D" (for "Levo-" and
"Dextro-," respectively) isomers are mirror images of each other
(Fig. 1-10C). Glycine is an exception, the R is only a hydrogen
atom (NH2-CH₂-COOH) in which the α-carbon does not represent
a chiral center. Accordingly, it does not have two "L" or "D" forms.
In contrast to the carbohydrates where only D-glucose is utilized
for energy production, the human body recognizes only the "L"
isomers of the amino acids in most of its reactions. "D" amino
acids are cleared through renal filtration.

Proteins are linear polymers built from L-α-amino acids and
are mostly folded in various three dimensional structures in biological fluids. The attachment between two amino acids, called
peptide bond, is a dehydration reaction between the carboxyl and
the amino group of two consecutive amino acids, called then resi-

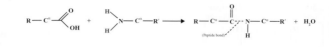

A.

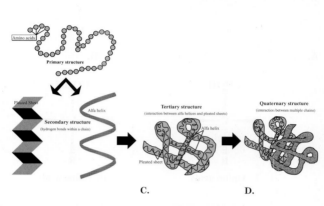

B.   **C.**   **D.**

Figure 1-11.   Peptide bond and protein formation. (A) A peptide bond is a liaison combining two amino acids together through a dehydration reaction (liberation of one molecule of water, H_2O). (B) Primary protein is the structure in which all amino acids are attached together through peptidic bonding only. It is a linear chain with no special folding. Through hydrogen interactions between different amino acid residues on the primary chain, two types of folding occur, an alfa helix form and a pleated sheet form, both coexist on a single chain. (C) In a tertiary structure, attractions occur between the alfa helices and the pleated sheets inducing more three dimensional folding. (D) Quaternary proteins are formed by the interaction of two or more tertiary structures. Thus, it includes more than one chain of amino acids.

dues in a protein chain (Fig. 1-11A). An oligopeptide consists of a protein length between 2 and 12 amino acids (i.e., dipeptide, tripeptide, tetrapeptide, pentapeptide, etc.). Proteins with higher number of amino acids units are called polypeptides or peptides. The protein will assume the three dimensional form by changing from the basic linear chain conformation (or primary protein structure; Fig. 1-11A) into a secondary (Fig. 1-11B) and then a tertiary structure (Fig. 1-11C) depending on various interactions between different residues and from different regions on the chain. The protein macromolecule can also be formed by more than one tertiary chain (chains can be similar or dissimilar), taking the name of quaternary protein structure (Fig. 1-11D).

A large number of molecules can follow the general formula for $NH_2CHRCOOH$ and be called amino acid. However, a limited variety appears in nature and only 20 amino acids are utilized and incorporated by human metabolism and nutrition. The synthesis of amino acids can be represented in two general schemes.

- Synthesis from amino acid precursors: this is done by addition of nitrogen to a carbon based backbone structure usually pyruvate, oxaloacetate, and glycolysis products of glucose or glycerol. In other terms, the nitrogen is added to the metabolic products of carbohydrates, proteins, and lipids.
- Synthesis from other amino acids: this involves usually the structural change of an amino acid without the need to add a nitrogen atom.

Amino acids have been divided into essential and nonessential amino acids. The essential status implies that nutritional supplementation is required because either these amino acids cannot be synthesized through any of the two pathways just mentioned or the quantity formed is not enough to maintain growth and function; they are also called indispensable amino acids. On the other hand the nonessential (or dispensable) amino acids can be created endogenously if they are not supplied in the diet. Traditionally 11 amino acids were considered nonessential: alanine, arginine, aspartic acid, asparagine, cysteine, glutamic acid, glutamine, glycine, proline, serine, and tyrosine. The remaining 9 are considered essential: isoleucine, leucine, lysine, methionine, phenylalanine, threonine, tryptophan, valine, and histidine. Some of the nonessential amino acids will become essential during special circumstances such as during childhood where higher growth rate is necessary, or in certain stress and disease conditions. These are named conditionally essential amino acids: arginine, cysteine, glutamine, and serine. The concept of conditional essentiality opens the way for further changes in subdividing the 20 amino acids and also affects the definition of the nutritional requirements of these amino acids.

Digestion and Absorption

In a typical western diet, 70 to 100 g of protein is ingested daily. An additional 35 to 200 g of protein joins this pool from endogenous sources (i.e., gastrointestinal secretions, desquamated intestinal cells, and plasma proteins). More than 95% of the total protein load delivered to the intestines is normally digested and absorbed.

No proteolysis occurs in the oral cavity of humans. Instead the digestion of proteins starts in the stomach. The gastric acidic milieu has a double effect on protein digestion; it denatures the structure of the macromolecule exposing it to the action of proteolytic enzymes and it converts pepsinogens (inactive) into pepsins (active). Pepsins are the proteolytic enzymes of the stomach; they work best in an acidic pH (pepsins are denatured in pH >5). They act on certain amino acids inside the peptide chain, thus called endopeptidases, yielding a mixture of oligopeptides. Of preference they cleave aromatic or neutral amino acids, that is, phenylalanine, tryptophan, and tyrosine. Pepsins have also an autocatalytic action inducing the activation of pepsinogens. The amount of proteins digested in the stomach is minimal; even people with total gastrectomy can digest and absorb protein normally. Even though the stomach contribution to effective proteolysis is minimal, gastric acid plays an important role in protein denaturation.

For example, the low pH of the stomach reduces food allergenicity by 10,000-fold favorably enhancing tolerance to allergic foods.

In the duodenum, the protein load is digested by proteolytic enzymes of the pancreas to approximately 60% when it reaches the proximal jejunum. These enzymes include mainly trypsinogen, chymotrypsinogen, proelastase, and pro-carboxypeptidases A and B. They all are secreted inactive as zymogens in the pancreatic juice. When they come in contact with the enterocyte, an enteropeptidase (or enterokinase) originating from the brush border of the duodenal epithelial cells activates trypsinogen to trypsin. Trypsin then activates all the proenzymes secreted by the pancreas (including trypsin). In contrast to pepsins, pancreatic enzymes do not require an acidic milieu for proper action. Trypsin operates at an optimum pH of 8 giving it a better activity in the duodenum and small intestine. Except for the carboxypeptidases, which are exopeptidases (cleave amino acids at the terminal end of a peptide), all pancreatic enzymes mentioned are endopeptidases (cleave amino acids within polypeptide chain). Trypsin cleaves at peptide bonds with lysine or arginine at one end but it refrains when the other end is occupied by proline. Chymotrypsin has similar specificity to pepsin (neutral amino acids or aromatic ones). Elastase has a relatively broader specificity attacking peptide bonds adjacent to small amino acids with aliphatic (linear) chains such as alanine, glycine, serine, and valine. Carboxypeptidase A splits aromatic amino acids from the terminal end of a peptide chain and carboxypeptidase B cleaves terminal arginine residues at the carboxyl end also. After the combined action of pancreatic enzymes approximately 70% of proteins are transformed into oligopeptides and 30% into free amino acids. Proline containing peptides are resistant to digestion by pancreatic proteases.

At the mucosal brush border, many cell surface peptidases produced by the enterocytes cleave more amino acids from the oligopeptide pool present at their contact, releasing free amino acids. Several surface peptidases hydrolyze proline-containing bonds, thus compensating for the deficit in the pancreatic proteases mentioned earlier.

The outcome of the whole intraluminal and brush border digestive processes culminates in the release of free amino acids, dipeptides, and tripeptides that are absorbed across the apical cell membrane of enterocytes by specific transporters. Further hydrolysis of dipeptides and tripeptides into amino acids occurs inside the cell by several cytosolic peptidases. From a load of proteins entering the digestive lumen, only simple amino acids are transferred to the basolateral space of the enterocyte. As a general rule, proteins are successfully broken down into smaller size entities as they progress along the digestive tract, releasing only amino acids into the bloodstream. However, small amounts of some dietary proteins are absorbed as a whole. For example, during food allergy or specific idiosyncratic reactions, macromolecules similar to the ingested proteins could appear in the blood. In that case, internalization through vesicle uptake at the mucosal surface or leaks between epithelial cells junctions are described as possible mechanisms involved in the transport of certain complete proteins. Thus the gate-keeping function of a normal gastric digestion in delivering a lower proportion of complete proteins to the intestines works in favor of decreasing food allergies and idiosyncratic outcomes. Hence the importance of a complete and functional digestive apparatus in achieving a safe and accurate protein digestion implies a specific and indispensable role for each part of the gastrointestinal system.

Proteins in Nutrition and Biological Value

Protein metabolism, function, and balance are the results of the availability of amino acids in the bloodstream, especially the essential ones, as well as the efficiency of our endogenous biological machinery to produce enough and qualified proteins. While the internal process is able to adapt to different daily variations in our needs and at different ages, the resources for amino acids will rely on the amount and especially on the type of proteins provided by nutrition.

As already stated, protein digestion required the complete breakdown of peptides into single amino acids. These processes, however, are not always complete. The physical and chemical properties of a protein will affect its rate of digestion and absorption. Whey, a group of proteins derived from the liquid portion of milk curdling (processing milk in order to obtain dairy products), is often used as a nutritional supplement for body building; it is soluble in solutions independent of pH. On the other hand, casein the solid portion of milk curdling, accounting for nearly 80% of proteins in cow's milk, is precipitated by acids and contains a relatively high proportion of proline. In the digestive tract, whey is easily digested and absorbed. On the other hand, casein resists gastric denaturation (clots in low pH) and proximal intestinal digestion (higher content of proline). Accordingly, whey is considered as a fast protein while casein is slower and considered as having longer digestive momentum. Accordingly, whey ingestion by healthy adults induced a dramatic but short-term increase in plasma amino acids while casein ingestion resulted in a prolonged plateau of moderate hyperaminoacidemia.

In the postprandial period the regulation of protein metabolism is dependent on two major components. First, various hormones and organs work in concert to promote metabolism and storage of amino acids. Insulin inhibits proteolysis and stimulates muscle protein synthesis. Second, the amount and the availability of amino acids in the blood represent major regulatory factors for promotion of protein synthesis and inhibition of protein breakdown thus leading to maintenance of muscle mass. Other variables affecting nitrogen accretion include the method of delivery of proteins or amino acids (small repeated doses), the ratio of fast versus slow proteins in the diet, the structure (folding and configuration), and digestive rates of proteins used. The net result is significant alterations in the rates of protein synthesis and breakdown favoring higher anabolic gain and muscle mass maintenance for slow proteins.

Protein metabolism is also affected by the availability of other nutrients in the food. Gastric emptying and, accordingly, the digestive and absorptive rate for whey are actually slower in the presence of carbohydrates and lipids, as would happen during a meal. Also age-related decrease in gastric acid secretion might alter the clotting of casein which will be emptied and absorbed faster than the coagulated form. This has led investigators to report that protein gain is greater with fast than with slow protein in elderly subjects, placing an added role for our endogenous biological machinery in determining different behavioral phenotypes at various functional levels. Also, in patients with type 2 diabetes the higher increase in postprandial amino acidemia for fast proteins was associated with a higher β-cell stimulation and insulin secretion.

Selected Readings

Abete I, Parra D, Martinez JA. Energy-restricted diets based on a distinct food selection affecting the glycemic index induce different weight loss and oxidative response. Clin Nutr 2008;27:545–551.

Achour L, Meance S, Briend A. Comparison of gastric emptying of a solid and a liquid nutritional rehabilitation food. Eur J Clin Nutr 2001;55:769–772.

Ao Z, Simsek S, Zhang G, et al. Starch with a slow digestion property produced by altering its chain length, branch density, and crystalline structure. J Agric Food Chem 2007;55:4540–4547.

Asp NG, Tovar J, Bairoliya S. Determination of resistant starch in vitro with three different methods, and in vivo with a rat model. Eur J Clin Nutr 1992;46(Suppl 2):S117–S119.

Astrup A, Meinert Larsen T, Harper A. Atkins and other low-carbohydrate diets: hoax or an effective tool for weight loss? Lancet 2004; 364:897–899.

Augustin LS, Gallus S, Bosetti C, et al. Glycemic index and glycemic load in endometrial cancer. Int J Cancer 2003;105:404–407.

Axen KV, Axen K. Very low-carbohydrate versus isocaloric high-carbohydrate diet in dietary obese rats. Obesity (Silver Spring) 2006; 14:1344–1352.

Badiali D, Corazziari E, Habib FI, et al. Effect of wheat bran in treatment of chronic nonorganic constipation. A double-blind controlled trial. Dig Dis Sci 1995;40:349–356.

Ball SD, Keller KR, Moyer-Mileur LJ, et al. Prolongation of satiety after low versus moderately high glycemic index meals in obese adolescents. Pediatrics 2003;111:488–494.

Baur H, Heldt HW. Transport of hexoses across the liver-cell membrane. Eur J Biochem 1977;74:397–403.

Behall KM, Scholfield DJ, Canary J. Effect of starch structure on glucose and insulin responses in adults. Am J Clin Nutr 1988;47: 428–432.

Bernard C. Leçons de physiologie expérimentale appliquée à la médecine, faites au Collège de France. Paris: J.B. Baillière et fils; 1855.

Biolo G, Williams BD, Fleming RY, et al. Insulin action on muscle protein kinetics and amino acid transport during recovery after resistance exercise. Diabetes 1999;48:949–957.

Bodmer MW, Angal S, Yarranton GT, et al. Molecular cloning of a human gastric lipase and expression of the enzyme in yeast. Biochim Biophys Acta 1987;909:237–244.

Boirie Y, Dangin M, Gachon P, et al. Slow and fast dietary proteins differently modulate postprandial protein accretion. Proc Natl Acad Sci USEA 1997;94:14930–14935.

Boirie Y, Gachon P, Cordat N, et al. Differential insulin sensitivities of glucose, amino acid, and albumin metabolism in elderly men and women. J Clin Endocrinol Metab 2001;86:638–644.

Brand-Miller JC, Holt SH, Pawlak DB, et al. Glycemic index and obesity. Am J Clin Nutr 2002;76(Suppl):S281–S285.

Burr GO, Burr MM. On the nature and role of the fatty acids essential in nutrition. J Biol Chem 1930;86:587–621.

Calbet JA, MacLean DA. Role of caloric content on gastric emptying in humans. J Physiol 1997;498(Pt 2):553–559.

Chanvrier H, Uthayakumaran S, Appelqvist IA, et al. Influence of storage conditions on the structure, thermal behavior, and formation of enzyme-resistant starch in extruded starches. J Agric Food Chem 2007;55:9883–9890.

Chevreul ME. Recherches chimiques sur les corps gras d'origine animale. Paris: F.G. Levrault; 1823.

Cho E, Spiegelman D, Hunter DJ, et al. Premenopausal dietary carbohydrate, glycemic index, glycemic load, and fiber in relation to risk of breast cancer. Cancer Epidemiol Biomarkers Prev 2003;12: 1153–1158.

Cook RP. Cholesterol: chemistry, biochemistry, and pathology. New York: Academic Press, 1958.

Crick FH, Griffith JS, Orgel LE. Codes without Commas. Proc Natl Acad Sci USA 1957;43:416–421.

Cummings JH, Pomare EW, Branch WJ, et al. Short chain fatty acids in human large intestine, portal, hepatic and venous blood. Gut 1987;28:1221–1227.

Cust AE, Slimani N, Kaaks R, et al. Dietary carbohydrates, glycemic index, glycemic load, and endometrial cancer risk within the European Prospective Investigation into Cancer and Nutrition cohort. Am J Epidemiol 2007;166:912–923.

Dangin M, Boirie Y, Garcia-Rodenas C, et al. The digestion rate of protein is an independent regulating factor of postprandial protein retention. Am J Physiol Endocrinol Metab 2001;280:E340–E348.

Dangin M, Guillet C, Garcia-Rodenas C, et al. The rate of protein digestion affects protein gain differently during aging in humans. J Physiol 2003;549:635–644.

Ebbeling CB, Leidig MM, Feldman HA, et al. Effects of a low-glycemic load vs low-fat diet in obese young adults: a randomized trial. JAMA 2007;297:2092–2102.

Englyst HN, Kingman SM, Cummings JH. Classification and measurement of nutritionally important starch fractions. Eur J Clin Nutr 1992;46(Suppl 2):S33–S50.

Eyster KM. The membrane and lipids as integral participants in signal transduction: lipid signal transduction for the non-lipid biochemist. Adv Physiol Educ 2007;31:5–16.

Flakoll PJ, Kulaylat M, Frexes-Steed M, et al. Amino acids augment insulin's suppression of whole body proteolysis. Am J Physiol 1989; 257:E839–E847.

Folsom AR, Demissie Z, Harnack L. Glycemic index, glycemic load, and incidence of endometrial cancer: the Iowa women's health study. Nutr Cancer 2003;46:119–124.

Foster GD, Wyatt HR, Hill JO, et al. A randomized trial of a low-carbohydrate diet for obesity. N Engl J Med 2003;348:2082–2090.

Foster-Powell K, Holt SH, Brand-Miller JC. International table of glycemic index and glycemic load values: 2002. Am J Clin Nutr 2002;76:5–56.

Frost G, Leeds AA, Dore CJ, et al. Glycaemic index as a determinant of serum HDL-cholesterol concentration. Lancet 1999;353:1045–1048.

Fujii H, Miwa I, Okuda J. Anomeric preference of glucose phosphorylation and glycolysis in human erythrocytes. Biochem Int 1986;13:359–365.

Furst P, Stehle P. What are the essential elements needed for the determination of amino acid requirements in humans? J Nutr 2004;134(Suppl 6):S1558–S1565.

Gagne L. The glycemic index and glycemic load in clinical practice. Explore (NY) 2008;4:66–69.

Gardner CD, Kiazand A, Alhassan S, et al. Comparison of the Atkins, Zone, Ornish, and LEARN diets for change in weight and related risk factors among overweight premenopausal women: the A TO Z Weight Loss Study: a randomized trial. JAMA 2007;297:969–977.

Gardner M. Absorption of intact proteins and peptides. In: Johnson LR, ed. Physiology of the gastrointestional tract, 3rd ed. New York: Raven Press, 1994:1795–1820.

Gibson NR, Fereday A, Cox M, et al. Influences of dietary energy and protein on leucine kinetics during feeding in healthy adults. Am J Physiol 1996;270:E282–E291.

Giles GG, Simpson JA, English DR, et al. Dietary carbohydrate, fibre, glycaemic index, glycaemic load and the risk of postmenopausal breast cancer. Int J Cancer 2006;118:1843–1847.

Gnagnarella P, Gandini S, La Vecchia C, et al. Glycemic index, glycemic load, and cancer risk: a meta-analysis. Am J Clin Nutr 2008;87:1793–1801.

Goddard MS, Young G, Marcus R. The effect of amylose content on insulin and glucose responses to ingested rice. Am J Clin Nutr 1984;39:388–392.

Granfeldt Y, Liljeberg H, Drews A, et al. Glucose and insulin responses to barley products: influence of food structure and amylose-amylopectin ratio. Am J Clin Nutr 1994;59:1075–1082.

Haber GB, Heaton KW, Murphy D, et al. Depletion and disruption of dietary fibre. Effects on satiety, plasma-glucose, and serum-insulin. Lancet 1977;2:679–682.

Halyburton AK, Brinkworth GD, Wilson CJ, et al. Low- and high-carbohydrate weight-loss diets have similar effects on mood but not cognitive performance. Am J Clin Nutr 2007;86:580–587.

Hamosh M. Lingual and gastric lipases. Nutrition 1990;6:421–428.

Hare-Bruun H, Flint A, Heitmann BL. Glycemic index and glycemic load in relation to changes in body weight, body fat distribution, and body composition in adult Danes. Am J Clin Nutr 2006;84:871–879.

Hatonen KA, Simila ME, Virtamo JR, et al. Methodologic considerations in the measurement of glycemic index: glycemic response to rye bread, oatmeal porridge, and mashed potato. Am J Clin Nutr 2006;84:1055–1061.

Heinen MM, Verhage BA, Lumey L, et al. Glycemic load, glycemic index, and pancreatic cancer risk in the Netherlands Cohort Study. Am J Clin Nutr 2008;87:970–977.

Hermansen ML, Eriksen NM, Mortensen LS, et al. Can the Glycemic Index (GI) be used as a tool in the prevention and management of Type 2 diabetes? Rev Diabet Stud 2006;3:61–71.

Higginbotham S, Zhang ZF, Lee IM, et al. Dietary glycemic load and risk of colorectal cancer in the Women's Health Study. J Natl Cancer Inst 2004;96:229–233.

Hipsley EH. Dietary "fibre" and pregnancy toxaemia. Br Med J 1953; 2:420–422.

Hodge AM, English DR, O'Dea K, et al. Glycemic index and dietary fiber and the risk of type 2 diabetes. Diabetes Care 2004;27: 2701–2706.

Holmes MD, Liu S, Hankinson SE, et al. Dietary carbohydrates, fiber, and breast cancer risk. Am J Epidemiol 2004;159:732–739.

Hooper RH, Short AH. The hepatocellular uptake of glucose, galactose and fructose in conscious sheep. J Physiol 1977;264:523–539.

Institute of Medicine (U.S.). Panel on Macronutrients. Standing Committee on the Scientific Evaluation of Dietary Reference Intakes. Dietary reference intakes for energy, carbohydrate, fiber, fat, fatty acids, cholesterol, protein, and amino acids. Washington, DC: National Academies Press; 2005.

Jenkins DJ, Wolever TM, Taylor RH, et al. Glycemic index of foods: a physiological basis for carbohydrate exchange. Am J Clin Nutr 1981;34:362–366.

Jian R, Ruskone A, Filali A, et al. [Effect of the increase of the caloric load of a meal on gastric emptying of its solid and liquid phases]. Gastroenterol Clin Biol 1986;10:831–836.

Johnson KJ, Anderson KE, Harnack L, et al. No association between dietary glycemic index or load and pancreatic cancer incidence in postmenopausal women. Cancer Epidemiol Biomarkers Prev 2005; 14:1574–1575.

Jonas CR, McCullough ML, Teras LR, et al. Dietary glycemic index, glycemic load, and risk of incident breast cancer in postmenopausal women. Cancer Epidemiol Biomarkers Prev 2003;12:573–577.

Jones JR, Lineback DM, Levine MJ. Dietary reference intakes: implications for fiber labeling and consumption: a summary of the International Life Sciences Institute North America Fiber Workshop, June 1–2, 2004, Washington, DC. Nutr Rev 2006;64:31–38.

Joslin EP, Kahn CR, Weir GC. Joslin's diabetes mellitus. Philadelphia: Lea & Febiger; 1994.

Kasper H, Thiel H, Ehl M. Response of body weight to a low carbohydrate, high fat diet in normal and obese subjects. Am J Clin Nutr 1973;26:197–204.

Kelly S, Frost G, Whittaker V, et al. Low glycaemic index diets for coronary heart disease. Cochrane Database Syst Rev 2004; CD004467.

King DE, Mainous AG, 3rd, Egan BM, et al. Effect of psyllium fiber supplementation on C-reactive protein: the trial to reduce inflammatory markers (TRIM). Ann Fam Med 2008;6:100–106.

Kolset SO. Glycaemic index. Tidsskr Nor Laegeforen 2003;123: 3218–3221.

Lajous M, Boutron-Ruault MC, Fabre A, et al. Carbohydrate intake, glycemic index, glycemic load, and risk of postmenopausal breast cancer in a prospective study of French women. Am J Clin Nutr 2008;87:1384–1391.

Landry N, Bergeron N, Archer R, et al. Whole-body fat oxidation rate and plasma triacylglycerol concentrations in men consuming an ad libitum high-carbohydrate or low-carbohydrate diet. Am J Clin Nutr 2003;77:580–586.

Larsson SC, Friberg E, Wolk A. Carbohydrate intake, glycemic index and glycemic load in relation to risk of endometrial cancer: A prospective study of Swedish women. Int J Cancer 2007;120: 1103–1107.

Levitan EB, Cook NR, Stampfer MJ, et al. Dietary glycemic index, dietary glycemic load, blood lipids, and C-reactive protein. Metabolism 2008;57:437–443.

Liu S, Manson JE, Stampfer MJ, et al. Dietary glycemic load assessed by food-frequency questionnaire in relation to plasma high-density-lipoprotein cholesterol and fasting plasma triacylglycerols in postmenopausal women. Am J Clin Nutr 2001;73:560–566.

Liu S, Willett WC, Stampfer MJ, et al. A prospective study of dietary glycemic load, carbohydrate intake, and risk of coronary heart disease in US women. Am J Clin Nutr 2000;71:1455–1461.

Livesey G, Brown JC. Whole body metabolism is not restricted to D-sugars because energy metabolism of L-sugars fits a computational model in rats. J Nutr 1995;125:3020–3029.

Lodish HF. Molecular cell biology. New York: W. H. Freeman, 2008.

Ludwig DS, Majzoub JA, Al-Zahrani A, et al. High glycemic index foods, overeating, and obesity. Pediatrics 1999;103:E26.

Mahe S, Roos N, Benamouzig R, et al. Gastrojejunal kinetics and the digestion of [15N]beta-lactoglobulin and casein in humans: the influence of the nature and quantity of the protein. Am J Clin Nutr 1996;63:546–552.

Malaisse WJ. The anomeric malaise: a manifestation of B-cell glucotoxicity. Horm Metab Res 1991;23:307–311.

Malewiak MI, Griglio S, Moulin N, et al. Weight and metabolic changes induced by low carbohydrate-high fat diets in man and in rat. Biomedicine 1977;26:297–302.

Marlett JA, McBurney MI, Slavin JL. Position of the American Dietetic Association: health implications of dietary fiber. J Am Diet Assoc 2002;102:993–1000.

McCann SE, McCann WE, Hong CC, et al. Dietary patterns related to glycemic index and load and risk of premenopausal and postmenopausal breast cancer in the Western New York Exposure and Breast Cancer Study. Am J Clin Nutr 2007;86:465–471.

McCarl M, Harnack L, Limburg PJ, et al. Incidence of colorectal cancer in relation to glycemic index and load in a cohort of women. Cancer Epidemiol Biomarkers Prev 2006;15:892–896.

McMillan-Price J, Petocz P, Atkinson F, et al. Comparison of 4 diets of varying glycemic load on weight loss and cardiovascular risk reduction in overweight and obese young adults: a randomized controlled trial. Arch Intern Med 2006;166:1466–1475.

McMurry J. Organic chemistry. Pacific Grove, CA: Brooks/Cole, 1988.

McNamara DJ. Cholesterol intake and plasma cholesterol: an update. J Am Coll Nutr 1997;16:530–534.

Meyer KA, Kushi LH, Jacobs DR, Jr, et al. Carbohydrates, dietary fiber, and incident type 2 diabetes in older women. Am J Clin Nutr 2000;71:921–930.

Michaud DS, Fuchs CS, Liu S, et al. Dietary glycemic load, carbohydrate, sugar, and colorectal cancer risk in men and women. Cancer Epidemiol Biomarkers Prev 2005;14:138–147.

Michaud DS, Liu S, Giovannucci E, et al. Dietary sugar, glycemic load, and pancreatic cancer risk in a prospective study. J Natl Cancer Inst 2002;94:1293–1300.

Michels KB, Mohllajee AP, Roset-Bahmanyar E, et al. Diet and breast cancer: a review of the prospective observational studies. Cancer 2007;109:2712–2749.

Miwa I, Fukatsu H, Toyoda Y, et al. Anomeric preference of glucose utilization in human erythrocytes loaded with glucokinase. Biochem Biophys Res Commun 1990;173:201–207.

Morihara M, Aoyagi N, Kaniwa N, et al. Assessment of gastric acidity of Japanese subjects over the last 15 years. Biol Pharm Bull 2001; 24:313–315.

Mozaffarian D, Willett WC. Trans fatty acids and cardiovascular risk: a unique cardiometabolic imprint? Curr Atheroscler Rep 2007;9: 486–493.

Nestruck AC, Davignon J. Risks for hyperlipidemia. Cardiol Clin 1986;4:47–56.

Nielsen TG, Olsen A, Christensen J, et al. Dietary carbohydrate intake is not associated with the breast cancer incidence rate ratio in postmenopausal Danish women. J Nutr 2005;135:124–128.

Nilsson A, Granfeldt Y, Ostman E, et al. Effects of GI and content of indigestible carbohydrates of cereal-based evening meals on glucose tolerance at a subsequent standardised breakfast. Eur J Clin Nutr 2006;60:1092–1099.

Nitske WR, Wilson CM. Rudolf Diesel, pioneer of the age of power. Norman: University of Oklahoma Press; 1965.

Nothlings U, Murphy SP, Wilkens LR, et al. Dietary glycemic load, added sugars, and carbohydrates as risk factors for pancreatic cancer: the Multiethnic Cohort Study. Am J Clin Nutr 2007;86: 1495–1501.

Patel AV, McCullough ML, Pavluck AL, et al. Glycemic load, glycemic index, and carbohydrate intake in relation to pancreatic cancer risk in a large US cohort. Cancer Causes Control 2007;18:287–294.

Peairs AT, Rankin JW. Inflammatory Response to a High-fat, Low-carbohydrate Weight Loss Diet: Effect of Antioxidants. Obesity (Silver Spring) 2008;16:1573–1578.

Peters JC. Dietary fat and body weight control. Lipids 2003;38: 123–127.

Pittas AG, Das SK, Hajduk CL, et al. A low-glycemic load diet facilitates greater weight loss in overweight adults with high insulin secretion but not in overweight adults with low insulin secretion in the CALERIE Trial. Diabetes Care 2005;28:2939–2941.

Poulos A, Beckman K, Johnson DW, et al. Very long-chain fatty acids in peroxisomal disease. Adv Exp Med Biol 1992;318:331–340.

Priebe MG, van Binsbergen JJ, de Vos R, et al. Whole grain foods for the prevention of type 2 diabetes mellitus. Cochrane Database Syst Rev 2008;CD006061.

Rabast U, Kasper H, Schonborn J. Comparative studies in obese subjects fed carbohydrate-restricted and high carbohydrate 1,000-calorie formula diets. Nutr Metab 1978;22:269–277.

Rankin JW, Turpyn AD. Low carbohydrate, high fat diet increases C-reactive protein during weight loss. J Am Coll Nutr 2007;26: 163–169.

Reeds PJ. Dispensable and indispensable amino acids for humans. J Nutr 2000;130(Suppl 7):S1835–S1840.

Riccardi G, Rivellese AA, Giacco R. Role of glycemic index and glycemic load in the healthy state, in prediabetes, and in diabetes. Am J Clin Nutr 2008;87(Suppl 1):S269–S274.

Robyt JF. Essentials of carbohydrate chemistry. New York: Springer, 1998.

Rovira A, Garrote FJ, Valverde I, et al. Anomeric specificity of glucose-induced insulin release in normal and diabetic subjects. Diabetes Res 1987;5:119–124.

Salmeron J, Ascherio A, Rimm EB, et al. Dietary fiber, glycemic load, and risk of NIDDM in men. Diabetes Care 1997;20:545–550.

Salmeron J, Manson JE, Stampfer MJ, et al. Dietary fiber, glycemic load, and risk of non-insulin-dependent diabetes mellitus in women. JAMA 1997;277:472–477.

Saris WH. Sugars, energy metabolism, and body weight control. Am J Clin Nutr 2003;78(Suppl 4):S850–S857.

Schulze MB, Liu S, Rimm EB, et al. Glycemic index, glycemic load, and dietary fiber intake and incidence of type 2 diabetes in younger and middle-aged women. Am J Clin Nutr 2004;80:348–356.

Sears B, Lawren B. The zone: a dietary road map. New York: Regan Books; 1995.

Sieri S, Pala V, Brighenti F, et al. Dietary glycemic index, glycemic load, and the risk of breast cancer in an Italian prospective cohort study. Am J Clin Nutr 2007;86:1160–1166.

Silvera SA, Jain M, Howe GR, et al. Dietary carbohydrates and breast cancer risk: a prospective study of the roles of overall glycemic index and glycemic load. Int J Cancer 2005;114:653–658.

Silvera SA, Rohan TE, Jain M, et al. Glycaemic index, glycaemic load and risk of endometrial cancer: a prospective cohort study. Public Health Nutr 2005;8:912–919.

Silvera SA, Rohan TE, Jain M, et al. Glycemic index, glycemic load, and pancreatic cancer risk (Canada). Cancer Causes Control 2005; 16:431–436.

Sperry WM. Lipid excretion. III. Further studies of the quantitative relations of the fecal lipids. J. Biol. Chem. 1926;68:357–383.

Stamler J. Diet and coronary heart disease. Biometrics 1982;38 (Suppl):S95–S118.

Stamler J. Dietary and serum lipids in the multifactorial etiology of atherosclerosis. Arch Surg 1978;113:21–25.

Stevens J, Ahn K, Juhaeri, et al. Dietary fiber intake and glycemic index and incidence of diabetes in African-American and white adults: the ARIC study. Diabetes Care 2002;25:1715–1721.

Strayer L, Jacobs DR Jr, Schairer C, et al. Dietary carbohydrate, glycemic index, and glycemic load and the risk of colorectal cancer in the BCDDP cohort. Cancer Causes Control 2007;18:853–863.

Tay J, Brinkworth GD, Noakes M, et al. Metabolic effects of weight loss on a very-low-carbohydrate diet compared with an isocaloric high-carbohydrate diet in abdominally obese subjects. J Am Coll Cardiol 2008;51:59–67.

Terry PD, Jain M, Miller AB, et al. Glycemic load, carbohydrate intake, and risk of colorectal cancer in women: a prospective cohort study. J Natl Cancer Inst 2003;95:914–916.

Tessari P, Kiwanuka E, Cristini M, et al. Slow versus fast proteins in the stimulation of beta-cell response and the activation of the entero-insular axis in type 2 diabetes. Diabetes Metab Res Rev 2007;23:378–385.

Thomas DE, Elliott EJ, Baur L. Low glycaemic index or low glycaemic load diets for overweight and obesity. Cochrane Database Syst Rev 2007;CD005105.

Thorburn A, Muir J, Proietto J. Carbohydrate fermentation decreases hepatic glucose output in healthy subjects. Metabolism 1993;42: 780–785.

Trowell H, Southgate DA, Wolever TM, et al. Letter: Dietary fibre redefined. Lancet 1976;1:967.

Trowell H. Crude fibre, dietary fibre and atherosclerosis. Atherosclerosis 1972;16:138–140.

U.S. Department of Health and Human Services and U.S. Department of Agriculture. Dietary Guidelines for Americans, 2005, 6th ed. Washington, DC: U.S. Government Printing Office; January 2005.

Untersmayr E, Jensen-Jarolim E. The effect of gastric digestion on food allergy. Curr Opin Allergy Clin Immunol 2006;6:214–219.

van Amelsvoort JM, Weststrate JA. Amylose-amylopectin ratio in a meal affects postprandial variables in male volunteers. Am J Clin Nutr 1992;55:712–718.

van Dam RM, Seidell JC. Carbohydrate intake and obesity. Eur J Clin Nutr 2007;61(Suppl 1):S75–S99.

van Dam RM, Visscher AW, Feskens EJ, et al. Dietary glycemic index in relation to metabolic risk factors and incidence of coronary heart disease: the Zutphen Elderly Study. Eur J Clin Nutr 2000;54: 726–731.

Vega-Lopez S, Ausman LM, Griffith JL, et al. Interindividual variability and intra-individual reproducibility of glycemic index values for commercial white bread. Diabetes Care 2007;30:1412–1417.

Volpi E, Ferrando AA, Yeckel CW, et al. Exogenous amino acids stimulate net muscle protein synthesis in the elderly. J Clin Invest 1998;101:2000–2007.

Wang CS, Hartsuck JA. Bile salt-activated lipase. A multiple function lipolytic enzyme. Biochim Biophys Acta 1993;1166:1–19.

Wang CS, Dashti A, Downs D. Bile salt-activated lipase. Methods Mol Biol 1999;109:71–79.

Weijenberg MP, Mullie PF, Brants HA, et al. Dietary glycemic load, glycemic index and colorectal cancer risk: results from the Netherlands Cohort Study. Int J Cancer 2008;122:620–629.

Wolever TM, Vorster HH, Bjorck I, et al. Determination of the glycaemic index of foods: interlaboratory study. Eur J Clin Nutr 2003;57: 475–482.

Womack M, Rose WC. The role of proline, hydroxyproline, and glutamic acid in growth. J. Biol. Chem. 1947;171:37–50.

Yamazaki M, Sakaguchi T. Effects of D-glucose anomers on sweetness taste and insulin release in man. Brain Res Bull 1986;17:271–274.

Yang MU, Van Itallie TB. Composition of weight lost during short-term weight reduction. Metabolic responses of obese subjects to starvation and low-calorie ketogenic and nonketogenic diets. J Clin Invest 1976;58:722–730.

Zhang C, Liu S, Solomon CG, et al. Dietary fiber intake, dietary glycemic load, and the risk for gestational diabetes mellitus. Diabetes Care 2006;29:2223–2230.

Effects of Chronic Kidney Disease on Metabolism and Hormonal Function

Jonathan Himmelfarb, Ian de Boer, and Bryan Kestenbaum

INTRODUCTION

In health, blood is filtered continuously by the kidneys, resulting in near complete homeostasis in the chemical composition of the blood compartment over a wide range of nutrient and fluid intakes. Kidney function thus plays a critical role in maintaining circulatory and organ system functional homeostasis, and the loss of kidney function in chronic kidney disease (CKD) and especially end-stage renal disease (ESRD) leads to dysregulation of many metabolic pathways. This results clinically in the uremic syndrome, characterized by subtle dysfunction of many organ systems.

The kidney also regulates body homeostasis not only by excretory function but by several synthetic and degradative properties dependent on glomerular and tubular epithelial cell function. These properties include synthesis of hormones, degradation of peptides and low-molecular-mass proteins (less than 50 kilodaltons [kDa]), and metabolic events aimed at conserving energy and regulating the composition of body fluids. The kidney is the site of synthesis of a number of hormones (i.e., erythropoietin [EPO], 1,25-dihydroxyvitamin D_3 [1,25-dihydroxycholecalciferol], and renin) and is an important catabolic site for several polypeptide hormones (e.g., insulin, glucagon, and parathyroid hormone [PTH]) and glycoproteins (Table 2-1).

Solute Accumulation

In CKD, as glomerular filtration rate (GFR) decreases solutes that are excreted by the kidney (such as creatinine and urea) accumulate in body fluids, and the plasma concentration of these solutes increases. Other solutes, including phosphates, sulfates, uric acid, and hydrogen ions, also can accumulate in body fluids. Accumulation of hydrogen ions is because of impairment of both ammoniagenesis and hydrogen ion secretion in tubular cells, resulting in the development of metabolic acidosis. Although the most profound changes occur with severe impairment of GFR, many of these abnormalities with associated adaptive or maladaptive responses begin at GFR of 60 mL/min/1.73 m^2 or more. As CKD progresses, other compounds that are retained in body fluids include phenols, guanidines, organic acids, indols, myoinositol and other polyols, polyamines, β_2-microglobulin, certain peptides, urofuremic acids, and trace elements, such as aluminum, zinc, copper, and iron. The accumulation of these toxic substances can lead to hormonal deficiencies (testosterone, fetuin, etc.), inability to appropriately respond to stimuli (insulin resistance, EPO resistance, etc.), or overproduction (prolactin). As kidney function declines, patients' abilities to adapt to changes in

Table 2-1. Components of kidney function

Excretion of metabolic waste products (urea, creatinine, uric acid)
Elimination and detoxification of drugs and toxins
Maintenance of volume and ionic composition of body fluids
Acid–base regulation
Regulation of systemic blood pressure (renin, angiotensin,
    prostaglandins, nitric oxide, sodium homeostasis)
Production of erythropoietin
Control of mineral metabolism through endocrine synthesis
    (1,25-dihydroxycholecalciferol and 24,25-dihydroxycholecalciferol)
Degradation and catabolism of peptide hormones (insulin,
    glucagon, parathyroid hormone) and low–molecular-weight
    proteins (β_2-microglobulin and light chains)
Regulation of metabolic processes (gluconeogenesis, lipid
    metabolism)

dietary intake, particularly those involving sodium, potassium, phosphorus, and water, become more restricted. Solute and water excretion per nephron increases as kidney function decreases, but this is counterbalanced by the fewer number of functional nephrons. As kidney disease progresses, the capacity to respond to changes in the intake of sodium, other solutes, and water becomes less flexible, and eventually this loss of capacity can result in changes in the volume and composition of the extracellular fluid. Thus, dietary intake in patients with CKD often needs to be adjusted.

METABOLIC PATHWAYS FREQUENTLY ALTERED IN CHRONIC KIDNEY DISEASE

Chronic kidney disease is known to be associated with alterations in multiple metabolic pathways. Recent studies indicate that these alterations might lead to a milieu highly conducive to development of atherosclerosis and might explain, at least to some extent, the exaggerated cardiovascular disease risk in this patient population (Fig. 2-1).

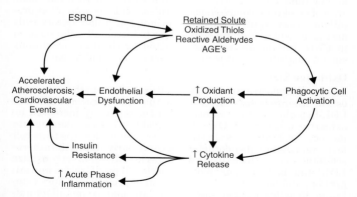

Figure 2-1. A proposed mechanism for uremia-induced CVD risk.

Inflammation

Acute-phase inflammation is a common feature of CKD and ESRD. It has been demonstrated that 30% to 50% of advanced patients with CKD have serologic evidence of an activated inflammatory response in cross-sectional studies. In longitudinal studies virtually all patients undergoing dialysis have evidence of intermittent inflammation. Elevated plasma levels of the proinflammatory cytokine interleukin 6 (IL-6) and the prototypical acute-phase protein C-reactive protein (CRP) have emerged as powerful independent predictors of cardiovascular events and mortality, often exceeding the prognostic value of traditional cardiovascular risk factors such as low-density lipoprotein (LDL) cholesterol. Moreover, plasma IL-6 and CRP levels do not change significantly over the course of time after initiation of dialysis therapy, suggesting that dialysis does not completely improve the inflammatory metabolic alterations associated with loss of kidney function. A plethora of additional inflammatory markers have been studied in kidney disease, including sICAM-1, Serum Amyloid A, IL-8, IL-18, myeloperoxidase, sCD40 ligand, and matrix metalloproteinase-9. Fibrinogen is also an important acute-phase reactant, and fibrinogen levels significantly predict cardiovascular events in patients with CKD undergoing peritoneal and hemodialysis.

The underlying etiology of the augmented inflammatory response in kidney disease remains poorly understood. The hemodialysis procedure itself contributes to a proinflammatory milieu by increasing the synthesis of fibrinogen, IL-6, and other proinflammatory peptides. This is primarily from bioincompatibility because of membrane and dialysate exposure during the extracorporeal procedure. Subclinical vascular access infections may also contribute to augmented inflammation in many patients undergoing dialysis. However, while multiple dialysis-related factors can contribute to maintenance of a chronic inflammatory response, recent data demonstrating that plasma IL-6 and CRP levels are already elevated in earlier stages of CKD suggest a more proximate relationship to loss of kidney function. Loss of kidney function is directly associated with reduced renal clearance of cytokines, complement peptides, oxidants, and other proinflammatory solutes. Biological priming of inflammatory cells may also be an important contributor to increased inflammation in CKD. Inflammation is exacerbated by comorbid conditions such as diabetes mellitus and inflammatory renal disease.

Oxidative Stress

Increased oxidative stress is known to contribute to the pathogenesis of atherosclerosis. According to the widely accepted oxidized LDL hypothesis, atherogenicity of LDL is greatly increased by oxidative modification. Oxidatively modified LDL is taken up into monocyte/macrophages via scavenger receptors, leading foam cell formation in the subendothelial space, an early step in the atherosclerotic process. Reactive oxygen species (ROS) directly oxidize LDL, stimulate vascular smooth muscle cell proliferation and migration, and potentiate the production of proinflammatory cytokines. Reactive oxygen species activate matrix metalloproteinases, which can lead to atherosclerotic plaque instability and rupture, as a precipitant of cardiovascular events. Reactive oxygen species also increase production of proinflammatory cytokines and acute phase proteins via activation of the transcription factor NF Kappa-B. NF-κB activation is controlled by the oxidation-reduction (redox) status of the cell, and generation of intracellular ROS may be a common step in all of the signaling pathways that lead to activation of NF-κB.

Uremia is now well recognized as an increased oxidative stress state. Increased oxidative stress in CKD and ESRD is characterized by excess formation and retention of lipid peroxidation products, alpha, beta unsaturated reactive aldehydes, and oxidized thiols. Levels of plasma F_2-isoprostanes, a lipid peroxidation end-product, are two to four times higher in patients undergoing hemodialysis than in age- and gender-matched healthy subjects. Levels of minimally oxidatively modified LDL are also higher in patients undergoing hemodialysis than healthy subjects. Several recent studies demonstrate that plasma levels of individual plasma oxidized solutes or antioxidants can predict subsequent cardiovascular mortality in patients undergoing dialysis. A linkage between increased oxidative stress and acute-phase inflammation in severely hypoalbuminemic dialysis patients has been described. Kidney transplantation, dialysis therapy, and antioxidant therapy may each have limited but beneficial effects on oxidative stress-related metabolic abnormalities.

Similar to assessment of inflammation in kidney disease, it has now become clear that the hemodialysis procedure itself is not the predominant cause of the increased oxidative stress observed in the ESRD population. The net effect of a single hemodialysis treatment on oxidative stress parameters is variable, as many oxidized solutes are removed, while there is likely a small increase in oxidant production. Even when cellulosic dialysis membranes that vigorously activate the alternative pathway of complement are used, it is difficult to detect an increase in oxidative stress over the course of the dialysis procedure. The best available evidence suggests that overall dialysis improves redox balance but does not have a long-term effect to mitigate oxidative stress.

Although the dialysis population is better-studied, data now convincingly demonstrates that patients with less severe degrees of CKD are also subject to high levels of oxidative stress. Multiple biomarkers of oxidative stress (and inflammation) are elevated in patients with moderate CKD compared with healthy subjects. Increases in lipid peroxidation end-products, protein carbonyls, advanced oxidation protein products (AOPPs), and changes in glutathione content have all been observed. Thus, there is a surprisingly high prevalence of inflammation and oxidative stress associated with the development of mild to moderate CKD.

The pathogenesis of uremic oxidative stress is not well understood; however, leukocyte activation clearly is an important contributor. Stimulated neutrophils and monocytes generate superoxide and hydrogen peroxide (after dismutation) and release the heme enzyme myeloperoxidase (MPO) during degranulation. MPO is one of the most abundant proteins in phagocytes, constituting approximately 5% neutrophil protein and 1% monocyte protein. MPO has the unique property of converting chloride in the presence of hydrogen peroxide to hypochlorous acid. A substantial body of evidence suggests that MPO is involved in uremic inflammation and oxidative stress. Catalytically active MPO can be released during the hemodialysis procedure, and 3-chlorotyrosine, an oxidative stress biomarker specific for MPO-catalyzed oxidation through hypochlorous acid, has been demonstrated in the plasma proteins of patients undergoing dialysis.

MPO can also directly modulate vascular inflammatory responses by functioning as a vascular nitric oxide oxidase, thereby regulating nitric oxide availability. Because MPO is released during acute inflammation, MPO-catalyzed oxidative injury and nitric oxide regulation provide a direct mechanistic linkage between inflammation, oxidative stress, and endothelial dysfunction. Other factors that contribute to increased oxidative stress in patients with CKD include dietary deficiency of antioxidants and scavenging systems, diabetes, inflammation, and age-related changes in antioxidant defenses.

Insulin Resistance

Glucose metabolism can be impaired by defects in insulin secretion from pancreatic beta cells and/or from defects in cellular sensitivity to insulin. Each mechanism may result in hyperglycemia and diminished glucose tolerance (defined by elevated circulating glucose concentrations after an oral or intravenous glucose challenge). There are several diagnostic techniques available for the assessment of insulin resistance. Fasting glucose measurements and oral glucose tolerance tests are routinely used to clinically identify disease, e.g., for the diagnosis of type 2 diabetes. More invasive diagnostic tests can be used to define underlying pathophysiology. These tests include glucose clamp studies and the intravenous glucose tolerance test (IVGTT). During the IVGTT, glucose and insulin concentrations are measured after a standard intravenous glucose bolus. The insulin response to the glycemic load reflects insulin secretion, while modeling relates glucose disappearance to insulin concentrations to calculate insulin sensitivity. Fasting insulin concentrations or indices calculated from fasting insulin and glucose (e.g., the Homeostasis Model Assessment [HOMA]), are also frequently used to estimate insulin sensitivity under basal conditions, particularly in large epidemiologic studies. The hyperinsulinemic euglycemic clamp procedure is the criterion standard for quantifying insulin sensitivity. During administration of exogenous insulin, an infusion of glucose is titrated to a rate that maintains peripheral glucose concentration at a normal fasting level. The glucose infusion rate equals the rate of glucose utilization by the body, providing a global measure of insulin sensitivity.

Glucose metabolism is frequently impaired in CKD, predominantly because of an extraordinarily high prevalence of insulin resistance (Fig. 2-2). In ESRD, insulin resistance was demonstrated to be the most profound disturbance using euglycemic and hyperglycemic clamp techniques. Specifically, ESRD is characterized by reduced insulin-mediated glucose uptake in skeletal muscle. Some patients with ESRD are able to compensate for insulin resistance by increasing insulin secretion. However, defects in insulin secretion are also common in ESRD. A recent epidemiologic study using data from the Third National Health

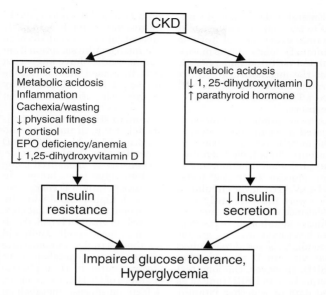

Figure 2-2.   Potential CKD-related alterations leading to insulin resistance.

and Nutrition Examination Survey (NHANES) reported that insulin resistance (elevated fasting insulin, hemoglobin A1c, and HOMA-insulin resistance score) was also associated with CKD in its earlier stages. It is not clear whether impaired glucose metabolism contributes to the pathogenesis of CKD and its progression (in the absence of overt diabetes), whether impaired kidney function causes impaired glucose metabolism, or both. In mild to moderate CKD, there is a high prevalence of insulin resistance, which is strongly associated with the degree of adiposity.

Impaired glucose metabolism is an established risk factor for cardiovascular events and mortality and thus represents an important potential therapeutic target pathway in CKD. In the Modification of Diet in Renal Disease Study, participants with stage 3–4 CKD without diabetes who had higher hemoglobin A1C levels had increased mortality over long-term follow-up. Other smaller observational studies have correlated the extent of insulin resistance in mild to moderate CKD with cardiovascular and all cause mortality risk. Among ESRD patients with diabetes, several studies have observed that higher hemoglobin A1c levels are associated with increased mortality, although this association was apparent only for very high levels. Insulin resistance and frank hyperglycemia may lead to cardiovascular risk and mortality risk through endothelial dysfunction, activation of the renin-angiotensin-aldosterone system, increasing dyslipidemia, and by amplifying oxidative stress and inflammatory pathways.

Emerging data suggest that vitamin D deficiency may contribute to the high prevalence of insulin resistance in CKD. In early seminal experimental work, administration of cholecalciferol to vitamin D-deficient rats more than doubled insulin secretion from isolated perfused pancreas. Subsequent studies have suggested that the mechanism for this effect is increased insulin release through stimulation of intracellular free calcium. Vitamin D may also affect insulin sensitivity through direct actions on insulin receptors.

A large number of cross-sectional human studies have demonstrated associations of vitamin D deficiency with impaired glucose metabolism. For example, circulating 25-hydroxyvitamin D concentrations have been directly correlated with glucose tolerance, beta-cell function, and insulin sensitivity, measured using oral glucose tolerance tests and hyperglycemic clamps. In NHANES III, lower circulating 25-hydroxyvitamin D concentrations were independently associated with higher HOMA-insulin resistance scores, the metabolic syndrome, and overt diabetes. Glucose metabolism in response to activated vitamin D (calcitriol) has been examined as an outcome in several small studies in hemodialysis patients. Collectively these studies demonstrate that vitamin D therapy may improve glucose metabolism in ESRD. However, the long-term effects of vitamin D on glucose metabolism in ESRD (and in earlier stages of CKD), are not clear, and data on whether vitamin D effects on glucose metabolism can translate into clinical benefit are lacking.

Endothelial Dysfunction

Endothelium plays a key role in the maintenance of vascular tone, structure, and hemostasis. This occurs primarily through the secretion of several vasodilating factors, among which the most important is nitric oxide (NO). Endothelium-derived NO has potent antiatherogenic properties that are mediated through inhibition of platelet aggregation, prevention of smooth muscle cell proliferation, and reduction of endothelial adhesion molecule expression. Low production of NO has been found in patients with CKD and could contribute to the development of hypertension, atherosclerosis, and the progression of kidney disease. NO abnormalities may also contribute to intradialytic hypotension in patients receiving hemodialysis therapy. Several endogenous inhibitors of NO synthesis have been identified that accumulate in CKD, of which asymmetric dimethylarginine (ADMA) and symmetric dimethylarginine (SDMA) and homocysteine have received the most attention. ADMA is a naturally occurring methylated form of the amino acid arginine that competes with arginine as a substrate for all three isoforms of nitric oxide synthase. SDMA competitively inhibits uptake of arginine by endothelial cells, thereby decreasing substrate availablility for nitric oxide synthesis. Patients with CKD and ESRD have high plasma levels of ADMA and SDMA, which have been closely associated with cardiovascular risk. Hyperhomocysteinemia is also highly prevalent in patients with CKD. Homocysteine circulates predominantly as a oxidized dimer (e.g., as homocystine or a mixed disulfide), and considerable experimental data suggest that plasma homocysteine levels are an independent risk factor for cardiovascular disease. Homocysteine has proatherogenic effects by inhibiting endothelial cell growth and promoting vascular smooth muscle cell proliferation. Conversely, a recent randomized clinical trial failed to show any benefit of folic acid supplementation to reduce cardiovascular and overall mortality in patients with stage 4 and 5 CKD. Oxidative stress is also closely linked with endothelial dysfunction in CKD. In increased oxidative stress states, superoxide anion produced via NADPH oxidase reacts extremely rapidly with nitric oxide, resulting in loss of nitric oxide bioactivity. The end-product of this reaction is peroxynitrite, itself a highly reactive and toxic reactive nitrogen species.

ALTERATIONS IN RENAL METABOLISM OF PEPTIDE HORMONES

The kidney is a major site for the catabolism of plasma proteins with a molecular mass less than 50 kDa but not for proteins with a molecular mass greater than 68 kDa (e.g., albumin and immunoglobulins). Because most polypeptide hormones have molecular masses greater than 30 kDa, they are metabolized by the kidney to a variable extent. Renal metabolism of polypeptide hormones often involves the binding of the hormone to specific receptors in the basolateral membrane of tubular epithelia or alternatively glomerular filtration and tubular reabsorption. Degradation results in the generation of amino acids, which are reabsorbed and returned to the circulation. Removal of peptide hormones by filtration depends on the molecular mass, shape, and charge of the molecule; for example, growth hormone, with a molecular mass of 21.5 kDa, has a filtration coefficient of 0.7, whereas insulin, with a molecular mass of 6 kDa, is freely filtered. Binding of a hormone to large proteins prevents its filtration. Other factors, including impaired renal and extrarenal degradation of a hormone or abnormal secretion, are also operative in kidney disease. Most filtered peptides are reabsorbed in the proximal tubule, so that less than 2% of filtered polypeptides appear in the urine. In experimental animals, nephrectomy prolongs the plasma half-life of insulin, proinsulin, glucagon, PTH, and growth hormone. Consequently, the circulating levels of numerous peptide hormones are elevated in advanced chronic kidney disease (see Table 2-2). In most instances, successful kidney transplantation rapidly restores the circulating levels of many peptide hormones to normal levels.

Insulin, Proinsulin, and C-Peptide

The major sites of insulin degradation are the kidney and the liver. In humans, less than 1% of the filtered insulin is excreted in the urine, and catabolism of insulin in the kidney involves both filtration-reabsorption and peritubular uptake. The kidney also catabolizes proinsulin and C-peptide. Renal extraction of all these peptides appears to be proportional to their arterial concentrations. Ligation of the renal pedicle of experimental animals results in a 75% increase in the levels of plasma insulin and a 300% increase in the levels of proinsulin and C-peptide. The kidney accounts for most of the catabolism of the insulin precursor, proinsulin. Conversely, the kidney accounts for only one third of the metabolic clearance rate of insulin; liver and muscle account for

Table 2-2.   Circulating levels of hormones and related peptides in advanced chronic kidney disease

Increased	Decreased
Insulin, proinsulin, C-peptide	Erythropoietin
Glucagon	1,25-dihydroxycholecalciferol
Growth hormone	Progesterone
Parathyroid hormone	Testosterone
Calcitonin	Thyroxine
Gastrin	Triiodothyronine
FGF-23	Renalase
Prolactin (particularly in women)	
Vasopressin	
Luteinizing hormone	
Follicle-stimulating hormone	
Luteinizing hormone–releasing hormone	
Secretin	
Cholecystokinin	
Vasoactive intestinal peptide	
Gastric inhibitory peptide	

two thirds of the disappearance of this peptide. In patients with advanced CKD, high plasma levels of immunoreactive insulin probably represent a greater contribution of proinsulin and C-peptide rather than of the active insulin. Consequently, when kidney function is decreased, dissociation can occur between the insulin level indicated by radioimmunoassay and the amount of biologically active insulin actually present.

Glucagon

The kidney accounts for about one third of the metabolic clearance of glucagon. Glomerular filtration is the major route of glucagon removal. The filtered hormone is degraded in the brush-border membrane of the proximal tubule and, to a lesser extent, by reabsorption and subsequent intracellular degradation of the intact hormone, so that glucagon excretion in the urine is less than 2% of the amount filtered (some peritubular removal of glucagon occurs). Plasma glucagon levels are increased in patients with advanced CKD, and the metabolic clearance rate of injected glucagon is markedly prolonged. Glucagon secretion in response to stimulants is exaggerated in these patients, but the high plasma glucagon levels in uremia are apparently caused by decreased metabolic clearance rather than hypersecretion of the hormone. Immunoreactive glucagon in the circulation of patients with CKD is heterogeneous: approximately 20% of the total immunoreactive hormone is the biologically active, 3.5 kDa species; another 60% is a 9 kDa species with little or no biologic activity; and the remainder is a high–molecular-mass form in excess of 40 kDa. The 9 kDa species is rarely present in the plasma of healthy subjects; thus, both biologically active and inactive forms of glucagon accumulate in patients with advanced CKD. These patients also show an altered physiologic response to glucagon; they demonstrate a three- to fourfold increase in the hyperglycemic response to this hormone. Over the long term, hemodialysis corrects some of these abnormalities.

Growth Hormone and Insulin-like Growth Factor I

The kidney accounts for approximately 40% to 70% of the metabolic clearance rate of growth hormone in experimental animals. Growth hormone (molecular mass, 21.5 kDa) has a somewhat restricted filtration rate of approximately 70%, compared with the rate for insulin. It is reabsorbed along the nephron, and less than 1% of filtered hormone is excreted in the urine. In advanced renal insufficiency, the metabolic clearance of growth hormone is markedly decreased, and plasma levels of the immunoreactive hormone are increased; but excess growth hormone production also contributes to the high growth hormone levels observed in subjects with uremia. Some of the biologic effects of growth hormone are mediated by insulin-like growth factors I and II (IGF-I and IGF-II). Growth hormone stimulates the synthesis and release of IGFs, and circulating IGFs exert a negative effect on growth hormone secretion, thereby forming a hormonal axis.

Recent evidence indicates that IGF-I plays a role in compensatory renal hypertrophy. Administering IGF-I increases GFR and kidney weight in intact animals. After uninephrectomy, IGF-I levels increase in the contralateral kidney, even though IGF-I receptor levels are unchanged. In patients with ESRD, plasma levels of IGF-I are normal, but the levels of IGF-II are elevated. Interestingly, the biologic effects of IGF-I and IGF-II are blunted when assayed in the presence of uremic serum, suggesting that a uremic factor (or factors) interferes with the biologic activity of IGF-I and perhaps IGF-II. However, long-term administration of supraphysiologic amounts of growth hormone to humans increases plasma IGF-I, improves nitrogen balance, and can have an anabolic effect. Clinical trials, mainly in children with renal insufficiency, have shown that administering growth hormone improves both the rate of growth and the amount of growth. For this reason, growth hormone is routinely administered to children with CKD or after kidney transplantation. The use of growth hormone in adults with CKD as a therapeutic for malnutrition is under active investigation.

Parathyroid Hormone

In response to hypocalcemia, hyperphosphatemia, decreased levels of 1,25-dihydroxycholecalciferol, alterations in the vitamin D and calcium sensor receptors, or some combination of these factors, the circulating level of PTH (a 9.1 kDa peptide of 84 amino acids) rises. This response stems from increased secretion of PTH by the parathyroid glands and impaired degradation of this hormone in the liver and kidney. Clinical measurement of PTH must be interpreted with caution; carboxy-terminal fragments of PTH are more elevated than amino-terminal fragments in the circulation of CKD patients, because carboxy-terminal fragments depend on filtration for their catabolism, whereas amino-terminal fragments are degraded by both filtration and peritubular uptake. The level of intact PTH depends on the balance between its production and removal by glomerular filtration and peritubular uptake. The circulating metabolic fragments of PTH are the result of enzymatic breakdown of intact PTH in the liver and, to a lesser extent, in the parathyroid glands. The kidney appears to be the only site where the carboxy-terminal fragments of the PTH molecule are degraded. Thus, the liver and the kidney are the principal sites of degradation, accounting for 60% and 30%, respectively, of intact PTH removal. A 7-84 amino acid degradation product is also present, which has no apparent biologic activity but is measured by some radioimmunoassay. In summary, assays directed against the carboxy-terminal portion of PTH or other fragments of the molecule reveal extremely high levels of immunoreactive PTH in the circulation, but these levels are out of proportion with true biologic activity.

Calcitonin

Calcitonin is a peptide with a molecular mass of 3.5 kDa. The kidney accounts for about two thirds of its metabolic clearance. Calcitonin receptors are located at both peritubular sites and the brush borders of tubular cells, and the hormone is degraded at the brush-border membrane of tubular cells and intracellularly in lysosomes. Chronic kidney disease decreases the metabolic clearance rate of calcitonin, leading to increased levels of the hormone in plasma. The calcitonin species that accumulates in the plasma of patients with CKD is a high–molecular-weight form that may or may not have biologic activity. The clinical consequences of elevated levels of calcitonin in these patients are unknown.

Gastrin

The plasma concentration of gastrin in humans is increased after nephrectomy. The hypergastrinemia seen in patients with CKD is most likely caused by reduced degradation of this hormone by the kidney.

Catecholamines

Plasma levels of norepinephrine are within normal limits in patients with mild to moderate CKD, but high levels are found in patients with stage 4 and 5 CKD. In these patients, a threefold increase in plasma norepinephrine levels occurs when patients assume an upright position, and this response exceeds that measured in healthy subjects. Patients with CKD metabolize norepinephrine abnormally because the activity of tyrosine hydroxylase, the critical enzyme involved in the synthesis of norepine-phrine in certain organs (e.g., heart and brain), is reduced. However, the norepinephrine level in patients with CKD does not appear to be caused by increased synthesis but rather by decreased degradation.

Prolactin

Approximately 16% of circulating prolactin is extracted during passage through the kidney. This hormone, which has a molecular mass of 23 kDa, is filtered to a modest extent and then is reabsorbed by the proximal tubules (less than 1% appears in the urine). Very likely, the kidney contributes to the metabolic clearance of prolactin, although adequate studies in humans are lacking. Elevated plasma prolactin levels occur in approximately 80% of women but in only 30% of men with CKD. Notably, the increase in prolactin is not modified by the administration of dopamine or bromocriptine. Patients with CKD experience a prolonged increase in prolactin levels after administration of thyroid-releasing factor, indicating that a pituitary gland disorder, plus a defect in the peripheral metabolism of the hormone, is present. The metabolic clearance of prolactin is diminished to about one third in patients with moderate to severe CKD. Apart from galactorrhea, other biologic effects of prolactin in patients with CKD are not clearly established.

Antidiuretic Hormone (Vasopressin)

Antidiuretic hormone (ADH) is metabolized in the liver and the kidney. ADH is filtered at the glomerular level, and the kidney accounts for approximately 60% of the total metabolic clearance of ADH. Whether vasopressin is filtered and reabsorbed in the proximal tubule with intracellular degradation or is degraded at the brush-border membrane of proximal tubular cells remains unclear. In patients with CKD and especially with long-term hemodialysis, removal of ADH is decreased, which results in high circulating levels of vasopressin.

Glucocorticoids

Plasma levels of cortisol are normal or high in patients with advanced CKD, especially in patients undergoing dialysis. The response of the adrenal gland to adrenocorticotropin (ACTH) is decreased, but the response of ACTH to stimulatory agents such as hypoglycemia is nearly normal. Thus, the normal or high cortisol level found might be the consequence of reduced clearance by the diseased kidney or in response to increased physiologic stress. The net effect is that adrenal function remains normal, and the expected diurnal variation remains unaltered in patients with CKD. Metabolic acidosis has been reported to increase glucocorticoid production.

Aldosterone

Aldosterone is the major mineral corticoid produced by the adrenal gland and, to a lesser extent, by endothelial and vascular smooth muscle cells. As a result, systemic and local production of aldosterone can each produce target organ effects. Aldosterone levels are elevated in most patients with CKD and in most animal models of CKD. Increasing evidence suggests that aldosterone participates in the development of fibrosis, proteinuria, and cardiomyopathy. These conditions may therefore respond therapeutically to aldosterone blockade.

Thyroid Hormones

Abnormalities of thyroid function are present in patients with CKD, because kidney disease affects the metabolism of thyroid hormones at different steps. Levels of both serum total thyroxine (TT_4) and free thyroxine index (FT_4I), measured as the product of TT_4 and the triiodothyronine (T_3) resin uptake are frequently low. Plasma iodide levels are usually high, and the plasma level of thyroid-stimulating hormone (TSH) is in general within normal limits, but the response to thyroid-releasing factor is blunted, especially when metabolic acidosis is present. The prevalence of goiter in patients with CKD is high compared with that in the general population. Individuals with CKD are subject to easy fatigability, lethargy, and cold intolerance; however, these changes are not accompanied by alterations in the basal metabolic rate or in the relaxation time for tendon reflexes (indicators of the biologic function of thyroid hormone). Low circulating levels of thyroid hormones in patients with ESRD may have a protective action on protein catabolism. Recent data has associated low levels of triiodothyronine with a poor outcome in patients with CKD and ESRD, which may be because of an inverse association with levels of inflammation. Thyroid supplementation is not advisable unless firm evidence of hypothyroidism exists.

Leptin

Leptin, a 16-kDa protein, is synthesized predominately in adipocytes under the control of the *ob* gene. Leptin's main target is the hypothalamus, where binding to the leptin receptor induces satiety, decreased food intake, increased energy expenditure, and weight loss. Leptin is mainly cleared by the kidney in the setting of normal kidney function, though nonrenal clearance is also evident and may increase in importance in CKD. Levels of free leptin are generally increased (when corrected for body mass) in patients with CKD and also correlate with low EPO levels and insulin resistance. Leptin may play a role in the cachexia and anorexia associated with uremia, but this remains controversial.

Sex Hormones

The kidney is a major site for the removal of glycoprotein hormones and their metabolites, including luteinizing hormone (LH), follicle-stimulating hormone (FSH), and human chorionic gonadotropin. Studies in animals suggest that the kidney accounts for 95% and 78% of the metabolic clearance rate of LH and FSH, respectively. Sexual dysfunction is a bothersome disorder for patients with advanced CKD. Sexual dysfunction is manifested clinically by impotence, decreased libido, testicular atrophy, and reduced sperm count in men and amenorrhea, dysmenorrhea, and decreased libido in women. Its cause is frequently related to dysfunction of the hypothalamic–pituitary–adrenal axis, characterized by elevated circulating levels of LH, FSH, prolactin, and LH-releasing hormone. These changes lead to lower levels of progesterone or testosterone in women and men, respectively. Contributory roles have been suggested for PTH, anemia, decreased levels of nitric oxide, and zinc deficiency in the pathogenesis of these abnormalities. Androgen therapy was used as an adjunctive therapy for anemia in CKD for many years, but androgen therapy for anabolic indications in patients with CKD remains controversial. Increased levels of prolactin can cause galactorrhea, whereas high levels of LH can cause gynecomastia. Many of these abnormalities are reversed or markedly improved after successful kidney transplantation.

HORMONAL DEFICIENCIES IN CHRONIC KIDNEY DISEASE

Erythropoietin

Although resistance of the bone marrow to EPO can occur, decreased synthesis of EPO by the diseased kidney is the major cause of anemia in patients with CKD. Patients with CKD have lower EPO levels than comparable persons with anemia who have normal renal function when adjusted for the hemoglobin concentration. Uncomplicated anemia of kidney disease is characterized as normocytic and normochromic. Administering pharmacologic doses of recombinant human EPO to patients with CKD can correct the anemia, reduce the need for blood transfusions, and improve quality of life. Results of several recent clinical trials have led to controversies concerning when in the course of kidney disease erythropoietic stimulating agents should be initiated and what the target hemoglobin should be.

Renalase

Renalase is a novel flavin–adenine–dinucleotide-dependent amine oxidase that circulates after synthesis and secretion in the kidney. Under basal conditions, circulating renalase lacks amine oxidase activity (prorenalase), and conversion from prorenalase to renalase occurs after exposure to norepinepherine. Active renalase metabolizes and degrades circulating catecholamines, and renalase activity has been demonstrated to be altered in animal models and human CKD. It has been hypothesized that abnormal renalase activity may contribute to hypertension, increased sympathetic activity, and increased cardiac risk in CKD by reducing catecholamine clearance. This hypothesis may be testable with renalase replacement therapy.

25-Hydroxycholecalciferol and 1,25-Dihydroxycholecalciferol (Calcitriol)

In healthy individuals, cutaneous synthesis is the predominant source of vitamin D, with smaller quantities coming from diet. Cholecaliferol and ergocalciferol from these sources are converted in the liver to 25-hydroxyvitamin D (25-OHD), and circulating 25-OHD reflects cutaneous and dietary vitamin D intake. 25-OHD is filtered at the glomerulus and actively reabsorbed into renal tubular cells via megalin and cubulin, where it is converted to the potent hormone 1,25-dihydroxyvitamin D (calcitriol) by the enzyme 1-α hydroxylase.

Vitamin D metabolism is profoundly disordered in CKD. Abnormalities begin during early CKD stages (i.e., stage 3 or sooner) and progress as kidney function declines. The central feature of this process is a decline in circulating calcitriol, which occurs early and is because of diminished 1-α hydroxylase substrate, mass, and activity (Fig. 2-3). While CKD is not an independent risk factor for 25-OHD insufficiency, it is clear that low 25-OHD concentrations are common in all CKD stages. Contributing factors may include decreased cutaneous synthesis (because of older age, comorbidities, and decreased physical activity), decreased dietary intake of fortified dairy products, obesity, and renal 25-OHD losses, which are most severe with heavy proteinuria. Di-

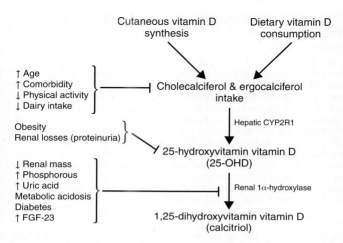

Figure 2-3.   Vitamin D metabolism and factors that influence its homeostasis in CKD.

minished 1-α hydroxylase activity is probably the most important cause of declining calcitriol levels in CKD. Hyperphosphatemia, hyperuricemia, metabolic acidosis, and diabetes are associated with decreased 1-α hydroxylase activity. Elevated levels of fibroblast growth factor-23, which act to maintain serum phosphorous concentration as GFR falls, potently suppress 1-α hydroxylase activity.

The main function of calcitriol is maintenance of calcium and bone homeostasis, which is accomplished through regulation of dietary calcium absorption, parathyroid hormone secretion, and osteoclast activity. However, vitamin D receptors are present throughout the body in diverse tissues, and hundreds of human genes contain vitamin D response elements. Thus, potential pleiotropic actions of vitamin D have recently attracted increasing interest. These actions may include suppression of the renin-angiotensin-aldosterone system, blood pressure reduction, modulation of immune function and cellular proliferation, prevention of myocyte hypertrophy, albuminuria reduction, and prevention of glomerulosclerosis. In observational studies, treatment with calcitriol or an activated vitamin D analogue in the setting of CKD has been associated with decreased risk for mortality and cardiovascular events.

Selected Readings

Annuk M, Zilmer M, Lind L, et al. Oxidative stress and endothelial function in chronic renal failure. J Am Soc Nephrol 2001;12: 2747–2752.

DeFronzo RA, Tobin JD, Rowe JW, et al. Glucose intolerance in uremia. Quantification of pancreatic beta cell sensitivity to glucose and tissue sensitivity to insulin. J Clin Invest 1978;62:425–435.

Dusso AS, Brown AJ, Slatopolsky E. Vitamin D. Am J Physiol Renal Physiol 2005;289:F8–F28.

Himmelfarb J, Stenvinkel P, Ikizler TA, et al. The elephant in uremia: oxidant stress as a unifying concept of cardiovascular disease in uremia. Kidney Int 2002;62:1524–1538.

Kalantar-Zadeh K, Ikizler TA, Block G, et al. Malnutrition-inflammation complex syndrome in dialysis patients: causes and consequences. Am J Kidney Dis 2003;42:864–881.

Levin A, Bakris GL, Molitch M, et al. Prevalence of abnormal serum vitamin D, PTH, calcium, and phosphorus in patients with chronic kidney disease: results of the study to evaluate early kidney disease. Kidney Int 2007;71:31–38.

Liu S, Quarles LD. How fibroblast growth factor 23 works. J Am Soc Nephrol 2007;18:1637–1647.

Mak RH. Intravenous 1,25 dihydroxycholecalciferol corrects glucose intolerance in hemodialysis patients. Kidney Int 1992;41:1049–1054.

Oberg BP, McMenamin E, Lucas FL, et al. Increased prevalence of oxidant stress and inflammation in patients with moderate to severe chronic kidney disease. Kidney Int 2004;65:1009–1016.

Siew ED, Ikizler TA. Determinants of insulin resistance and its effects on protein metabolism in patients with advanced chronic kidney disease. Contrib Nephrol 2008;161:138–144.

Stenvinkel P. Inflammation in end-stage renal disease: the hidden enemy. Nephrology (Carlton) 2006;11:36–41.

Teng M, Wolf M, Ofsthun MN, et al. Activated injectable vitamin D and hemodialysis survival: a historical cohort study. J Am Soc Nephrol 2005;16:1115–1125.

Vallance P, Leone A, Calver A, et al. Accumulation of an endogenous inhibitor of nitric oxide synthesis in chronic renal failure. Lancet 1992;339:572–575.

Zimmermann J, Herrlinger S, Pruy A, et al. Inflammation enhances cardiovascular risk and mortality in hemodialysis patients. Kidney Int 1999;55:648–658.

Zoccali C, Tripepi G, Cutrupi S, et al. Low triiodothyronine: a new facet of inflammation in end-stage renal disease. J Am Soc Nephrol 2005;16:2789–2795.

Calcium, Phosphorus, and Vitamin D in Kidney Disease

Ishir Bhan and Ravi Thadhani

CHANGES IN CALCIUM AND PHOSPHOROUS METABOLISM IN CHRONIC KIDNEY DISEASE

A host of metabolic changes occur as chronic kidney disease (CKD) progresses, particularly with respect to mineral metabolism. As glomerular filtration rate (GFR) declines it is accompanied by a fall in the activity of the renal vitamin D 1α-hydroxylase enzyme. As a result, conversion of vitamin D from its inactive form (25-hydroxyvitamin D) to the active 1,25-dihydroxyvitamin D is impaired. With reduced 1,25-dihydroxyvitamin D activity, the vitamin D-dependent calcium absorption from the gastrointestinal tract is limited and blood concentrations of calcium can fall. Phosphorous excretion, in contrast, becomes restricted in the setting of CKD because of decreased tubular function. Reduced phosphorous excretion appears also to trigger increased production of fibroblast growth factor-23 (FGF-23). This recently discovered phosphaturic hormone also suppresses 1α-hydroxylase, limiting the production of 1,25-dihydroxyvitamin D.

In addition to the effects of declining kidney function and FGF-23 on production of 1,25-dihydroxyvitamin D, its synthesis may also be limited by a reduction in substrate for 1α-hydroxylase. Indeed, deficiency of 25-hydroxyvitamin D is common in CKD. This may result at least in part from the urinary loss of the vitamin D binding protein (DBP) and 25-hydroxyvitamin D bound to DBP in individuals with proteinuria. In addition, the ability of the skin to produce vitamin D in response to ultraviolet radiation appears to be impaired in CKD. Protein malnutrition in this population may also play a role in promoting 25-hydroxyvitamin D deficiency.

One of the roles of 1,25-dihydroxyvitamin D is to suppress the production of parathyroid hormone (PTH) gene transcription. Not only is 1,25-dihydroxyvitamin D synthesis impaired in CKD, but the amount of vitamin D receptor (VDR) in the parathyroid gland is also reduced. Furthermore, in advanced CKD the binding of 1,25-dihydroxyvitamin D to VDR and of VDR to vitamin D response elements (VDRE) in DNA are also decreased. As a result of decreased vitamin D action, including reduced serum calcium from decreased gastrointestinal absorption, PTH production increases in a counterregulatory attempt to release calcium from bone stores. Unfortunately, the accompanying phosphate release further exacerbates the hyperphosphatemia of CKD, which promotes further production of PTH.

The net result of these metabolic changes is a progressive and persistent increase in PTH levels. Although extremely high levels of PTH have been associated with worsened survival in patients with end-stage renal disease (ESRD) on hemodialysis, PTH and bone minerals are not established surrogates of mortality. The principal association of hyperparathyroidism has been an increased risk of CKD-related bone disease.

BONE DISEASE AND CHRONIC KIDNEY DISEASE

The hyperparathyroidism of CKD has been most closely linked to the form of bone disease known as osteitis fibrosa cystica, characterized by markedly increased rates of bone turnover. Mineralization is preserved and bone volume is variable. The disease is often accompanied by bone marrow fibrosis, although a milder form of hyperparathyroid bone disease can also occur. The persistently high turnover seen in this disease is associated with a replacement of lamellar bone by woven bone, which is less resilient to stress. As a result, individuals with osteitis fibrosa cystica may be predisposed to fractures out of proportion to their bone density. While hyperparathyroidism is felt to be the strongest contributor to the development of osteitis fibrosa cystica, there may also be a contribution from 1,25-dihydroxyvitamin D deficiency itself.

The use of vitamin D replacement in CKD has been largely driven by the goal of preventing osteitis fibrosa cystica. Early studies demonstrated improvement in bone histology of osteitis fibrosa cystica after treatment with 25-hydroxyvitamin D. More recent studies have noted the ability of intravenous calcitriol to increase osteoblastic osteoid while reducing marrow fibrosis in patients on hemodialysis. Because of these findings, along with the physiology supporting suppression of PTH, vitamin D is considered to be an increasingly important therapy, particularly in patients on maintenance dialysis.

Increased use of vitamin D analogs may not come without risk, particularly with respect to bone disease. Adynamic bone disease, characterized by markedly reduced bone turnover, is the other major form of bone disease seen in CKD. Though mineralization is preserved, bone volume is usually low. As with osteitis fibrosa cystica, this disease has been linked to increased skeletal fragility. The prevalence of adynamic bone disease appears to be growing over time, especially in patients on peritoneal dialysis. This may be, at least in part, the result of increased use of active vitamin D analogs, as the development of adynamic bone disease has been reported in patients with osteitis fibrosa cystica treated with these agents.

The osteomalacia of CKD, characterized by a reduction in bone turnover and low to normal bone volume, is a third form of bone disease. Unlike adynamic bone disease, bone mineralization is markedly abnormal in osteomalacia. The distinguishing characteristic is an abundance of unmineralized osteoid, which is not typically seen in either adynamic bone disease or osteitis fibrosa cystica. The primary cause of osteomalacia is thought to be accumulation of aluminum and other heavy metals in bone, which can disrupt normal mineralization of the bone matrix. As aluminum-based phosphate binders have greatly declined in use, osteomalacia in CKD has faded from prominence.

MANAGING MINERAL METABOLISM IN CHRONIC KIDNEY DISEASE

The changes in calcium, phosphorous, and PTH that accompany CKD can be modified through the use of several therapeutic strategies, including an increasingly broad range of medications.

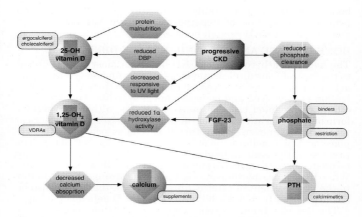

Figure 3-1.   Changes in vitamin D and mineral metabolism associated with progressive chronic kidney disease. CKD, chronic kidney disease; FGF-23, fibroblast growth factor 23; PTH, parathyroid hormone; VDRA, vitamin D receptor antagonists.

Phosphate Restriction and Binders

Phosphate control is a critical component in the management of CKD because of the protean effects of phosphate retention and hyperphosphatemia on a range of metabolic processes. As PTH promotes phosphate wasting, hyperphosphatemia can drive the development of hyperparathyroidism and osteitis fibrosa cystica. Phosphate retention promotes the production of the phosphatonin FGF-23, leading to suppression of 1α-hydroxylase and reduced production of 1,25-dihydroxyvitamin D (Fig. 3-1). Chronic elevation in serum phosphate, at least in patients with ESRD, also contributes to calcium phosphate deposition in tissues and vessel walls. In chronic hemodialysis patients, serum phosphorous levels above 6.5 mg/dL have been linked to an increased risk of early mortality. The importance of hyperphosphatemia in early stage CKD mortality is still a topic of investigation.

Given the wide-ranging deleterious effects of hyperphosphatemia, control of phosphate levels is an important focus of CKD management. Kidney Disease Outcomes Quality Initiative (K/DOQI) guidelines recommend maintaining serum phosphate between 2.7 mg/dL and 4.6 mg/dL in stage 3–4 CKD and between 3.5 mg/dL and 5.5 mg/dL in stage 5 CKD.

Dietary phosphate restriction is a reasonable initial approach with mild hyperphosphatemia, although it may have limited efficacy and practicability in some patients. K/DOQI guidelines recommend an intake of 800–1,000 mg daily for patients exceeding the target range for serum phosphate. Dairy products, beans, and meats are common sources of dietary phosphate but also important sources of protein. Thus, excessive focus on reducing dietary phosphorous could lead to inadvertent and excessive reduction in dietary protein. This may be particularly important in the dialysis population, where nutritional status has been linked to patient outcomes. There are few studies directly evaluating the effects of dietary phosphate restriction alone on either serum phosphate or PTH levels. A detailed description of food and meal choices regarding phosphorus restriction is reviewed in Chapter 19.

Given the limitations of dietary phosphate restriction, the addition of oral phosphate binders is often necessary to achieve adequate control of serum phosphate. These agents are taken with food to reduce absorption of phosphate from the gastrointestinal tract.

Calcium-based phosphate binders include calcium acetate and calcium carbonate. Calcium citrate, a calcium supplement used in the non-CKD population, can increase absorption of aluminum and is not recommended for use as a phosphate binder. These agents are popular because of their low cost and providers' familiarity with them. Although the calcium content of these drugs may seem beneficial in balancing the hypocalcemia of CKD, there has been concern about the propensity of this calcium exposure to promote vascular calcification. Thus, the K/DOQI guidelines have recommended restricting dietary elemental calcium to less than 2000 mg daily. In addition, the K/DOQI guidelines recommend against the use of calcium-based phosphate binders in individuals with corrected serum calcium levels over 10.2 mg/dL given the risk of worsening hypercalcemia. Additional side effects of calcium-based binders include gastrointestinal effects such as constipation.

Sevelamer hydrochloride is a nonabsorbed polymer that avoids the risk of excess calcium load of the calcium-based binders. However, randomized trials failed to show a significant difference between calcium-based binders and sevelamer on either the progression of coronary artery calcification or all-cause mortality. Despite this, use of sevelamer might be preferred in patients with known hypercalcemia or metastatic calcification. An additional concern with the use of sevelamer hydrochloride is the potential for worsening metabolic acidosis, particularly in the nondialysis population; a newer formulation of this agent, sevelamer carbonate, appears to abrogate this risk.

Lanthanum is an element with the ability to bind phosphate and has been used in its carbonate form as a phosphate binder in CKD. This newer agent has the potential advantage of both sevelamer (lower calcium load) without the increase in metabolic acidosis risk. Despite the potential appeal of this agent, the long-term risks are still not well studied, and gadolinium, another lanthanide element, has been linked to the development of nephrogenic systemic fibrosis. As with sevelamer, the higher cost of lanthanum compared with the calcium-based binders is a potential downside.

Aluminum-based phosphate binders such as aluminum hydroxide were first-line agents for hyperphosphatemia in the past because of their high efficacy. However, they have fallen out of favor because of the long-term risks of aluminum toxicity, particularly osteomalacia and neurotoxicity. Short-term use of aluminum compounds (e.g., one 4-week course) is still considered rea-

Table 3-1.   Kidney Disease Outcomes Quality Initiative Guidelines for vitamin D receptor agonists use with thresholds for serum phosphorous and calcium levels

		Avoid Therapy If	
CKD Stage	PTH Goal (pg/mL)	Serum Phosphorous (mg/dL)	Serum Calcium (mg/dL)
3	30–70	≥4.6	≥9.5
4	70–110	≥4.6	≥9.5
5	150–300	≥5.2	≥10.2

CKD, chronic kidney disease; PTH, parathyroid hormone.

sonable for individuals with persistent severe hyperphosphatemia.

Vitamin D Receptor Agonists for Hyperparathyroidism

Given the risk of hyperparathyroidism and consequent osteitis fibrosa cystica as well as the underlying deficiency of 1,25-dihydroxyvitamin D that accompanies progressive CKD, treatment with active vitamin D and its analogs plays a central role in patients with ESRD and, to a lesser extent, in predialysis CKD. These analogs, generally referred to as vitamin D receptor agonists (VDRAs), include the native calcitriol as well as newer agents such as paricalcitol, doxercalcitriol, falecalcitriol, 22-oxacalcitriol, and alfacalcidol (1-hydroxyvitamin D, converted to 1,25-dihydroxyvitamin D in the liver); the last four agents are not available in the United States at this time. Because the focus of these agents has been on the treatment of hyperparathyroidism, K/DOQI guidelines have focused on target PTH values to guide therapy (Table 3-1). These guidelines recommend deferring or withholding therapy for predialysis individuals with corrected serum calcium >9.5 mg/dL or serum phosphorous >4.6 mg/dL or for dialysis patients with calcium >10.2 mg/dL or phosphorous >5.5 mg/dL (Table 3-1).

PTH goals are higher in the more advanced stages of CKD because of the development of PTH resistance in bone. Because of the inability to directly measure bone PTH activity and the impracticality of routine bone biopsy, PTH levels have remained as the primary, albeit imperfect, guide to VDRA treatment. Given the potential role of vitamin D beyond the control of hyperparathyroidism (see below), the focus may shift away from PTH levels in the future.

There has been much interest in the potential of newer VDRAs to suppress PTH while minimizing promotion of calcium and phosphate absorption from the gastrointestinal tract. This is supported by some animal data and limited human studies but remains a topic of active investigation. Use of one VDRA over another cannot be strongly recommended at this time.

Nutritional Vitamin D

Nutritional forms of vitamin D include the plant-derived ergocalciferol and the animal-based cholecalciferol. These must be hydroxylated by both the hepatic 25-hydroxylase and the renal 1α-hydroxylase; the utility of these agents in CKD has therefore been thought to be limited. However, recent data suggest that treatment of 25-hydroxyvitamin D deficiency with ergocalciferol is effective at reducing PTH in stage 3 CKD. The presence of extrarenal 1α-hydroxylase also points to the potential importance of these nutritional forms. The role for this form of vitamin D therapy remains a topic of active research.

Calcimimetics

The recent advent of calcimimetic drugs has added a more direct pathway for the suppression of PTH. This class of drugs binds to the calcium-sensing receptor (CaSR) on the parathyroid gland, thus simulating a hypercalcemic state in the setting of a normal serum calcium levels. Consequently, PTH production is decreased. In addition, increased stimulation of the CaSR may be helpful in minimizing parathyroid gland hyperplasia. Only one calcimimetic, cinacalcet, is currently available. Cinacalcet offers the potential to control PTH without the risk of hypercalcemia or hyperphosphatemia associated with VDRAs. Because of the underlying mechanism of action, cinacalcet should be avoided in patients with a serum calcium level below 7.5 mg/dL.

A meta-analysis of three randomized controlled trials of cinalcet versus placebo demonstrated a greater likelihood of achieving K/DOQI targets for PTH, calcium, phosphorous, and the calcium-phosphorous product in the cinacalcet groups. Cinacalcet is approved for use in the maintenance dialysis population. Use in predialysis CKD is not Food and Drug Administration (FDA) approved for management of hyperparathyroidism and remains controversial given the potential for severe hypocalcemia.

VITAMIN D AND SURVIVAL

Although much of the focus on VDRA use has centered on management of PTH, calcium, and phosphorus, there has been increasing attention on potential effects of VDRAs on improved outcomes in CKD. A retrospective study in over 60,000 maintenance hemodialysis patients demonstrated a 16% reduction in all-cause mortality associated with paricalcitol over calcitriol. This reduction persisted despite adjustment for a wide range of clinical characteristics, including levels of calcium, phosphorous, and PTH, suggesting that any mortality benefits may result from actions beyond the traditional axis of mineral metabolism. In a later study, the same group found a 26% 2-year reduction in mortality in patients who received any form of active vitamin D compared with those who did not receive the therapy.

Although retrospective cohort studies such as these cannot prove a causative link, several other studies have now emerged with similar results in a wide range of patient populations. Intriguingly, one study suggests that the dialysis survival benefit associated with black race may be explained by increased use of VDRAs in this population.

While the bulk of research examining the influence of VDRAs on survival has been done in maintenance dialysis cohorts, two recent studies suggest that these agents may play a similar role in patients with stage 3–5 CKD with reduction in the risk of death ranging from 26% to 65% in patients receiving oral calcitriol compared with those who did not receive it.

Potential Mechanisms of a Survival Benefit of Vitamin D Receptor Agonists

Because cardiovascular mortality is the leading cause of death in CKD and the risk of cardiovascular disease is dramatically increased in this population, the potential actions of vitamin D on the cardiovascular system have been a topic of great interest. These mechanisms have largely been explored through animal models. VDRAs appear to suppress renin production, thus potential mitigating the risk of heart failure. An animal model at high risk of developing left ventricular hypertrophy and heart failure demonstrated improved cardiac function following treatment with paricalcitol, and observational data has suggested that similar benefits may exist in humans. Although high doses of vitamin D have been implicated in vascular calcification in animals, newly elucidated pathways suggest that vitamin D has the potential to reduce this calcification at lower doses. Randomized trials of VDRAs actions on cardiac structure and function in both the dialysis and predialysis CKD populations are currently underway and may significantly alter the indications for VDRAs.

Although cardiovascular disease has been the focus of research on the link between VDRAs and improved patient outcomes, recent research tying vitamin D to expression of antimicrobial peptides raises the possibility of an effect on infectious disease as well, which represents the second-leading cause of death in dialysis. At this time, these actions in humans remain speculative but are active areas of investigation.

It should be noted that in the absence of data from randomized controlled trials, routine use of VDRAs in the hope of improving patient outcomes cannot be definitively substantiated by existing research. Observational studies such as those described above are helpful for generating testable hypothesis and guiding further research. Despite the fact that these studies adjusted for potential confounding from mineral levels and patient health, there is always the potential for residual confounding from unmeasured factors.

CONCLUSION

A cascade of changes in the metabolism of calcium, phosphorous, and vitamin D lead to a disordered state of mineral metabolism that accompanies the progression of CKD. Given the risk of metabolic bone disease associated with hyperparathyroidism, attempts to normalize levels of calcium and phosphorous and regulate the level of PTH have been central to the management of CKD. This may be achieved through modification of diet or use of phosphate binders, calcimimetics, and VDRAs. The choice of agents is dictated in part by levels of minerals and PTH. Importantly, calcium, phosphorous, and PTH have not been established as surrogate outcomes of survival, and emerging data on the diverse actions of VDRAs suggests that this class of agents may influence mortality independently of these levels. New randomized trials over the next several years may have a significant impact on the indications for management of mineral metabolism disorders in patients with CKD.

Selected Readings

Andress D, Norris KC, Coburn JW, et al. Intravenous calcitriol in the treatment of refractory osteitis fibrosa of chronic renal failure. N Engl J Med 1989;321:274–279.

Block GA, Klassen PS, Lazarus JM, et al. Mineral metabolism, mortality, and morbidity in maintenance hemodialysis. J Am Soc Nephrol 2004;15:2208–2218.

Bodyak N, Ayus JC, Achinger S, et al. Activated vitamin D attenuates left ventricular abnormalities induced by dietary sodium in Dahl salt-sensitive animals. Proc Natl Acad Sci USA 2007;104:16810–16815.

Foundation NK. K/DOQI clinical practice guidelines for bone metabolism and disease in chronic kidney disease. Am J Kidney Dis 2003; 42:S1–S201.

Goodman WG, Ramirez JA, Belin TR, et al. Development of adynamic bone in patients with secondary hyperparathyroidism after intermittent calcitriol therapy. Kidney Int 1994;46:1160–1166.

Ishimura E, Nishizawa Y, Inaba M, et al. Serum levels of 1,25-dihydroxyvitamin D, 24,25-dihydroxyvitamin D, and 25-hydroxyvitamin D in nondialyzed patients with chronic renal failure. Kidney Int 1999;55:1019–1027.

LaClair RE, Hellman RN, Karp SL, et al. Prevalence of calcidiol deficiency in CKD: a cross-sectional study across latitudes in the United States. Am J Kidney Dis 2005;45:1026–1033.

Moe SM, Chertow GM, Coburn JW, et al. Achieving NKF-K/DOQI bone metabolism and disease treatment goals with cinacalcet HCl. Kidney Int 2005;67:760–771.

Qunibi W, Moustafa M, Muenz LR, et al. A 1-year randomized trial of calcium acetate versus sevelamer on progression of coronary artery calcification in hemodialysis patients with comparable lipid control: the Calcium Acetate Renagel Evaluation-2 (CARE-2) study. Am J Kidney Dis 2008;51:952–965.

Suki WN, Zabaneh R, Cangiano JL, et al. Effects of sevelamer and calcium-based phosphate binders on mortality in hemodialysis patients. Kidney Int 2007;72:1130–1137.

Teng M, Wolf M, Lowrie E, et al. Survival of patients undergoing hemodialysis with paricalcitol or calcitriol therapy. N Engl J Med 2003;349:446–456.

Teng M, Wolf M, Ofsthun MN, et al. Activated injectable vitamin D and hemodialysis survival: a historical cohort study. J Am Soc Nephrol 2005;16:1115–1125.

Wolf M, Betancourt J, Chang Y, et al. Impact of Activated Vitamin D and Race on Survival among Hemodialysis Patients. J Am Soc Nephrol 2008;19:1379–1388.

Zhou C, Lu F, Cao K, et al. Calcium-independent and 1,25(OH)(2)D(3)-dependent regulation of the renin-angiotensin system in 1alpha-hydroxylase knockout mice. Kidney Int 2008;74:170–179.

Zisman AL, Hristova M, Ho LT, et al. Impact of ergocalciferol treatment of vitamin D deficiency on serum parathyroid hormone concentrations in chronic kidney disease. Am J Nephrol 2007;27: 36–43.

4

Management of Lipid Abnormalities in the Patient with Kidney Disease

Christoph Wanner and Vera Krane

To understand dyslipidemia in chronic kidney disease (CKD) stages 1 through 5, knowing some general aspects of lipid metabolism is useful. In general, all five major lipoprotein classes (chylomicrons, very low-density lipoproteins [VLDL], intermediate-density lipoproteins [IDL], low-density lipoproteins [LDL], high-density lipoproteins [HDL]) consist of lipids (cholesterol, triglycerides, and phospholipids) and apolipoproteins. Apolipoproteins (A-I, A-II, B-48, B-100, C-I, C-II, C-III, and E) are found in different distributions among the various lipoproteins and serve as cofactors for enzymes and ligands for receptors. Levels of chylomicrons, the largest lipoprotein particle, increase after eating and are almost absent in the fasting state. These lipoproteins are formed in the intestinal epithelial cells; their main lipid content, triglycerides, is synthesized from re-esterification of dietary monoglycerides and fatty acids. Triglycerides represent 90% of chylomicrons and are hydrolyzed by lipoprotein lipase (LPL) present in adipose and vascular tissue. The residual particles, also called chylomicron remnants, are usually removed rapidly by the liver. In addition to dietary-derived chylomicrons, the liver has the capacity to produce endogenous lipoproteins from excess hepatocyte cholesterol and triglycerides. These lipids are synthesized and are secreted as triglyceride-rich VLDL. The triglycerides present in VLDL are gradually removed by LPL (with apoC-II acting as a cofactor), resulting in IDL. IDL, also named *VLDL remnants*, represents a transition step in the lipolysis of VLDL to LDL, the main cholesterol-carrying lipoprotein, which accounts for 70% of circulating cholesterol (Fig. 4-1). The characteristics of the various lipoproteins and their lipid and apolipoprotein composition in healthy humans are given in Figure 4-1.

Lipoprotein(a) [Lp(a)], another apolipoprotein, should not be neglected in patients with kidney disease, because high levels are especially atherogenic. Lp(a) contains a structural protein called [apo(a)]. Apo(a) exhibits a high homology to plasminogen and an extreme size polymorphism, with the apo(a) isoproteins ranging in size from 420 to 840 kD. Inherited in an autosomal-codominant fashion, the apo(a) isoprotein is an important factor that determines plasma Lp(a) concentrations, with an inverse correlation between the size of apo(a) isoprotein and the plasma Lp(a) concentration. The distribution of plasma Lp(a) levels is highly skewed toward lower concentrations, with more than two thirds of the population having levels lower than 20 mg per dL. High plasma concentrations of Lp(a) (more than 20 mg per dL) are associated with the risk for premature coronary atherosclerosis, cerebrovascular atherosclerosis, and saphenous vein bypass graft stenosis.

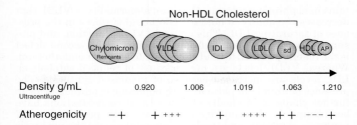

Figure 4-1. Classification of major lipoprotein particle density classes. (From Quaschning T, Krane V, Metzger T, et al. Abnormalities in uremic lipoprotein metabolism and its impact on cardiovascular disease. Am J Kidney Dis 2001;38(Suppl. 1):S14–S19, with permission.)

TYPES OF DYSLIPIDEMIA IN DIFFERENT STAGES OF CHRONIC KIDNEY DISEASE AND RENAL REPLACEMENT THERAPY

General Aspects

Qualitative characteristics of dyslipoproteinemia are similar in early renal insufficiency and in advanced kidney failure. The main metabolic abnormality is hypertriglyceridemia and delayed catabolism of triglyceride-rich lipoproteins resulting in increased concentrations of very low density lipoproteins (VLDLs) and intermediate density lipoproteins (IDLs) and reduced levels of HDL. Plasma cholesterol concentration is usually normal, even reduced, and only occasionally elevated. Dyslipidemia is detected in an early stage of chronic kidney disease (CKD, stage 2) when diagnosed and characterized by abnormalities in the composition of apolipoproteins. Increased levels of apoC-III and decreased levels of the apoA-I/apoC-III ratio are considered to be the hallmarks of an altered profile in kidney disease.

Chronic Kidney Disease and Proteinuria: Impact on Serum Lipids and Lipoproteins

Dyslipidemia is present in 70% to 90% of patients with nephrotic syndrome and most often expressed as both an increase in the serum total cholesterol and/or LDL cholesterol and increased serum triglycerides (50%). One third of patients have an exclusive elevation of LDL cholesterol, whereas only 4% of patients show pure hypertriglyceridemia. Changes in the composition of lipoprotein particles also have been described, with cholesterol enrichment in IDL but not LDL. The levels of HDL cholesterol may vary. This could be because of high serum lipoprotein(a) [Lp(a)] contaminating the HDL samples when cholesterol is assayed. The reasons why patients with nephrotic syndrome present different accumulations of triglycerides and cholesterol may include factors such as genetic apolipoprotein phenotypes, concomitant drug therapy, and the catabolic state of the individual. Delayed catabolism and over synthesis of lipoproteins are operative. Two separate processes impede the removal of triglyceride-rich lipoproteins in nephrotic syndrome. One is an abnormality in VLDL that decreases the ability to bind to endothelial surfaces in the presence of saturating LDL. This defect in VLDL function, and presumably structure, results from proteinuria. The second defect is the inability of LDL to bind effectively to vascular endothelium. Whereas VLDL levels are high because of reduced catabolism, LDL levels are increased because of increased synthesis. The presence of uremia in patients with nephrotic syndrome leads to further changes. Markedly elevated Lp(a) concentrations have been found in the majority of patients with proteinuria and nephrotic syndrome and resolve when remission of the nephrotic syndrome is induced. There are data to suggest that increased synthesis, rather than decreased catabolism, causes elevated plasma Lp(a) concentrations in nephrotic syndrome.

Hemodialysis and Dyslipidemia

Dyslipidemia in patients undergoing hemodialysis is more frequent than in the general population and is characterized by hypertriglyceridemia and low levels of HDL. Levels of total cholesterol and LDL usually are normal. This translates into the most characteristic feature of the end-stage renal disease (ESRD)-associated dyslipidemia represented by an accumulation of triglyceride-rich lipoproteins (VLDL remnants) and IDL. Catabolism of IDL and LDL is severely impaired, resulting in a markedly prolonged residence time of both particles. Additionally, qualitative changes of LDL with formation of small dense LDL are found. By the level of apolipoproteins, the dyslipidemia can also be classified as an accumulation of apoB-containing triglyceride-rich lipoprotein particles containing apoC-III and Lp(a) or lipoprotein B complex particles.

Besides a defect in postprandial chylomicron remnant clearance, abnormal HDL apoA-I and apoA-II kinetics have been described, with increased catabolism of apoA-I and decreased production rate of apoA-II resulting in reduced plasma levels of both apolipoproteins.

Continuous Ambulatory Peritoneal Dialysis and Dyslipidemia

Patients undergoing continuous ambulatory peritoneal dialysis (CAPD) present with higher plasma cholesterol, triglyceride, LDL, and Lp(a) levels than patients undergoing hemodialysis. This additional increase is most likely because of two factors: (i) loss of protein (7–14 g/day) into the peritoneal dialysate, mimicking nephrotic syndrome, and (ii) absorption of glucose (150–200 g/day) from the dialysis fluid. This was in part reflected in the data from Prinsen et al., who reported that VLDL-1 apoB100 and VLDL-2 apoB100 pool sizes were increased because of disturbances in both synthesis and catabolism. VLDL-1 apoB100 production is at least partially explained by increased free fatty acid availability secondary to peripheral insulin resistance; thus, insulin resistance might be a potential therapeutic target in patients undergoing peritoneal dialysis. In general, qualitative lipoprotein abnormalities are similar to those found in patients undergoing hemodialysis, and most mechanisms altering lipoprotein metabolism are probably also qualitatively the same, even though a study in normolipidemic CAPD patients demonstrated less pronounced abnormalities of cholesterol transport than observed in patients undergoing hemodialysis.

Lipid Abnormalities after Kidney Transplantation

Posttransplant dyslipidemia is qualitatively and quantitatively dependent on age, gender, body weight and type, and dose of immunosuppressive agents. The prevalence of lipid changes in kidney transplant recipients is very high. Particularly common are increases in cholesterol and LDL. HDL is usually normal, and triglycerides are often increased.

DYSLIPIDEMIA AND IMPACT ON CARDIOVASCULAR DISEASE

The overall risks of cardiovascular morbidity and mortality are profoundly increased in patients with CKD, and the majority of patients with CKD die of cardiac and vascular events before reaching ESRD.

Nephrotic Syndrome

There is no reason to doubt that the severe, persistent elevations of cholesterol, LDL, IDL, and Lp(a) do not represent a highly atherogenic condition. However, relatively little and conflicting information has been published on the risk of atherosclerotic vascular disease in patients with CKD. All of these studies were retrospective, however, and flawed by small sample numbers, selection bias, and lack of control for other atherosclerotic risk factors. Some studies included patients with minimal change disease, and most of these patients would most likely resolve their nephrotic syndrome and hence not remain at risk for the long-term complications of hyperlipidemia. According to Ordonez et al., the adjusted relative risks of myocardial infarction and coronary death in nephrotic syndrome are 5.5 and 2.8, respectively. Data were obtained for 142 patients matched with healthy controls and followed prospectively for 5.6 and 1.2 years.

Dialysis

Cardiac and vascular disease is the leading cause of morbidity and mortality in patients undergoing hemodialysis; cardiac disease accounts for 44% of overall mortality. Approximately 22% of these deaths from cardiac causes are attributed to acute myocardial infarction but are only 10% of all-cause mortality. In patients who survive a myocardial infarction, the mortality from cardiac causes is 59% at 1 year, 73% at 2 years, and nearly 90% at 3 years. After adjusting for age, gender, race, and diagnosis of diabetes mellitus, mortality from cardiovascular disease (CVD) is far greater in patients undergoing hemodialysis than in the general population. It ranges from 500-fold in individuals aged 25 to 35 years to fivefold in individuals aged >85 years. This might be because of an increased prevalence of traditional and kidney disease-related risk factors. In this context, lipid abnormalities have been suggested as a major cause of vascular disease in hemodialysis patients. Whereas the log-linear relation between risk of coronary artery disease and blood cholesterol is well-established in the general population, most cross-sectional studies with longitudinal follow-up have failed to demonstrate that plasma total cholesterol, LDL cholesterol, and triglycerides are associated with increased cardiovascular mortality in patients undergoing hemodialysis. Even inverse associations were observed among patients undergoing hemodialysis between serum cholesterol concentrations and all-cause or cardiovascular mortality. The relationship between serum cholesterol and mortality has been described as U-shaped and, recently, as a J-shaped curve. The risk of death is 4.3 times greater in patients undergoing hemodialysis with serum cholesterol of <100 mg/dL (<2.6 mmol/L) than in those with values between 200 and 250 mg/dL (5.2–6.5 mmol/L). Concomitant chronic illnesses accompanied by inflammation or infection that induce a compensatory decrease in cholesterol synthesis are also associated with an increased risk of death, producing artifactual negative associations (confounding) between cholesterol and mortality. This hypothesis is supported by Liu et al., who demonstrated that hypercholesterolemia was an independent risk factor for all-cause and cardiovascular mortality in a subgroup of patients with ESRD without serologic evidence of inflammation or malnutrition but not in patients with inflammation. In another prospective study of 1167 hemodialysis patients, low serum cholesterol levels were associated with all-cause mortality in patients with low serum albumin. These effects may limit the extent to which standard observational studies can identify the true impact of serum cholesterol on the development of vascular disease in this and other populations. In the largest and longest study to date, 419 dialysis patients were followed prospectively over a 21-year period. During this time 49% died of CVD and 23% experienced fatal or nonfatal ischemic events. Smoking, hypertension, and hypertriglyceridemia were identified as independent risk factors for CVD. Another "positive" study in a group of 196 patients with diabetes receiving hemodialysis demonstrated elevated cholesterol levels with high LDL/HDL ratios that were associated with an increased risk of cardiac death during a 45-month follow-up. Data on the effects of lipids on cardiovascular risk in patients receiving peritoneal dialysis are sparse. Only two studies that examined the relationship between dyslipidemia and CVD were identified. Both had major design limitations.

Kidney Transplantation

Kidney transplant recipients suffer from a high morbidity and mortality because of premature CVD. Several observational studies have reported a positive association between total cholesterol and CVD, but unfortunately few of them have examined the relationship between LDL cholesterol and CVD. Lower levels of HDL were associated with CVD in most studies. In about half of the studies, higher levels of triglycerides were associated with CVD. Recently, the findings of an observational study of 1200 patients up to 15 years after kidney transplantation were in line with these results, showing associations between diabetes, prior transplant, body mass index at the time of transplant, cholesterol level, and LDL level with early acute coronary syndrome. Another recent observational study did not prove these findings. There was no significant association between triglyceride and total cholesterol levels with patient mortality. Similarly, no associations were found with allograft loss. This study was done in a much smaller cohort (154 patients) with clearly shorter follow-up (6.1 years).

CARDIOVASCULAR ENDPOINT STUDIES ON LIPID-LOWERING THERAPY IN PATIENTS WITH CHRONIC KIDNEY DISEASE

Chronic Kidney Disease Stages 1 to 4

Until now, no prospective, randomized, controlled trials on lipid lowering therapy in patients with CKD stages 1–4 have been published. The effect of lipid-lowering therapy on cardiovascular, cerebrovascular, and renal outcomes in patients with CKD stages 2 and 3 was investigated in post hoc analyses of the Pravastatin Pooling Project. In this trial, a total of 12,333 subjects with estimated glomerular filtration rates (GFRs) determined by the Cockcroft-Gault equation of 60 to 89.9 mL/min/1.73 m^2 and 4491 subjects with estimated GFRs of 30–59.9 mL/min/1.73 m^2 were analyzed; the results showed that 40 mg/day pravastatin produced a significant 23% relative risk reduction for the combined risk of nonfatal myocardial infarction, coronary mortality, and coronary revascularization in people with moderate CKD. Similar results were obtained in patients with mild CKD. In the subgroup of patients with diabetes (i.e., the patients with the highest baseline risk), the highest absolute risk reduction was observed (6.4%). Furthermore, a prespecified subgroup analysis of 6517 patients with kidney dysfunction from the ASCOT study revealed that atorvastatin significantly reduced the risk of the combined primary endpoint of nonfatal myocardial infarction and cardiac death. Of the 1329 patients with serum creatinine levels of 110–200 μmol/L who entered the Heart Protection Study, 182 of those who received simvastatin and 268 of those in the placebo group experienced a vascular event, indicating a proportional risk reduction with simvastatin treatment of about one fourth. Finally, a recent pooled analysis of 30 double-blind, randomized trials testing fluvastatin versus placebo in patients with moderate (creatinine clearance of ≥50 mL/min) to severe (creatinine clearance of ≤50 mL/min) renal insufficiency described 41% and 30% relative reductions in the risk of cardiac death and nonfatal myocardial infarction in patients with severe and moderate renal impairment. The analysis of adverse effects in the above-mentioned trials showed no special safety concerns in patients with CKD. Serum lipids were adequately lowered. Other lipid-lowering agents to be considered are fibrates. Gemfibrozil was shown to lower the risk of coronary death or nonfatal myocardial infarction in 1046 patients of the VA-HIT trial with impaired renal function, but the risk of sustained increases in serum creatinine was elevated in participants treated with gemfibrozil compared with placebo. In conclusion, there is indirect evidence that patients with CKD stages 2 and 3 may benefit from statin therapy with respect to cardiovascular events to a higher extent than subjects with normal kidney function. Patients with stage 4 CKD (GFR of <30 mL/min/1.73 m^2) were either absent or their numbers were too small to be analyzed.

Chronic Kidney Disease Stage 5: Dialysis

In light of the findings described above, the results of the 4D study came as a surprise. A total of 1255 patients with type 2 diabetes on maintenance hemodialysis were randomized to receive 20 mg atorvastatin or matching placebo. After a median follow-up of 4 years, a nonsignificant 8% relative risk reduction in the primary composite endpoint (cardiac death, nonfatal myocardial infarction, and stroke) was observed. Atorvastatin reduced the rate of all cardiac events combined (relative risk, 0.82; 95% confidence interval, 0.68–0.99; $p = 0.03$, nominally significant) but did not reduce the rate of all cerebrovascular events combined or the total mortality. Of note, there was a higher incidence of fatal stroke in the atorvastatin group compared with placebo (27 versus 13; relative risk, 2.03; $p = 0.04$). The overall incidence of adverse events was comparable between groups. According to these data, we would not recommend initiation of statin treatment in patients with type 2 diabetes mellitus undergoing hemodialysis and with LDL levels of <190 mg/dL at the present time. Large-scale randomized controlled trials on lipid-lowering therapy in patients receiving peritoneal dialysis and nondiabetic hemodialysis patients are currently under way: The AURORA study, comparing rosuvastatin with placebo in more than 2750 hemodialysis patients, will be analyzed by 2009. Results from the SHARP trial, which is a randomized study of 9489 patients with CKD (not including kidney transplant recipients) partly on dialysis treatment (hemodialysis and peritoneal dialysis) and receiving either simvastatin in combination with ezetimibe or a placebo, will be presented early in 2011.

Chronic Kidney Disease Stages 1 to 4, Kidney Transplant Recipients

The final CKD subpopulation considered in this chapter is kidney transplant recipients. The ALERT study was the first large scale cardiovascular outcome trial to be conducted in kidney transplant recipients and compared fluvastatin with placebo in 2102 patients followed for 5 to 6 years. Fluvastatin (40–80 mg/day) showed no significant reduction in the composite primary endpoint of cardiac death, nonfatal myocardial infarction, and coronary intervention procedure. The reductions observed in two of three subcomponents of the primary endpoint, cardiac death or nonfatal myocardial infarction, were interpreted as a great success for this therapy. Notably, the overall incidence of adverse events and study discontinuations with fluvastatin treatment was similar to placebo. The authors suggested that the trial was too small to detect a significant effect on the composite primary endpoint because the event rate was lower than expected. Therefore, an extension study was performed in which 1652 patients were treated with open-label fluvastatin for 2 years. A 31% relative reduction in major adverse cardiac events and a 29% relative reduction in cardiac death or definite nonfatal myocardial infarction were found. Total mortality and graft loss did not differ significantly between groups. Another subgroup analysis supported an early introduction of fluvastatin therapy in kidney transplant recipients and suggested a greater benefit with respect to cardiac death and myocardial infarction in patients treated earlier.

Clearly, studies in patients who have received kidney transplants require a high number-needed-to-treat in their design, in line with primary prevention trials. In summary, the results of the 4D and ALERT studies do not necessarily cast doubt on the validity of the subgroup analyses done for patients with CKD stages 2 and 3, in whom statins appear to be just as effective as in patients with normal kidney function. The issue remains undecided whether statins are still effective for reducing cardiovascular risk in those with more advanced stages of CKD.

RENAL ENDPOINT STUDIES OF LIPID-LOWERING THERAPY IN PATIENTS WITH CHRONIC KIDNEY DISEASE

In addition to the effects of lipid-lowering drugs on cardiac and vascular, including cerebrovascular outcomes, there are data that suggest that lipid lowering may slow the rate of decline in kidney function and lower urinary protein excretion. Recently, a meta-analysis of 27 studies, including 39,704 participants with a baseline mean GFR of 41–99 mL/min, addressed these questions. It showed that statin therapy leads to a small reduction in the rate of kidney function loss in patients with CVD (loss of estimated GFR, 1.22 mL/min/year slower in statin recipients) but not a significant effect based on studies of subjects with diabetic or hypertensive kidney disease or glomerulonephritis. Proteinuria appeared to be modestly reduced. Gemfibrozil did not exert a clinically relevant effect on rates of kidney function loss in a comparable analysis.

TREATMENT GUIDELINES

General Remarks

Guidelines for management of dyslipidemia in CKD have been issued, including the European Best Practices Guidelines (EBPG) and the U.S. National Kidney Foundation's Kidney Disease Outcomes Quality Initiative (K/DOQI) guidelines. Guidelines on lipid-lowering therapy in patients with CKD were difficult to define because of the lack of randomized controlled interventional trials showing that the treatment of dyslipidemia reduces the incidence of vascular events. Meanwhile, the issue of safety has been resolved in patients with CKD or patients after transplantation. When these guidelines were prepared, the 4D and ALERT trials were still underway. In the following section, the main aspects of the EBPG guidelines for the treatment of hemodialysis patients and the K/DOQI guidelines are summarized but reflect that they are mainly opinion based.

Principles of Lipid-Lowering Therapy for Patients with Chronic Kidney Disease

Because patients with CKD have a very high prevalence of dyslipidemia and CVD, the EBPG working group concluded that hemodialysis patients should be treated according to existing guidelines of lipid-lowering therapy for the general population, applying a high-risk strategy. The K/DOQI working group recommended that the NCEP/ATP III guidelines were generally applicable to patients with CKD stages 1 to 4. Some additional specific aspects of the management of dyslipidemias in CKD should be considered. These include the following:

- CKD should be classified as a CVD risk equivalent.
- Complications of lipid-lowering therapies resulting from reduced kidney function should be anticipated.
- Indications for the treatment of dyslipidemia other than preventing CVD should be considered when deciding on specific treatment strategies.
- Treatment of proteinuria as an alternative treatment of dyslipidemia may prove beneficial.
- In conjunction with dyslipidemia, the assessment and management of other modifiable, conventional risk factors (hypertension, smoking, obesity, and diabetes) should be performed.

Assessment and Diagnosis of Dyslipidemia

A complete fasting lipid profile with total cholesterol, LDL, HDL, and triglycerides is recommended for patients with CKD. For patients with stage 5 CKD, dyslipidemia should be evaluated upon presentation, at 2 to 3 months after a change in treatment, or with other conditions known to cause dyslipidemia (change in proteinuria, GFR, and so forth) and at least annually thereafter. The EBPG advises measurement of cholesterol, HDL, and triglycerides more frequently. LDL should be calculated according to the Friedewald formula if triglycerides are <400 mg/dL; otherwise, direct LDL measurement is recommended. If triglycerides are >800 mg/dL, no LDL measurement needs to be performed. Whenever possible in patients with CKD stage 5, lipid profiles should be measured after an overnight fast, because eating increases especially triglycerides and also total cholesterol. However, it is better to obtain nonfasting lipid profiles than to forgo evaluation altogether. In patients receiving hemodialysis, blood should be taken either before dialysis or on nondialysis days, at least 12 hours after hemodialysis treatment, because the hemodialysis procedure may acutely alter plasma lipids. Patients with dyslipidemia should be evaluated for secondary causes. Acute medical conditions (e.g., serious infections or myocardial infarction) may alter plasma lipids. It is best to wait until these conditions have resolved. Immunosuppressive medications may cause dyslipidemia. The recommendation is to assess the lipid profile 2 to 3 months after starting or stopping an agent that is known to influence plasma lipids.

Treatment of Dyslipidemia

Three patient groups are to be distinguished:

- In adults with stage 5 CKD and fasting triglycerides of ≥500 mg/dL (≥5.65 mmol/L) that cannot be ameliorated by correcting an underlying cause, treatment with therapeutic lifestyle changes (TLC) and a triglyceride-lowering agent should be considered to prevent acute pancreatitis. Only when triglycerides are <500 mg/dL (<5.65 mmol/L) should attention be focused on LDL cholesterol reduction. According to EBPG, in patients with triglycerides of >800 mg/dL (>9 mmol/L) who are resistant to any intervention, the administration of fish

oil and/or a switch to low molecular-weight heparin as antico-
agulant during hemodialysis therapy should be considered.
- For adults with stage 5 CKD and LDL of ≥100 mg/dL (≥2.59
  mmol/L), treatment should be considered to reduce LDL to
  <100 mg/dL (<2.59 mmol/L).
- For adults with stage 5 CKD and LDL of <100 mg/dL (<2.59
  mmol/L), fasting triglycerides of ≥200 mg/dL (≥2.26 mmol/
  L), and non-HDL cholesterol (total cholesterol minus HDL
  cholesterol) of ≥130 mg/dL (≥3.36 mmol/L), treatment should
  be considered to reduce non-HDL cholesterol to <130 mg/dL
  (<3.36 mmol/L). The EBPG chose a lower threshold for initiation of therapy with triglycerides, ≥180 mg/dL (≥2 mmol/L).

Treatment of Very High Triglycerides

TLC is the therapy of first choice and includes diet, weight control, increased physical activity, abstinence from alcohol, and
treatment of hyperglycemia, if present. For patients with fasting
triglycerides of ≥1000 mg/dL (≥11.29 mmol/L), the NCEP/ATP
III diet recommendations include a very low fat diet (<15% total
calories), medium-chain triglycerides, and fish oils. Diet should
be used judiciously, if at all, in individuals who are malnourished
or inflamed. If TLC is not sufficient to reduce triglycerides to
<500 mg/dL (<5.65 mmol/L), treatment with a fibrate or nicotinic
acid should be considered. Statins cause less triglyceride lowering, and bile acid sequestrants (BASs) may actually increase triglyceride levels. In any case, the benefits of drug therapy for hypertriglyceridemia should be weighed against the increased risks
(particularly for myositis and rhabdomyolysis) in CKD.

Treatment of High Low-Density Lipoprotein—Treatment with Therapeutic Lifestyle Changes

It may be possible to reduce the level of proteinuria and thereby
improve a patient's lipid profile. For patients with LDL of
100–129 mg/dL (2.59–3.34 mmol/L), it is reasonable to attempt
dietary changes for 2 to 3 months before beginning drug treatment. Diet changes should be used judiciously, if at all, however,
when there is evidence of protein–energy malnutrition, because
there have been no randomized trials that have examined the
safety and efficacy of a low-fat, low-cholesterol diet in patients
with CKD. There are data that suggest exercise improves cardiovascular function in patients undergoing hemodialysis and decreases triglycerides in patients with CKD. The role of weight
reduction in patients with CKD is unclear. Additional studies are
needed to define the role of diet, exercise, and weight reduction
in patients with CKD.

Treatment of High Low-Density Lipoprotein—Treatment with a Statin

In patients who cannot reduce LDL to <100 mg/dL (<2.59 mmol/
L) by TLC, a statin should be added because of the strong evidence
from studies in the general population that statins reduce CVD
and all-cause mortality and the lack of any strong evidence to
the contrary in patients with CKD. Whether statins cause hepato-
toxicity is controversial. EBPG recommends liver function tests
every 6 weeks. Patients should be monitored for signs and symp-

toms of myopathy. Creatine kinase monitoring is mandatory if muscle symptoms develop. The risk of myopathy from statins is increased by CKD, advanced age, small body frame, and concomitant medications. Patients who develop muscle pain or tenderness should discontinue statin therapy immediately and have a creatine kinase level determined. Doses of lovastatin, fluvastatin, or simvastatin are recommended to be reduced by approximately 50% in patients with CKD stages 4 and 5 according to K/DOQI, whereas the EBPG states that statin doses are usually the same in patients receiving hemodialysis as in the general population. Medications known to increase statin blood levels should either be avoided or the statin should be reduced or stopped. Cyclosporine has been shown to increase the blood levels of virtually every statin. Even fluvastatin and pravastatin, which are not metabolized by cytochrome P450 3A4, show two- and five-fold increased plasma levels. Accumulating evidence suggests that statins can be used safely with cyclosporine if the dose of the statin is reduced. The addition of a third agent that is also metabolized by the cytochrome P450 system increases the risk of myositis and rhabdomyolysis. Such combinations should be avoided. Because of the lack of sufficient data, it should also be assumed that tacrolimus may cause elevations in statin blood levels. Everolimus has minimal effects on blood levels of atorvastatin and pravastatin. The effects of sirolimus on statins are not well known.

Adding a Second Low-Density Lipoprotein-Lowering Agent to a Statin

There are very few data on the safety and efficacy of combination therapies in patients with CKD. The K/DOQI guidelines state that in general, it is wise to avoid the use of a fibrate together with a statin. EBPG recommended avoiding combining a fibric acid analog with a statin because of the high risk of rhabdomyolysis. BASs can be considered in combination with a statin in patients with LDL of ≥100 mg/dL (≥2.59 mmol/L) despite TLC and optimal treatment with a statin. They are contraindicated in patients with triglycerides of ≥400 mg/dL (≥4.52 mmol/L) because they may increase triglycerides in some patients. Sevelamer hydrochloride lowers lipid levels by mechanisms similar to those of BASs. Furthermore, nicotinic acid can be considered an alternative second agent in combination with a statin for patients with high triglycerides or for those not tolerating a BASs. There are no data on the use of a combination therapy with a statin and nicotinic acid in patients with CKD.

Treating High Low-Density Lipoprotein in Patients Who Cannot Take a Statin

Patients with minor adverse effects from a statin may tolerate a reduced dose or a different statin; sometimes a second-line agent needs to be used. BASs, nicotinic acid, and sevelamer are possible alternatives.

Use of Bile Acid Sequestrants in Kidney Transplant Recipients

Using BASs in kidney transplant recipients may be difficult because of a possible interference with the absorption of immunosuppressive medications that bind to lipids. Even though two small studies did not find a reduction in cyclosporine levels, it may be prudent to avoid administering a BAS from 1 hour before until 4 hours after the administration of cyclosporine and to monitor blood levels of cyclosporine. For many patients, the potential risk of transplant rejection resulting from poor absorption of immunosuppressive medication may outweigh the benefits of a further reduction in LDL. For kidney transplant recipients who have LDL levels of ≥100 mg/dL (≥2.59 mmol/L) despite maximal medical management, consideration should be given to changing the immunosuppression protocol. In deciding whether to change immunosuppressive agents, the risk of rejection should be weighed against the risk of CVD. Moreover, the effects of immunosuppression on overall CVD risk should be taken into account, not just their effects on dyslipidemia. For example, different immunosuppressive agents have different effects on blood pressure and post-transplant diabetes, both of which can affect the incidence of CVD.

Treating Non–High-Density Lipoprotein Cholesterol in Patients with High Triglycerides

Non-HDL cholesterol is defined as total cholesterol minus HDL. High fasting triglyceride levels (180–499 mg/dL; 2–5.7 mmol/L) are not used as goals of therapy, but they are markers of increased coronary risk and should be treated in the absence of increased LDL.

The finding that elevated triglycerides were an independent cardiovascular risk factor in some studies suggests that some triglyceride-rich lipoproteins are atherogenic. The latter are partially degraded VLDL, commonly called remnant lipoproteins. Non-HDL cholesterol was demonstrated to remain one of the strongest predictors for intima media thickness in 897 patients receiving hemodialysis. Non-HDL cholesterol also was a predictor of aortic atherosclerosis in a cohort of 205 hemodialysis patients. Therefore, non-HDL cholesterol is an independent factor affecting arterial wall thickening and stiffness. Recent data suggest that non-HDL cholesterol may actually be a better predictor of coronary mortality than LDL. Non-HDL cholesterol is also a reasonable surrogate marker for apoB, the major apolipoprotein of all atherogenic lipoproteins. In one study, patients receiving hemodialysis showed higher levels of VLDL and IDL and lower levels of HDL than age- and sex-matched controls with similar levels of plasma triglycerides. However, so far no evidence has linked low HDL, high fasting triglycerides, and increased non-HDL cholesterol directly to CVD in patients with CKD. Clearly, additional studies are needed to establish whether therapy targeting lower levels of VLDL and IDL is safe and effective in patients with CKD.

Therapeutic Lifestyle Changes for High Triglycerides and Non–High-Density Lipoprotein Cholesterol

There are virtually no studies on the effects of alcohol consumption in patients with CKD. Even if studies from the general population have produced conflicting results as to whether intensive glycemic control reduces the risk for CVD patients with CKD who have low HDL and/or high triglycerides should be assessed for diabetes, and patients with diabetes who have this lipid profile should have as good glycemic control as possible without causing excessive hypoglycemia. Obesity is associated with low HDL and/or high triglycerides. There are a few studies demonstrating successful weight reduction in obese patients with CKD. A limited number of studies suggest that low-fat diets and increased physical activity may be effective in patients with CKD. A few studies have examined the effects of fish oil supplements on lipoproteins in patients with CKD; their results have been inconclusive.

Drug Therapy for High Triglycerides and Non–High–Density Lipoprotein Cholesterol

Patients who are not already receiving a statin for treatment of LDL cholesterol who have fasting triglycerides of ≥200 mg/dL (≥2.26 mmol/L) (K/DOQI) or ≥180 mg/dL (≥2 mmol/L) (EBPG) and non-HDL cholesterol of ≥130 mg/dL (≥3.36 mmol/L) and who do not have liver disease should be started on a statin along with TLC. The safety and efficacy of statins for preventing CVD have been more conclusively established in randomized trials in the general population. If a statin cannot be used, a fibrate may be considered. The blood levels of bezafibrate, clofibrate, and fenofibrate are increased in patients with decreased kidney function compared with controls with normal kidney function. In contrast, blood levels of gemfibrozil do not appear to be altered by decreased kidney function. Bezafibrate, ciprofibrate, fenofibrate, and gemfibrozil have been reported to cause increased serum creatinine and blood urea nitrogen levels. Because dose modification for decreased kidney function is not required for gemfibrozil, unlike other fibrates, gemfibrozil should probably be considered the fibrate of choice for most patients with CKD. Nicotinic acid can be used in place of fibrates for patients with elevated triglycerides. However, there are almost no data on blood levels of nicotinic acid in patients with CKD. Furthermore, the use of polysulfone or polyamide high-flux dialysis has been shown to ameliorate hypertriglyceridemia in some patients. Treatment of renal anemia with erythropoietin in patients receiving hemodialysis has beneficial effects on plasma lipid concentrations.

Isolated Low High-Density Lipoprotein Cholesterol

Patients with isolated low HDL cholesterol should be treated with TLC. Pharmacologic treatment of isolated low HDL cholesterol is not recommended because the risks of pharmacologic therapy to raise HDL probably outweigh the benefits.

Other Lipid-Lowering Agents

Ezetimibe was approved after publication of the above-presented guidelines. There is accumulating evidence on ezetimibe treatment in patients with CKD stages 3, 4, and 5 on peritoneal dialysis or hemodialysis treatment as in the ongoing SHARP study as well as in kidney transplant recipients that it is an effective lipid-lowering agent when added to other lipid lowering therapies. It has been shown to be safe in patients with reduced kidney function and in patients who do not tolerate statin therapy.

At this time, there are no data about its effects on cardiovascular events.

Selected Readings

Baigent C, Burbury K, Wheeler D. Premature cardiovascular disease in chronic renal failure. Lancet 2000;356:147–152.

European Best Practice guidelines for haemodialysis (part 1). Section VII. Vascular disease and risk factors. Nephrol Dial Transplant 2002;17(Suppl 7):88–109.

Executive Summary of The Third Report of The National Cholesterol Education Program (NCEP) Expert Panel on Detection, Evaluation, And Treatment of High Blood Cholesterol In Adults (Adult Treatment Panel III). JAMA 2001;285:2486–2497

Heart Protection Study Collaborative Group. MRC/BHF Heart Protection Study of cholesterol lowering with simvastatin in 20,536 high-risk individuals: a randomised placebo-controlled trial. Lancet 2002;360:7–22.

Holdaas H, Fellstrom B, Jardine AG, et al. Assessment of LEscol in Renal Transplantation (ALERT) Study Investigators. Effect of fluvastatin on cardiac outcomes in renal transplant recipients: a multicentre, randomised, placebo-controlled trial. Lancet 2003; 361:2024–2031.

Kasiske BL. Hyperlipidemia in patients with chronic renal disease. Am J Kidney Dis 1998;32:S142–S156.

National Kidney Foundation Kidney Disease Outcomes Quality Initiative (K/DOQI). Clinical practice guidelines for nutrition in chronic renal failure. Am J Kidney Dis 2000;35:S1–S140.

National Kidney Foundation. K/DOQI clinical practice guidelines for managing dyslipidemias in chronic kidney disease. Am J Kidney Dis 2003;41(Suppl 3):S1–S92.

National Kidney Foundation. KDOQI Clinical Practice Guidelines and Clinical Practice Recommendations for Diabetes and Chronic Kidney Disease Am J Kidney Dis 2007;49(Suppl 2):S88–S95.

Wanner C, Krane V, Marz W, et al. German Diabetes and Dialysis Study Investigators. Atorvastatin in patients with type 2 diabetes mellitus undergoing haemodialysis. N Engl J Med 2005;353: 238–248.

Nutritional Support in Acute Renal Failure

Wilfred Druml

Previously, acute kidney injury (AKI) was regarded in terms of "simple" organ dysfunction, which is easily supported by modern renal replacement therapies (RRT). Currently, AKI is recognized as a systemic inflammatory syndrome, a pro-oxidative, proinflammatory, and hypermetabolic state exerting a profound impact on the course of the disease that is associated with AKI. Despite modern dialytic techniques, AKI is still associated with a high mortality.

Because dialysis does not provide a cure, the nutritional and metabolic management must present a cornerstone in the care of these patients. Nutrition support now provides much more than a merely quantitative approach to providing energy and nitrogen and, instead, is a more qualitative type of metabolic intervention aimed at modulating the inflammatory state, correcting the oxygen radical scavenger system, and promoting immunocompetence. The goals of nutritional therapy are not only to replace the macro- and micronutrient requirements but also to take advantage of specific pharmacologic effects of various nutrients. Similar considerations are applicable in the prevention and treatment of AKI.

In patients with AKI, the metabolic environment is complex; it is not only affected by the acutely uremic condition per se but also by the underlying disease process(es) with the associated complications. The type and intensity of RRT must also be considered. Depending on the severity of associated illnesses, nutrient requirements can differ widely among individual patients and during the course of disease. A nutritional program for a patient with AKI is not fundamentally different from the regimens proposed for other critically ill patients, but it is more complicated because the regimen must be devised in the context of the complex alterations in metabolism and nutrient balances that occur with acute loss of kidney function. In addition, the nutritional program has to be coordinated with RRT. Patients with AKI are extremely prone to developing metabolic complications during nutritional support. A major problem is a patient's lack of tolerance to administering fluids and electrolytes because of impaired excretory function and because metabolic processing of nutrients is altered. Clearly, nutritional therapy for patients with AKI must be more closely monitored than patients with other acute disease states.

For many years, parenteral nutrition was the preferred route for supporting nutritional demands of patients with AKI. This is now changed as enteral nutrition has become the preferred principal route for nutritional support of these patients. It is important to recognize, however, that enteral and parenteral nutrition should not be viewed as opposed therapies but rather as complementary methods of nutritional support. Since meeting the nutritional requirements by the enteral route alone is often not possible, supplementary parenteral nutrition is necessary but the benefits of enteral nutrition are not lost.

METABOLIC ALTERATIONS CHANGE NUTRITIONAL REQUIREMENTS IN ACUTE KIDNEY INJURY

Rarely is AKI an isolated disease process; instead, it often complicates sepsis, trauma or conditions leading to multiple-organ failure. In short, the metabolic responses of critically ill patients with AKI are determined not only by impaired kidney function but also by the underlying disease process and complications, including severe infections and multiple organ dysfunction. The type and intensity of RRT can exert a profound effect on metabolism and nutrient balances. It is clear that AKI by itself induces and/or augments a systemic inflammatory response with multiple downstream consequences, including decreased immunocompetence. In short, the acute loss of kidney function not only affects water, electrolyte, and acid-base metabolism, but also it can induce important changes in the "milieu interieur" (Table 5-1).

Protein and Amino Acid Metabolism and their Requirements in Acute Kidney Injury

The hallmark of metabolic alterations in AKI is the activation of protein catabolism, which releases excessive amounts of amino acids from skeletal muscle thereby increasing hepatic gluconeogenesis and ureagenesis. This results in sustained negative nitrogen balance and, hence, loss of somatic protein stores. Besides accelerated protein breakdown, the utilization of amino acids in the processes of protein synthesis is defective. For example, in the liver, the synthesis and secretion of acute phase proteins are stimulated. These processes can lead to imbalances in the pools of amino acids in both the plasma and the intracellular fluid of muscle. In addition, the clearance of most amino acids that support gluconeogenesis is enhanced by AKI. Finally, several amino acids (e.g., arginine or tyrosine), conventionally considered as nonessential amino acids, become "conditionally indispensable" when their metabolism is altered by AKI.

Table 5-1. Important metabolic abnormalities induced by acute kidney injury

---

- Induction of a proinflammatory state
- Activation of protein catabolism
- Peripheral glucose intolerance / increased gluconeogenesis
- Inhibition of lipolysis and altered fat clearance
- Oxidative Stress
  - Activation of ROS
  - Depletion of the antioxidant system
- Impairment of immunocompetence
- Endocrine abnormalities: hyperparathyroidism, insulin resistance, EPO resistance, resistance to growth factors, anabolic hormones

---

EPO, erythropoietin; ROS, reactive oxygen species.

Table 5-2.   Protein catabolism in acute kidney injury: contributing factors

Impairment of metabolic functions by uremic toxins

Endocrine factors
  Insulin resistance
  Increased secretion of catabolic hormones (catecholamines,
    glucagon, glucocorticoids)
  Hyperparathyroidism
  Suppression of release / resistance to growth factors

Acidosis

Acute phase reaction—Systemic inflammatory response syndrome
  (activation of cytokine network)

Release of proteases

Inadequate supply of nutritional substrates

Renal replacement therapy
  Loss of nutritional substrates
  Activation of protein catabolism

The etiology of hypercatabolism in AKI is complex; in addition to the loss of kidney function, the induction of an inflammatory state, the stresses of concurrent illnesses, and the type and intensity of RRT all contribute to the process (Table 5-2). A major stimulus of the acceleration of muscle protein catabolism by AKI is the development of insulin resistance. Interestingly, AKI glucose formation is not suppressed by excessive substrate as occurs in healthy subjects or patients with chronic kidney disease (CKD). When insulin resistance develops, there is depressed protein synthesis and increased protein degradation. Consequently, providing insulin to maintain normoglycemia can be beneficial to patients with AKI by acting to suppress excessive muscle protein catabolism, although this potential benefit of intensive glucose control has recently been questioned in large studies.

Acidosis is another important factor that stimulates muscle protein breakdown. The accumulation of acid activates the catabolism of protein and the oxidation of amino acids in muscle, independently of azotemia. In patients with CKD, there is evidence that correcting the degree of acidosis can eliminate the increase in muscle protein degradation to improve nitrogen balance. Clinical experience suggests that correcting acidosis is associated with improved nitrogen balance in patients with AKI.

Additional catabolic factors causing loss of protein stores include the release of inflammatory mediators, such as tumor necrosis factor-α (TNF-α) and interleukin-1 and -6, which are associated with hypercatabolism in many animal models and human disease states. In addition, secretion of hormones with catabolic properties such as catecholamines, glucagon, and glucocorticoids; development of hyperparathyroidism; suppression of and decreased sensitivity to growth factors; and the release of proteases from activated leukocytes can separately (or together) stimulate protein breakdown. Finally, the type and frequency of RRT can

Table 5-3.   Metabolic effects renal replacement therapy in acute kidney injury

Intermittent hemodialysis
  Loss of water soluble molecules
    Amino acids
    Water soluble vitamins
    L-carnitine
  Activation of protein catabolism:
  Impairment of insulin/IGF-1 signalling leading to activation of muscle protein degradation
  Loss of amino acids, protein and blood inducing release of proinflammatory cytokines (IL-1, IL-6, and TNF-α)
  Inhibition of protein synthesis
  Increase in ROS production
    Loss of antioxidants
    Stimulation of ROS formation through bioincompatibility
Continuous renal replacement therapy (CRRT)
  Heat loss
  Excessive load of substrates (lactate, citrate, glucose)
  Loss of nutrients (amino acids, vitamins, selenium etc.)
  Loss of electrolytes (phosphate, magnesium)
  Elimination of (short-chain) proteins (hormones, mediators?, but also albumin)
  Metabolic consequences of bio incompatibility (induction/ activation of mediator-cascades, of an inflammatory reaction, stimulation of protein catabolism)

IGF-1, insulin-like growth factor-I; IL-1, interleukin-1; IL-6, interleukin-6; ROS, reactive oxygen species; TNF-α, tumor necrosis factor-α.

affect protein balance (Table 5-3). During hemodialysis, protein catabolism is accelerated, a process mediated in part by the loss of nutritional substrates plus the activation of catabolic pathways mentioned above (see Chapter 11).

Last but not least, inadequate nutritional support can contribute to the loss of protein mass in patients with AKI. In experimental animals, starvation aggravates the catabolic response to AKI, and clinical experience suggests that pre-existing malnutrition is a major determinant of complications and mortality in patients with AKI.

AMINO ACID AND PROTEIN REQUIREMENTS IN PATIENTS WITH ACUTE RENAL FAILURE

Despite the well-established highly protein catabolic state of AKI, few studies have attempted to define the optimal requirements for protein or amino acids in these patients. In noncomplicated, nonhypercatabolic patients with AKI, a protein intake of 0.97 to 1.3 g/kg b.w./day was shown to lead to a positive nitrogen balance during the polyuric phase of AKI. It should be pointed out, however, that measuring nitrogen balance in patients who are experiencing rapid changes in accumulated nitrogen waste products is difficult and subject to considerable error.

In complicated critically ill patients with AKI, especially in ones who are treated with continuous renal replacement therapy (CRRT), the estimated protein catabolic rate is reportedly at 1.4 to 1.75 g/kg b.w./day. There also appears to be an inverse relation between protein and energy provision and protein catabolic rate. On the basis of these measurements, an amino acid/protein intake of about 1.5 g/kg b.w./day is recommended. It also recommended that amino acid/protein intake should not exceed 1.7 g/kg b.w./day. Higher amino acid or protein intakes (e.g., 2.5 g/kg b.w./day) have been suggested, but there is no convincing evidence that the higher intakes are beneficial. In addition, excessive intake of amino acids/proteins will definitely increase the accumulation of unexcreted waste products. This in turn, will induce adverse metabolic complications such as hyperammonemia while aggravating uremic complications and increasing the need for dialysis by stimulating muscle protein degradation. Unfortunately, the dialysis procedure itself is catabolic, and therefore, providing amounts of amino acid/protein above 1.5 g/kg b.w./day and increasing the frequency of dialysis could be counterproductive. In short, hypercatabolism cannot be overcome by simply increasing protein or amino acid intake; even in patients with normal kidney function who have sepsis or burns, providing more than 1.5 g protein (or amino acids)/kg b.w./d does not improve catabolism.

It is recommended that unless AKI will be brief and there are no associated catabolic illnesses, the intake of protein or amino acids should not be less than 0.8 g/kg b.w./day. But when patients with AKI are catabolic, they should receive approximately 1.2 g to 1.5 g protein (or amino acids)/kg b.w./day. This recommendation is in accordance with those for critically ill patients. The recommended level of amino acid/protein intake includes the amount needed for the amino acid and protein losses that occur with hemodialysis, CRRT, or peritoneal dialysis.

POTENTIAL METABOLIC INTERVENTIONS OF CONTROLLING CATABOLISM

Unfortunately, no effective methods have been identified that will reduce or stop the hypercatabolism associated with AKI. Consequently, "upstream" therapeutic interventions aimed at mitigating underlying metabolic abnormalities, especially inflammation, have been attempted.

- Nutritional substrates: It is not possible to reverse hypercatabolism and the hepatic gluconeogenesis that is stimulated by AKI simply by providing conventional nutritional substrates (see subsequent sections for details on nutritional supplementation in AKI). It is speculated that novel substrates (e.g., glutamine, leucine or its keto-acid, or structured triglycerides) might exert a more pronounced anti-inflammatory, hence anticatabolic response.

- Endocrine: Experimentally, therapy with anabolic hormones (insulin, insulin-like growth factor-I [IGF-I], recombinant human growth hormone [rHGH]) or hormone antagonists (antiglucocorticoids) can be partially effective in suppressing hypercatabolism in critical illness. But clinical results with the administration of IGF-I and rHGH (described later in this chapter) have been rather disappointing and in certain circumstances deleterious (e.g., the increased mortality of critically ill patients treated with rHGH).

- Anti-inflammatory interventions: Proinflammatory cytokines such as IL-1, IL-6, and TNF-α can cause excessive release of amino acids from skeletal muscle while activating hepatic amino acid uptake and gluconeogenesis. Various nutritional supplements such as specific amino acids (glutamine, glycine, arginine), omega-3-fatty acids, or antioxidants can modify the inflammatory response in animal models, but they have not been tested clinically in critically ill patients with AKI. The same is true for proinflammatory cytokine antagonists (IL-1 receptor, IL-6, and TNF-α receptor antagonists).
- Interventions to block catabolic pathways: Correcting acidosis is simple and clearly can suppress muscle protein catabolism by blocking the ubiquitin–proteasome proteolytic system.

Energy Metabolism and Energy Requirements

In patients with uncomplicated AKI, oxygen consumption is similar to that in healthy subjects. In patients with AKI with sepsis or the multiple-organ dysfunction syndrome, however, oxygen consumption increases to 20% to 30% above the calculated basal energy expenditure (BEE). In short, energy expenditure in patients with AKI is determined by the underlying disease and its associated complications rather than by the acute loss of kidney function.

Previously, energy requirements for patients with AKI were grossly overestimated, and excessive energy intakes were advocated. The adverse effects of an exaggerated nutrient intake are now established. The energy supply should never exceed actual energy requirements; complications from slightly "underfeeding" calories are less deleterious than those caused by overfeeding calories. Increasing energy intake of patients with AKI from 30 kcal/kg b.w./day to 40 kcal/kg b.w./day merely increases the frequency of metabolic complications such as hyperglycermia and hypertriglyceridemia.

Unfortunately, direct measurements of energy requirements of individual patients with AKI is generally unavailable, so energy requirements are calculated using a standard formula based on the BEE from the Benedict–Harrison equation multiplied by a "stress factor." On average, patients with AKI should receive 20 to 30 kcal/kg b.w./day; even when they are in a hypermetabolic state because of other underlying diseases (i.e., sepsis or multiple-organ failure), the energy expenditure rarely exceeds 130% of calculated BEE, and we recommend that the energy intake should not exceed 30 kcal/kg b.w./day in any patient with AKI.

CARBOHYDRATE METABOLISM

Frequently, AKI is associated with hyperglycemia because of insulin resistance of stress, which is further exacerbated as a complication of the loss of kidney function. The condition is recognized if there is a high plasma insulin concentration, a 50% decrease in the maximal insulin-stimulated glucose uptake by skeletal muscle and impaired glycogen synthesis in muscle. AKI-induced abnormalities in glucose metabolism also include accelerated hepatic gluconeogenesis because of excessive conversion from amino acids released during protein catabolism. Notably, hepatic gluconeogenesis in patients with AKI cannot be suppressed by exogenous glucose infusion. Besides resistance to the hypoglycemic effects of insulin, the rate of endogenous insulin secretion in patients with AKI is low in the basal state and during glucose infusion. Because the kidney is the main organ of insulin disposal, insulin degradation is decreased in AKI. Surprisingly, insulin catabolism in the liver is also consistently reduced in AKI, which may simply be a response to nonphysiologic hyperglycemia.

The importance of insulin resistance in AKI is further emphasized by studies showing improved patient and kidney survival in critically patients with strict normalization of blood glucose levels (80 to 110 mg/dL [4.4 to 6.1 mmol per liter]) versus conventional therapy (insulin administered when the blood glucose level exceeded 215 mg/dL [12 mmol per liter], with the infusion tapered when the level fell below 180 mg/dL [10 mmol per liter]). Because nutritional supplementation is a critical determinant of plasma glucose concentrations, appropriate therapy is important. Most recent studies also indicate a significant increase in hypoglycemic episodes in critically ill patients receiving strict blood glucose control regimens, adding some controversy to the subject. For these reasons, we recommend that while normoglycemia should be the goal during nutritional support of patients with AKI, the target glucose concentrations to be considered as "normoglycemia" must be adjusted according to the risk/benefit profile of the patient with particular attention to prevention of hypoglycemic events.

LIPID METABOLISM

There are also profound alterations of lipid metabolism in patients with AKI. The triglyceride content of plasma lipoproteins, especially very low-density lipoproteins (VLDL) and low-density lipoproteins (LDL) are increased; total cholesterol and HDL-cholesterol in particular, are decreased. The major cause of lipid abnormalities in AKI is impaired lipolysis because the activities of the lipolytic systems, peripheral lipoprotein lipase, and hepatic triglyceride lipase are decreased to values 50% below normal values. These changes contrast with those in most other acute disease states, which are usually associated with enhanced lipolysis. Metabolic acidosis can contribute to the impairment of lipolysis in AKI by inhibiting lipoprotein lipase. Notably, artificial lipid emulsions provided in parenteral nutritional solutions are degraded similar to endogenous VLDL. Thus, the impaired lipolysis of AKI leads to a delay in eliminating intravenously infused lipid emulsions: the elimination half-life is doubled and the clearance of fat emulsions is reduced by more than 50%. Finally, intestinal lipid absorption is delayed, complicating the responses to enteral nutrition.

METABOLISM AND REQUIREMENTS OF MICRONUTRIENTS

Because of vitamin losses occurring during RRT, serum levels of water-soluble vitamins are low in patients with AKI; patients with AKI require more of the water-soluble vitamins. An exception is ascorbic acid (vitamin C), a precursor of oxalic acid. Vitamin C intake should be less than 250 mg per day to avoid second-ary oxalosis and oxalate precipitation in soft tissues.

As in patients with CKD, vitamin D activation and plasma levels of 25(OH) vitamin D_3 and 1, 25-(OH) vitamin D_3 are low in patients with AKI. Serum concentrations of vitamin A and vitamin E, unlike those in patients with CKD, are decreased in patients with AKI, while serum vitamin K levels are normal or even elevated. Even though fat-soluble vitamins are not lost via hemodialysis, requirements for these vitamins, with the excep-tion of vitamin K, are increased because of AKI. Most commer-cially available multivitamin preparations for parenteral infu-sions contain the recommended daily allowances (RDA) of vitamins and can be safely given to patients with AKI. Neverthe-less, vitamin C and K administration must be closely monitored.

There are limited reports about trace element metabolism in patients with AKI. The available information includes low plasma levels of iron, selenium, and zinc but increased levels of copper. These findings may in part represent "acute phase reac-tion" responses. Nevertheless, selenium concentrations in plasma and erythrocytes are severely decreased in patients with AKI, and there are relevant selenium losses during continuous RRT (CRRT). In critically ill patients, preliminary reports indicate that selenium replacement reduces the incidence of AKI and im-proves the clinical outcome.

Parenteral administration of trace elements to patients with AKI should be undertaken with care, however, because gastroin-testinal absorption, the main regulator of trace element homeo-stasis, is bypassed, and renal excretion is impaired. The combina-tion of these factors raises the risk of toxicity. Micronutrients are part of the patient's defense against oxygen free radical–induced injury to cellular components. A profound depression in antioxi-dant status occurs in patients with AKI, and adequate supple-mentation with antioxidants must be provided by nutritional support.

ELECTROLYTES

Derangements in electrolyte balance in patients with AKI are affected by a spectrum of factors in addition to kidney failure. These include the underlying diseases and the degree of hyperca-tabolism, the type and intensity of RRT, the provision of drugs, and the timing, type, and composition of nutritional support. Electrolyte requirements vary considerably among patients, and they can change radically during the course of AKI. Conse-quently, there are no "standard" recommendations for electro-lytes. Nutritional support, especially parenteral nutrition in which there is low electrolyte content, can induce hypophos-phatemia and hypokalemia during therapy (the "refeeding syn-drome"). For these reasons, electrolyte requirements have to be evaluated in patients with AKI on a day-to-day basis with oral intake and supplementation adjusted accordingly.

Metabolic Impact of Acute Kidney Injury

Critical illness and the metabolic changes induced by AKI repre-sent potential therapeutic targets for improving outcomes. There is release of a cascade of potent inflammatory mediators into the systemic circulation, followed temporally by a compensatory anti-inflammatory response. In critically ill patients with AKI, pro- and anti-inflammatory cytokines are simultaneously markedly elevated in the presence or absence of sepsis. Critically ill patients with AKI also have impaired monocyte cytokine production closely resembling other critically ill patients without AKI. These studies suggest that strategies designed to reduce inflammation in critically ill patients with established AKI should be attempted with caution so as not to exacerbate risk of infectious complications.

Hyperglycemia and intensive insulin therapy designed to maintain blood glucose at or below 110 mg/dL can reduce morbidity and mortality in surgical or medical intensive care units, although the benefits of this therapy has been recently challenged. Whether hyperglycemia and/or hyperinsulinemia contribute directly to adverse events in critically ill patients with AKI or are simply a marker of metabolic injury severity has not been established.

Oxidative stress is a pathogenic mechanism associated with ischemic and toxic renal tubular injuries. Kidney disease itself is now recognized as an additional stimulus for increased oxidative stress. Consequently, critically ill patients with AKI manifest a marked increase in oxidative stress biomarkers.

Metabolic Impact of Dialysis Therapy

Hemodialysis therapy affects metabolism in many ways (see also Chapter 11). Protein catabolism is stimulated not only by substrate losses but also by activation of pathways of protein breakdown mediated in part by release of leukocyte-derived proteases and inflammatory mediators following blood–membrane interactions, endotoxin release, or both. Notably, these responses persist for at least several hours after ending the dialysis treatment. In addition, water soluble substances, such as amino acids and vitamins, are lost during hemodialysis, while the generation of reactive oxygen species is augmented. All of these factors can stimulate protein breakdown in muscle and other tissues.

CRRT, including continuous (venovenous) hemofiltration and continuous hemodialysis, is often used for patients with AKI, especially in critically ill patients. Relevant metabolic consequences of CRRT result from prolonged therapy and the high fluid turnover (see Table 5-3). A major consequence of CRRT is that small- and medium-sized molecules are eliminated. This is important because amino acid losses are estimated from the volume of the filtrate and the average plasma concentrations of amino acids. The total loss varies from 5 to 15 g amino acid per day or about 10% to 15% of amino acid intake. Amino acid losses during continuous hemofiltration and continuous hemodialysis are of a comparable magnitude. Depending on the type of therapy and the membrane material used, additional losses of protein can account for up to 10 g/day.

Water soluble vitamins (folic acid, vitamin B_1, vitamin B_6, and vitamin C) are also eliminated by CRRT, and an intake above the RDA is required to maintain plasma concentrations of these vitamins. Selenium losses during CRRT can amount to twice the amount needed to achieve the RDA.

Glucose balance during CRRT depends on the glucose concentration of the substitution fluid. For this reason, peritoneal dialysis solutions should not be used as the dialysate for CRRT, because they lead to excessive glucose uptake. Dialysate glucose concentrations should range between 1 to 2 g/dL to maintain a zero glucose balance. Lactate is present in most substitution fluids to buffer the acid generated. During CRRT, lactate uptake is substantial and when lactate formation is increased (e.g., during cardiogenic shock), or if lactate clearance is impaired (liver insufficiency), bicarbonate-based dialysates must be used. Bicarbonate is preferred because citrate metabolism can be reduced in patients with liver disease; it is usually unimpaired in critically ill patients with AKI.

Impact of Nutritional and Endocrine Interventions on Renal Regeneration in Acute Kidney Injury

Starvation accelerates protein breakdown and impairs protein synthesis in the kidney. In experimental animals, nutritional strategies can accelerate tissue repair and the recovery of kidney function. In patients with AKI, however, a benefit from nutritional therapy has been much more difficult to prove. Only one report concludes there is a positive effect of parenteral nutrition on the resolution of kidney damage.

Amino acids (infused either before or during ischemia, or when nephrotoxicity occurs) exacerbates the degree of tubular damage and will accelerate the loss of kidney function in rodent models of AKI. This "therapeutic paradox" is related in part to the increase in metabolic work that is linked to kidney transport processes that are activated. Because oxygen supply is limited, provision of nutrients aggravates the degree of ischemic injury. Similar observations have been made with the infusion of glucose during renal ischemia. Therefore, avoiding hyperglycemia can help to prevent evolution of AKI. Certain amino acids may exert kidney protection: glycine and, to a lesser degree, alanine and taurine, can limit tubular injury in ischemic or nephrotoxic models of AKI. Arginine reportedly preserves renal perfusion and tubular function during both nephrotoxic and ischemic injury. This may involve production of nitric oxide because inhibitors of nitric oxide synthase exert an opposite effect. Parenterally infused amino acids or an enteral supply of amino acids or protein can increase both renal perfusion and excretory renal function ("renal functional reserve"). In cirrhotic patients with functional kidney failure, intravenous infusion of amino acids can improve renal plasma flow (approximately 25%) and glomerular filtration rate (GFR). Whether a similar benefit systematically occurs with an improvement in kidney function in patients with AKI is unknown. Results of a pilot study, however, suggest that amino acid infusions can help increase GFR and reduce the requirements for diuretics in patients with AKI.

In experimental models of AKI, various endocrine-metabolic interventions (e.g., thyroxine, rHGH, epidermal growth factor [EGF], IGF-1, hepatocyte growth factor [HGF]) have been shown to accelerate tubular regeneration. In clinical studies, however, these beneficial effects have not been confirmed. A multicenter study, in which IGF-I was administered to patients with AKI, was terminated early because of the lack of benefit. In a pilot study of five patients with AKI, rHGH improved various indices of protein metabolism. But administering rHGH to critically ill patients, many of whom also had AKI, actually increased patient mortality. Administering triiodothyronine to upregulate the EGF receptor expression is ineffective in patients with AKI and increased mortality. To date, HGF has not been sufficiently evaluated in humans to recommend its use.

Nutrient Administration

Patient Selection

Ideally, a nutritional program should be designed for each patient with AKI, but in clinical practice, three major groups of patients with AKI can be identified. The differences are largely based on the severity of disease and the extent of protein catabolism (Table 5-4).

- Group I includes patients without excess protein catabolism and a urea nitrogen appearance rate (UNA) <6 g of nitrogen above the nitrogen intake. In these patients, AKI is usually limited to risk or injury (by Acute Kidney Injury Network [AKIN] criteria) and is caused by nephrotoxins such as aminoglycosides and contrast media. They rarely present major nutritional problems and in most cases, they can be fed orally; their prognosis is good.

- Group II consists of patients with moderate hypercatabolism and a UNA exceeding nitrogen intake by 6 to 12 g nitrogen per day. These patients frequently suffer from complicating infections or moderate other organ injury in association with AKI. Tube feeding, intravenous nutritional support, or both are generally required, and dialysis or CRRT often becomes necessary to limit waste product accumulation.

- Group III includes patients in whom AKI is associated with severe trauma, burns, or overwhelming infections in the context of multiple-organ failure syndrome. UNA is markedly elevated (more than 12 g of nitrogen above nitrogen intake). Treatment strategies are usually complex and include enteral nutrition, parenteral nutrition, or both; hemodialysis or CRRT plus blood pressure and ventilatory support are commonly needed. Mortality in this group of patients exceeds 60% to 80%. The severity of the underlying illness, together with the untoward systemic consequences of AKI, accounts for the poor prognosis.

ORAL FEEDING

Oral feeding should be used in all patients who can tolerate it (usually, this category is restricted to patients who are nonhypercatabolic [group I]). Energy is provided by simple carbohydrates (sugar, jellies, and other sweets) or glucose polymers given at regular intervals. Initially, 40 g per day of high-quality protein is given (0.6 g/kg b.w./d), and protein intake is gradually increased to 0.8 g/kg b.w./d as long as the blood urea nitrogen (BUN) remains below 80 mg/dL. For patients treated with hemodialysis, protein intake should be increased to 1.0 to 1.2 g/kg b.w./d to make up for amino acids lost during dialysis and for the potential

Table 5-4.   Patient classification and nutrient requirements in patients with acute renal failure

	Extent of Catabolism		
	Mild	Moderate	Severe
Excess urea appearance (above N intake)	>5 g	5–10 g	>10 g
Clinical setting (examples)	Drug toxicity	Elective surgery ± Infection	Sepsis, ARDS MODS
Mortality	20%	40% to 60%	>60%
Dialysis/ CRRT - frequency	Rare	As needed	Frequent
Route of nutrient administration	Oral	Enteral and/or parenteral	Enteral and/or parenteral
Energy Recommendations (kcal/kg b.w./day)	20–25	20–30	25–35
Energy substrates	Glucose	Glucose + fat	Glucose + fat
Glucose (g/kg b.w./day)	3.0–5.0	3.0–5.0	3.0–5.0
Fat (g/kg b.w./day)		0.6–1.0	0.8–1.2
Amino acids/ protein (g/kg/day)	0.6–1.2	1.0–1.4	1.2–1.5 (1.7)
	EAA(+NEAA)	EAA + NEAA	EAA + NEAA
Nutrients used oral/ enteral	Food, sip feeds	Enteral formulas	Enteral formulas
Parenteral		Glucose 50% to 70% Lipids 10% to 20% AA 6.5% to 10%* Micronutrients†	Glucose 50% to 70% Lipids 10% to 20% AA 6.5% to 10%* Micronutrients†

*AA, amino acid solution: general or special, "nephro" solutions (EAA + specific NEAA)
†Multivitamin and multitrace element preparations
ARDS, acute respiratory distress syndrome; CRRT, continuous renal replacement therapy; EAA, essential amino acids; MODS, multiple organ dysfunction syndrome, NEAA, nonessential amino acids.

catabolic effects of the dialytic process. For patients undergoing peritoneal dialysis, protein intake should be raised to 1.4 g/kg b.w./d to counteract losses of both amino acids and protein. A supplement of water-soluble vitamins is recommended.

ENTERAL NUTRITION (TUBE FEEDING)

During the last decade, enteral nutrition has become the standard method of providing nutritional support for critically ill patients. There are well-documented advantages of enteral nutrition, including the fact that even small amounts of luminal nutrients maintain gastrointestinal function and support the barrier function of the intestinal mucosa. Enteral nutrition also helps to preserve the structural integrity of the mucosal layer and prevent the development of mucosal ulcerations that lead to translocation of bacteria and systemic infections.

Enteral nutrition may have specific advantages in patients with AKI. In models of AKI, enteral nutrition augments renal plasma flow and can improve kidney function. In two clinical studies, enteral nutrition was a factor associated with an improved prognosis in patients with AKI. Unfortunately, few systematic studies of enteral nutrition for patients with AKI have been conducted. In the largest study, the feasibility of and tolerance to enteral nutrition was examined in 182 patients with AKI. Side effects of enteral feeding were more common in patients with AKI than in those with normal renal function, but, in general, enteral nutrition was safe and effective in both groups.

As noted, critically ill patients with AKI can have impaired gastrointestinal motility making it impossible to meet requirements by the enteral route alone. For such patients, parenteral nutrition can be added. Enteral and parenteral nutrition should be viewed as complementary types of nutritional support because even small amounts of enteral diets given regularly (i.e., 50 to 100 mL of polymeric diets given 6 times each day) can help maintain intestinal functions.

ENTERAL FORMULAS

Three types of enteral formulas have been used in patients with AKI, but these formulas were not specifically developed to counteract specific metabolic and nutritional abnormalities akin to this patient population.

- Elemental powder diets: The concept of a low-protein diet supplemented with essential amino acids (EAA) in the oral nutrition of patients with CKD has been extended to enteral nutrition for patients with AKI. Some formulas contain the eight EAA plus histidine. Therefore, they must be supplemented with energy substrates, vitamins, and trace elements. Major disadvantages are the limited spectrum of nutrients and a high osmolality. These formulations should be replaced by "ready-to-use" liquid products.
- Polymeric enteral formulas: These are designed for patients with AKI who are not in failure stage; many critically ill patients with AKI receive standard enteral formulas. Disadvantages of these formulas include the amount and type of protein and the high content of electrolytes (e.g., potassium and phos-

phate). Whether diets enriched in specific substrates such as glutamine, arginine, nucleotides, or omega-3-fatty acids ("immunonutrition") might exert beneficial effects in patients with AKI is not known.

• Specific enteral polymeric liquid formulas adapted to correct metabolic alterations of uremia: These ready-to-use liquid diets were designed for patients with compensated CKD. The diets have a reduced protein and electrolyte content. Other diets were created to meet the nutrient requirements of patients undergoing hemodialysis; there is a higher protein and a reduced electrolyte content, plus a high specific energy content of 1.5 to 2.0 kcal/mL. Some are supplemented with additional nutrients (e.g., histidine or carnitine). This category of formulas represents a reasonable approach to enteral nutrition of hypercatabolic patients with AKI.

PARENTERAL NUTRITION

If nutrient requirements cannot be met by the enteral route or if the enteral route cannot be used, supplementary or total parenteral nutrition should be used. Fluids are usually restricted in patients with AKI and parenteral nutritional solutions are hyperosmolar, so the formulas are infused through central venous catheters to avoid peripheral vein damage.

Components of Parenteral Nutrition

Carbohydrates

Glucose should be used as the main energy substrate, because it is metabolized by all organs even under hypoxic conditions. Glucose intake must be restricted to less than 3 to 5 g/kg b.w./day, because higher intakes are not metabolized but simply promote hyperglycemia, lipogenesis (including fatty infiltration of the liver and excessive carbon dioxide production), and increase the risk of infections. Because glucose tolerance in AKI is impaired, the use of these formulas generally requires supplemental insulin. Considering the well-known side effects of even short-term hyperglycemia, blood glucose levels must be maintained within the physiologic range to reduce complications and improve survival.

Because of the dangers of a high glucose intake, a portion of the energy requirement should be supplied with lipid emulsions. The most suitable means of providing the energy requirements in critically ill patients is not glucose or lipids but glucose and lipids. Other carbohydrates, including fructose, sorbitol, or xylitol, are available in some countries. These compounds should be avoided because of potential adverse metabolic effects.

Fat Emulsions

Advantages of intravenous lipids include their high specific energy content, a low osmolality, provision of essential fatty acids to prevent deficiency syndromes, a lower rate of hepatic lipid accumulation, a lower risk of inducing hyperglycemia, and reduced carbon dioxide production (especially relevant in patients with respiratory failure) and potentially, anitinflammatory properties of omega-3-fatty acids. Moreover, lipids are structural components of cell membranes and are precursors of regulatory molecules, such as hormones, prostanoids, and leukotrienes. Finally, because oxidation of fatty acids covers a large portion of the energy metabolism of critically ill patients, lipids are directly used and present an ideal energy substrate.

Parenteral lipid emulsions usually contain long-chain triglycerides that are mostly derived from soybean oil, but fat emulsions containing a various mixture of long- and medium-chain triglycerides (coconut oil) and/or olive oil and/or fish oil are available. Whether a lower content of polyunsaturated fatty acids yields the proposed advantages and a reduction in proinflammatory side effects is unknown. Administering medium-chain triglycerides does not increase their utilization for energy because AKI delays the elimination of both types of fat emulsions equally. The amount infused should be adjusted to meet the patient's capacity to use lipids. Generally, 1 g fat/kg b.w./day does not increase plasma triglycerides, so they can be used to supply approximately 20% to 30% of energy requirements. Lipids should not be given to patients with hyperlipidemia (plasma triglycerides >350 mg/ dL), with activated intravascular coagulation, with acidosis (pH <7.20), or with impaired circulation or hypoxemia.

Amino Acid Solutions

Three types of amino acid solutions have been used for parenteral nutrition in patients with AKI: (i) EAA alone; (ii) EAA plus nonessential amino acids (NEAA); or (iii) specifically designed "nephro" solutions of different proportions of EAA plus specific NEAA that might become "conditionally essential" for patients with AKI.

The use of solutions of EAA alone was based on principles established for treating patients with chronic kidney disease using a low-protein diet plus an EAA supplement. These solutions should no longer be used, because they are incomplete and do not contain several amino acids that become conditionally essential in patients with uremia (histidine, arginine, tyrosine, serine, and cysteine). The absence of these amino acids creates imbalances, resulting in serious derangements of plasma amino acid concentrations. Solutions including both EAA and NEAA in standard proportions or in special proportions designed to counteract the metabolic changes of kidney failure ("nephro" solutions) should be used in nutritional support for patients with AKI. Tyrosine has low water solubility, so dipeptides containing tyrosine (such as glycyltyrosine) are used in modern "nephro" solutions. The amino acid analogue N-acetyl tyrosine, which was used frequently as tyrosine source, cannot be converted to tyrosine in humans and should not be administered.

As for other amino acid solutions, an examination of a parenteral supplement of branched-chain amino acids (BCAA) given to patients with AKI failed to exert any benefits. In a study comparing a BCAA-enriched amino acid solution and a standard amino acid solution in critically ill patients with AKI treated with CRRT, no improvement using BCAA was seen in nitrogen balance or plasma protein concentrations.

Glutamine, an amino acid that is traditionally termed as nonessential, exerts important metabolic functions and can improve nitrogen metabolism and support immunocompetence and the antioxidative system while preserving gastrointestinal barrier function and potentially, kidney function. Because of these potential benefits, glutamine is regarded a conditionally indispensable for patients with catabolic illnesses. In one study, a standard parenteral nutrition was compared with a nutrition solution enriched with glutamine; long-term survival was improved in patients who received the additional glutamine. In a post hoc analysis, the improvement in prognosis was most pronounced in patients with AKI (4 of 24 survivors without glutamine, 14 of 23 with glutamine, p <0.02). Because free glutamine is not stable in aqueous solutions, glutamine-containing dipeptides (alanyl-glutamine or glycyl-glutamine) are contained in parenteral nutritional solutions.

Parenteral Solutions

Standard solutions with amino acids, glucose, and fat emulsions contained in a single bag are commercially available and have become the standard treatment approach (i.e., "three-chamber-bags"). Vitamins, trace elements, and electrolytes can be added to these solutions and are known as total nutritional admixtures or "all-in-one" solutions (Table 5-5).

The stability of fat emulsions in such mixtures must be assessed, and if the patient develops hyperglycemia, insulin should be added to the solution or administered separately.

As noted, electrolyte requirements are extremely variable in patients with AKI. Besides the obvious intra- and extracellular shifts in electrolyte concentration (e.g., potassium, amino acids) related to insulin, it should be emphasized that the "refeeding syndrome" consisting of hypokalemia and hypophosphatemia can develop because of infusion of insulin or glucose-stimulated insulin secretion. If phosphate or calcium are added to "all-in-one" solutions containing lipid emulsions, organic salts such as glycerophosphate, glucose-1-phosphate, and calcium gluconate must be used to avoid incompatibilities with other ions and impaired stability of the fat emulsion.

To ensure maximal nutrient use and to avoid metabolic derangements, the parenteral nutrition infusion (similarly to enteral nutrition) should be started at a low rate (providing about 50% of requirements) and gradually increased over several days. Optimally, the solution should be infused continuously over 24 hours to avoid marked changes in substrate concentrations.

COMPLICATIONS AND MONITORING OF NUTRITIONAL SUPPORT

Technical problems and infectious complications originating from the central venous catheter or the enteral feeding tube as well as the metabolic complications of nutrition support and gastrointestinal side effects of enteral nutrition are similar in patients with AKI and in those who do not have kidney disease (Table 5-6). Metabolic complications frequently occur because the utilization of various nutrients is impaired or there is intolerance to the administration of excessive volumes of nutrients and electrolytes. There also is the sharp increase in the BUN (and hence, other nitrogen containing waste products) in patients with impaired kidney function who are infused with an exaggerated protein or amino acid intake. Glucose intolerance and decreased fat

Table 5-5. "Renal failure fluid"—"all-in-one solution"

Component	Quantity	Remarks	
Glucose	30% to 60%	500 m	Caution: insulin resistance! Strictly observe normoglycemia
Fat emulsion	10% to 20%	500 ml	Keep triglycerides <350 mg/dL modern PUFA-reduced emulsions?
Amino acids	6.5% to 10%	500 ml	General or special "nephro" amino acid solutions including EAA and NEAA addition of glutamine dipeptide?
Water soluble vitamins*	2 × RDA		Limit vitamin C intake <250 mg/day
Fat soluble vitamins*	RDA		Increased vitamin E requirements?
Trace elements*	RDA		Caution: toxic effects Selenium 200–500 µg/d?
Electrolytes	As required		Caution: hypophosphatemia or hypokalemia after initiation of TPN
Insulin	As required		Added directly to the solution or given separately

"All in one solution" with all components contained in a single bag, start infusion rate initially at 50% of requirements, to be increased over a period of 3 days to satisfy requirements. For details, see text.
*Combination products containing the recommended daily allowances (RDA)
EAA, essential amino acids; NEAA, nonessential amino acids; PUFA, polyunsaturated fatty acids; TPN, total parenteral nutrition.

Table 5-6. A minimal suggested schedule for monitoring of nutritional support

Variables	Patient Metabolically	
	Unstable	Stable
Blood glucose, potassium	1–6× daily	Daily
Osmolality	Daily	1× weekly
Electrolytes (sodium, chloride)	Daily	3× weekly
Calcium, phosphate, magnesium	Daily	3× weekly
BUN/BUN rise/day	Daily	Daily
UNA	Daily	1× weekly
Triglycerides	Daily	2× weekly
Blood gas analysis/pH	Daily	1× weekly
Ammonia	2× weekly	1× weekly
Transaminases + bilirubin	2× weekly	1× weekly

BUN, blood urea nitrogen; UNA, urea nitrogen appearance rate.

clearance can cause hyperglycemia and hypertriglyceridemia, respectively. Nutritional therapy for patients with AKI requires a tighter schedule of monitoring of metabolic parameters than needed for other patient groups. Table 5-6 summarizes laboratory tests needed to monitor nutritional support to avoid developing metabolic complications. The frequency of testing will depend on the metabolic stability of the patient, but levels of plasma glucose, potassium, and phosphate should be monitored repeatedly after initiation of nutritional therapy.

CONCLUSION

- AKI presents a protein and energy catabolic, pro-oxidative, and pro-inflammatory syndrome. The metabolic environment in patients with AKI is complex, being affected by the acute loss of kidney function and by the underlying disease process and by the type and intensity of renal replacement therapy.
- Renal replacement therapies exert a profound impact on electrolyte and nutrient balances. This is especially true for continuous replacement modalities because of the prolonged therapy duration and the recommended high fluid turnover.
- Although a nutritional program for patients with AKI is not fundamentally different from that in patient without renal dysfunction, the multiple metabolic consequences of AKI, of RRT and the underlying disease process and/ or associated complications must be considered.
- In the critically ill patient with AKI nutritional support should be initiated early and be both qualitatively and quantitatively sufficient.
- Enteral nutrition is the preferred type of nutritional support in patients with and without AKI. Even small amounts of a diet entering the intestines can support gastrointestinal functions. Potentially, enteral nutrition might exert specific beneficial effects on renal function and recovery.
- Despite its obvious advantages, many patients have severe

limitations to enteral nutritional supplementation and will require supplementary or even total parenteral nutrition. Enteral and parenteral nutrition should not be viewed as competing but rather considered as complementary types of nutrition support. In select patients with AKI, the combination of enteral with parenteral nutrition may enable an optimal nutrient intake.

- Because of the limited tolerance to fluids and electrolytes and the altered processing of several nutrients, side effects and complications of nutrition support are much more frequent in patients with AKI compared with other patient groups. This requires careful monitoring of patients with AKI.

- Modern nutrition therapy has discarded a merely quantitatively oriented approach for covering nitrogen and energy requirements. Currently, a more qualitative type of metabolic intervention is used to modulate the inflammatory state, the oxygen radical scavenger system, the support of immunocompetence, and endothelial functions. These goals require taking advantage of specific pharmacologic effects of various nutrients (such as glutamine, fish oil, selenium, antioxidants). A reduction of the distressingly high mortality rate of patients with AKI will depend on further improvements in metabolic care.

Selected Readings

Angstwurm MW, Engelmann L, Zimmermann T, et al. Selenium in Intensive Care (SIC): results of a prospective randomized, placebo-controlled, multiple-center study in patients with severe systemic inflammatory response syndrome, sepsis, and septic shock. Crit Care Med 2007;35:118–126.

Artinian V, Krayem H, DiGiovine B. Effects of early enteral feeding on the outcome of critically ill mechanically ventilated medical patients. Chest 2006;129:960–967.

Basi S, Pupim LB, Simmons EM, et al. Insulin resistance in critically ill patients with acute renal failure. Am J Physiol Renal Physiol 2005;289:F259–F264.

Berger MM, Shenkin A, Revelly JP, et al. Copper, selenium, zinc, and thiamine balances during continuous venovenous hemodiafiltration in critically ill patients. Am J Clin Nutr 2004;80:410–416.

Biolo G, De Cicco M, Lorenzon S, et al. Treating hyperglycemia improves skeletal muscle protein metabolism in cancer patients after major surgery. Crit Care Med 2008;36:1768–1775.

Cano N, Fiaccadori E, Tesinsky P, et al. ESPEN Guidelines on Enteral Nutrition: Adult renal failure. Clin Nutr 2006;25:295–310.

Cianciaruso B, Bellizzi V, Napoli R, et al. Hepatic uptake and release of glucose, lactate, and amino acids in acutely uremic dogs. Metabolism 1991;40:261–269.

Dissanaike S, Shelton M, Warner K, et al. The risk for bloodstream infections is associated with increased parenteral caloric intake in patients receiving parenteral nutrition. Crit Care 2007;11:R114.

Druml W, Fischer M, Sertl S, et al. Fat elimination in acute renal failure: long-chain vs medium-chain triglycerides. Am J Clin Nutr 1992;55:468–472.

Druml W, Mitch W. Enteral nutrition in renal disease. In: Rolandelli RH, Bankhead R, Boullata JI, et al., eds. Clinical Nutrition: Enteral and Tube Feeding. Philadelphia: WB Saunders; 2004.

Druml W, Schwarzenhofer M, Apsner R, et al. Fat-soluble vitamins in patients with acute renal failure. Miner Electrolyte Metab 1998; 24:220–226.

Druml W. Acute renal failure is not a "cute" renal failure! Intensive Care Med 2004;30:1886–1890.

Druml W. Metabolic aspects of continuous renal replacement therapies. Kidney Int Suppl 1999;72:S56–S61.

Fiaccadori E, Lombardi M, Leonardi S, et al. Prevalence and clinical outcome associated with preexisting malnutrition in acute renal failure: a prospective cohort study. J Am Soc Nephrol 1999;10: 581–593.

Fiaccadori E, Maggiore U, Giacosa R, et al. Enteral nutrition in patients with acute renal failure. Kidney Int 2004;65:999–1008.

Heidegger CP, Romand JA, Treggiari MM, et al. Is it now time to promote mixed enteral and parenteral nutrition for the critically ill patient? Intensive Care Med 2007;33:963–969.

Himmelfarb J, McMonagle E, Freedman S, et al. Oxidative stress is increased in critically ill patients with acute renal failure. J Am Soc Nephrol 2004;15:2449–2456.

Jeejeebhoy KN. Permissive underfeeding of the critically ill patient. Nutr Clin Pract 2004;19:477–480.

Leblanc M, Garred LJ, Cardinal J, et al. Catabolism in critical illness: estimation from urea nitrogen appearance and creatinine production during continuous renal replacement therapy. Am J Kidney Dis 1998;32:444–453.

Lecker SH, Goldberg AL, Mitch WE. Protein degradation by the ubiquitin-proteasome pathway in normal and disease states. J Am Soc Nephrol 2006;17:1807–1819.

Macias WL, Alaka KJ, Murphy MH, et al. Impact of the nutritional regimen on protein catabolism and nitrogen balance in patients with acute renal failure. JPEN J Parenter Enteral Nutr 1996;20: 56–62.

Metnitz GH, Fischer M, Bartens C, et al. Impact of acute renal failure on antioxidant status in multiple organ failure. Acta Anaesthesiol Scand 2000;44:236–240.

Mouser JF, Hak EB, Kuhl DA, et al. Recovery from ischemic acute renal failure is improved with enteral compared with parenteral nutrition. Crit Care Med 1997;25:1748–1754.

Scheinkestel CD, Kar L, Marshall K, et al. Prospective randomized trial to assess caloric and protein needs of critically ill, anuric, ventilated patients requiring continuous renal replacement therapy. Nutrition 2003;19:909–916.

Schetz M, Vanhorebeek I, Wouters PJ, et al. Tight blood glucose control is renoprotective in critically ill patients. J Am Soc Nephrol 2008;19:571–578.

Singer P. High-dose amino acid infusion preserves diuresis and improves nitrogen balance in non-oliguric acute renal failure. Wien Klin Wochenschr 2007;119:218–222.

Zager RA, Johnson AC, Lund S, et al. Acute renal failure: determinants and characteristics of the injury-induced hyperinflammatory response. Am J Physiol Renal Physiol 2006;291:F546–F556.

6

Requirements for Protein, Calories, and Fat in the Predialysis Patient

Tahsin Masud and William E. Mitch

GOALS OF NUTRITIONAL THERAPY

The goals of dietary therapy for patients with chronic kidney disease (CKD) are: (i) to diminish the accumulation of nitrogenous wastes and limit the metabolic disturbances characteristic of uremia; (ii) to prevent loss of protein stores; and (iii) to slow the progression of CKD. Protein-restricted diets improve uremic symptoms because they reduce the levels of uremic toxins, most of which result from the metabolism of protein. A low-protein diet also ameliorates specific complications of CKD, including metabolic acidosis, renal osteodystrophy, hyperkalemia, and hypertension. This occurs because a diet that is restricted in protein is invariably restricted in the quantities of sulfates, phosphates, potassium, and sodium eaten each day. Contrariwise, when the diet exceeds the daily protein requirement, the excess protein is degraded to urea and other nitrogenous wastes, and these products accumulate (Fig. 6-1). These considerations explain why dietary protein restriction has been used for decades to treat chronically uremic patients.

ASSESSING PROTEIN REQUIREMENTS

Nitrogen Balance and Protein Requirements

Nitrogen balance (Bn) is the criterion standard for assessing dietary protein requirements, because a neutral or positive Bn indicates that the body's protein stores are being maintained or increased. Although measuring Bn is time consuming and technically demanding, no readily acceptable alternative methods are available for assessing amino acid or protein requirements.

On the basis of Bn measurements, the average protein requirement for healthy adults who perform a moderate amount of physical activity and consume sufficient (but not excessive) calories is approximately 0.6 g protein/kg body weight/day (b.w./d). This level of dietary protein was based on Bn results from subjects who had been fed variable amounts of protein. By an extrapolation process, the World Health Organization determined that the average protein intake required to maintain neutral Bn was 0.6 g protein/kg b.w./day, and this value plus 2 standard deviations (approximately 0.75 g protein/kg b.w./day) was designated as the "safe level of intake." This amount meets the protein requirements of 97.5% or more for healthy adults. Dietary protein above these levels is converted to waste products that must be excreted by the kidney.

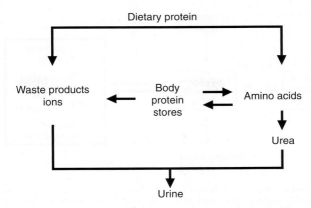

Figure 6-1. **A flow diagram illustrating the use of foods rich in protein by healthy adults and by patients with chronic kidney disease (CKD). The scheme indicates that dietary protein is converted to amino acids, which can be used to build new stores of body protein. Any excess is converted to urea, which must be excreted by the kidney, and hence, will accumulate with renal insufficiency.**

MECHANISMS RESPONSIBLE FOR NEUTRAL NITROGEN BALANCE

Healthy Subjects

For adults in Western societies, the protein intake usually exceeds the requirement. But consuming more protein does not increase muscle mass; instead, the body adapts by oxidizing any excess of amino acids from dietary protein. The nitrogen liberated by amino acid oxidation is converted to waste nitrogen (principally urea) and excreted by the kidney. When the intake of protein decreases, amino acid oxidation is reduced, allowing amino acids to be recycled and yielding more efficient use of dietary essential amino acids (EAA) (see Chapter 1).

Besides amino acid oxidation, protein synthesis and degradation determine the level of Bn. Note that the daily rates of protein synthesis and degradation are much larger than the rate of amino acid oxidation (Fig. 6-2); approximately 280 g of body protein are synthesized and degraded in a 70-kg adult each day. With fasting, however, body protein stores (principally skeletal muscle) are degraded to amino acids, which are used in the liver for gluconeogenesis. With feeding, protein degradation declines sharply, and protein synthesis repletes body protein stores. The net daily result is a neutral (or positive) Bn, and protein stores will be preserved as long as the diet is nutritionally adequate. A principal modulator of these changes in protein turnover is insulin, the principal anabolic hormone. In adult subjects, insulin mainly suppresses protein degradation. In summary, healthy adults successfully adapt to dietary protein restriction by: (i) suppressing catab-

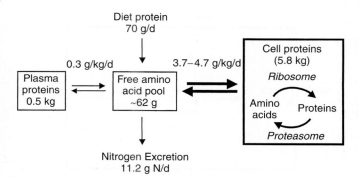

Figure 6-2. Results illustrated in this figure are the amounts of protein in the cellular pool and in plasma as well as the amount of free amino acids in the body of an adult weighing approximately 70 kg. A very large turnover of cellular proteins (3.7 to 4.7 g protein/kg b.w./day) occurs, amounting to the protein contained in 1 to 1.5 kg of muscle. This rate is 10-fold higher than the turnover of protein in the plasma pool.

olism of EAA, and (ii) inhibiting protein degradation and increasing protein synthesis with feeding.

Patients with Chronic Kidney Disease

Patients with advanced but uncomplicated CKD (glomerular filtration rate [GFR] approximately 5 to 15 mL per minute depending on the etiology of CKD) are remarkably efficient in adapting to dietary protein restriction. These patients reduce rates of amino acid oxidation and protein degradation in the same fashion as normal adults when their protein diet is restricted from 1.0 to 0.6 g/kg/day. The same adaptive metabolic responses are activated when the diet is restricted to only 0.3 g/kg/day and a supplement of essential amino acids or their nitrogen-free analogues (ketoacids) is given. Such a dietary regimen maintains both neutral Bn and indices of adequate nutrition during more than 1 year of observation. This happens because patients with CKD activate the same adaptive responses to dietary protein restriction as healthy adults. First, amino acid oxidation is decreased, resulting in both a lower requirement for and more efficient utilization of essential amino acids. Second, if protein or amino acid intake is barely sufficient, neutral Bn is achieved by a postprandial suppression of whole body protein degradation, with or without an accompanying increase in protein synthesis. But when protein (or amino acid) intake is inadequate, these compensatory response(s) are incomplete, leading to negative Bn and loss of lean body mass.

Dietary Protein Restriction and Nephrotic Syndrome

Patients with nephrotic syndrome (i.e., more than 3 g proteinuria per day) could have an increased risk for protein wasting. This issue is very important, because patients who are given a well-designed low-protein diet (LPD) have decreased proteinuria and increased serum albumin concentrations compared with patients fed excessive amounts of protein. Because the degree of proteinuria is closely related to the risk for progressive kidney and cardiovascular diseases, LPD could help prevent these problems. Fortunately, restricting dietary protein also activates adaptive responses in patients with nephrotic syndrome as determined by positive results in measurements of Bn and the components of protein turnover when they consumed a diet containing 0.8 or 1.6 g/kg b.w./day protein (plus 1 g/kg b.w./day dietary protein for each g proteinuria) and 35 kcal/kg b.w./day energy. In nephrotic and age- and gender-matched adults, a low-protein diet suppressed amino acid oxidation, and protein degradation decreased while protein synthesis increased during feeding. These responses resulted in neutral or positive Bn. The increase in amino acid oxidation induced by feeding was also blunted, suggesting that the urinary protein losses were closely associated with suppression of amino acid oxidation. Thus, proteinuria in CKD does not block the adaptive responses that are required to improve or maintain protein homeostasis. Evidence also suggests that diets containing less protein (<0.6 g/kg b.w./day) do not increase the risk for protein wasting in patients with the nephrotic syndrome.

In summary, patients with uncomplicated CKD, including those with nephrotic range proteinuria, activate normal compensatory responses to dietary protein restrictions by suppressing EAA oxidation and reducing protein degradation. Consequently, Bn is neutral and lean body mass is maintained during long-term dietary therapy.

Complications that Impair Adaptive Responses in Protein Turnover

Metabolic acidosis and insufficient insulin are complications of CKD, and both limit adaptive nutritional responses to an LPD. In muscle, acidosis and acute insulin deprivation stimulate the oxidation of EAA and accelerate the degradation of protein. Metabolic acidosis, in addition to causing negative Bn in adults and impairment of growth in children and infants, also causes insulin resistance in healthy adults. Fortunately, the risks for metabolic acidosis and insulin resistance are substantially reduced with an LPD.

The branched-chain amino acids, valine, leucine, and isoleucine, are catabolized by branched-chain keto acid dehydrogenase (BCKAD), and acidosis increases the activity of this enzyme in skeletal muscle. The activation includes an increase in the muscle levels of mRNAs that encode BCKAD enzyme complex, suggesting there is an increased capacity to degrade these amino acids. Acidosis also accelerates protein degradation by increasing the activity of the adenosine triphosphate (ATP)-dependent, ubiquitin–proteasome proteolytic pathway. As with BCKAD, the mRNAs that encode components of the pathway are increased. These cellular responses explain why metabolic acidosis counteracts the adaptive responses activated by a LPD.

Acid is generated during metabolism of animal-derived proteins, and there is a strong inverse relationship between a higher protein intake and reduced predialysis serum bicarbonate concentration. Similarly, a significant increase in serum bicarbonate level occurred in the Modification of Diet in Renal Disease (MDRD) study in patients with both stage 3 and 4 CKD when protein intake decreased by 0.2 g/kg b.w/day. As a general rule, the serum HCO_3 should be kept at 24 mmol/L or more to prevent the loss of muscle mass and to treat the bone, hormonal, and other complications of acidosis. Usually, two or three 650-mg sodium bicarbonate tablets (approximately 8 mEq of sodium and bicarbonate per tablet), given two to three times daily, are well tolerated and effective.

Amelioration of Insulin Resistance

Subjects with advanced CKD develop glucose intolerance, with fasting hyperglycemia and hyperinsulinemia, especially when metabolic acidosis complicates CKD. The major metabolic abnormality resides in peripheral tissues, including decreased glucose uptake by skeletal muscle and adipose tissue, both without and with insulin. In contrast, hepatic glucose production is normal and is appropriately suppressed in response to insulin. The abnormality involves defects after insulin interacts with its receptor (i.e., a postreceptor defect) apparently caused by suppression of phosphatidyl-inositol 3 kinase activity. Interestingly, diabetic patients with CKD treated with a low-protein diet displayed improvements in insulin sensitivity, fasting serum insulin levels, their need for daily insulin support, lower blood glucose levels, and a lower rate of endogenous glucose production.

OTHER ADVANTAGES OF LOW PROTEIN INTAKE

Amelioration of Hyperfiltration and Proteinuria

Both in experimental models and humans, high protein load acutely increases GFR, potentially contributing to the severity of microalbuminuria and, over the long term, glomerulosclerosis. A linear relationship between reduction in protein intake and decrease in proteinuria was first demonstrated in animals with CKD and was confirmed in several clinical trials. Levels of profibrotic compounds, such as transforming growth factor α (TGFα) and plasminogen activator inhibitor, can be reduced by an LPD, resulting in less severe renal injury and proteinuria compared with results with an uncontrolled diet.

Improvement of Lipid Profile

LPDs prescribed for patients with CKD are commonly designed by limiting animal sources of protein (e.g., meat and dairy products). As such, the intake of saturated lipids associated with animal proteins is decreased, resulting in an improved serum lipid profile. Reducing protein intake from 1.1 to 0.7 g/kg b.w/day for 3 months led to increased levels of serum lipoprotein A-1 and the apolipoprotein A-1:apoprotein B ratio.

Effect on Mineral and Bone Disorder

Phosphorus is an integral constituent of animal-derived proteins (1 g of protein contains about 13 mg of phosphorus), so reducing protein intake automatically reduces phosphate intake. Reduced phosphate accumulation will lower serum levels of parathyroid hormone and improve renal osteodystrophy. In fact, renal osteomalacia and osteofibrosis do improve after 12 months of an LPD supplemented with ketoanalogs. VLPD was also associated with a decrease in the urinary excretion and serum levels of urea nitrogen and phosphate.

Improvement in Blood Pressure

Another unexpected advantage of low protein intake is the improvement in blood pressure (BP); blood pressure decreased markedly (in the order of 15 mm Hg in systolic BP and 6 mm Hg in diastolic BP) in patients with CKD treated with a VLPD supplemented with ketoanalogs. Decreased protein intake of about 30% was associated with a 28% drop in sodium intake, but there was no change in BP or sodium intake in the two groups of patients whose protein intakes were not modified.

Amelioration of Erythropoietin Unresponsiveness

The relationship between the uremic state and erythropoiesis in patients with advance CKD (creatinine clearance ≤ 25 ml/mim/$1.73m^2$) was evaluated after randomization to either LPD (0.6 g/kg b.w/day) or VLPD (0.3 g/kg b.w/day) supplemented with ketoanalogs. The erythropoietin (EPO) dose to maintain hemoglobin was unchanged in patients treated with a LPD but progressively decreased in those treated with the VLPD.

CONCERNS ABOUT LOW-PROTEIN INTAKE DURING THE COURSE OF PROGRESSIVE CHRONIC KIDNEY DISEASE

Two observations have raised concerns about using LPDs. First, an association was observed in patients receiving hemodialysis therapy between hypoalbuminemia and increased mortality; second, patients with CKD starting dialysis with advanced CKD had worse outcome. Let's examine both of these issues in detail. The finding that dialysis patients often have low levels of serum proteins has led some to suggest that low-protein diets should be used cautiously or avoided in patients with CKD and that an "early start" of dialysis therapy should be considered. If patients with CKD are not properly instructed and supervised, a spontaneous decrease in protein intake and deterioration of some nutritional indices may indeed occur. Conversely, hypoalbuminemia in these patients is linked more closely to other factors such as inflammation and fluid status than to dietary inadequacy alone. In fact, patients with CKD who are not on maintenance dialysis treated with LPDs are shown to have increased serum protein concentrations at the initiation of maintenance dialysis therapy. An LPD is also associated with improved survival of patients with CKD who subsequently began maintenance dialysis. Further, there is abundant evidence that with proper implementation, an LPD yields neutral nitrogen balance and the maintenance of normal serum proteins and anthropometric indices during long-term therapy. After beginning dialysis, patients treated with supplemented very low-protein diet (SVLPD) were found to rapidly increase their protein intake with a gain in lean body mass in a study that followed patients with CKD treated with SVLPD for

5 years after beginning renal replacement therapy; the mortality was low and did not correlate with nutritional parameters measured at the end of SVLPD therapy. Finally, the conclusion that there is a negative impact of low residual renal function on survival are flawed by a failure to take into account "lead-time bias." This bias refers to the influence of measuring survival from the start of dialysis. This seems to increase the apparent survival of those who started with more residual renal function (i.e., earlier in the course of the disease) compared with those who start dialysis with less residual renal function. When lead-time bias was considered in patients with CKD followed from an estimated creatinine clearance (eC_{cr}) of 20 mL/minute to one of 8.3 mL/minute after being divided into early and late start groups, there was no survival benefit of survival from an earlier initiation of dialysis. More recently, a study examining data from the dialysis Morbidity Mortality Study Wave II to evaluate if beginning dialysis at higher levels of creatinine clearance or GFR (estimated from the MDRD formula) concluded that there is insufficient evidence to advocate early initiation of dialysis.

The greatest challenge for physicians and dieticians is compliance of patients with LPD. In MDRD study, the compliance rate for patients assigned to 0.6 g/kg b.w/day diet, did not exceed 35% in study A and 46% in study B. Clearly, a skilled dietician must be involved in the treatment of patients with CKD. The nutritionist must be familiar with the problems specific to patients with CKD and must have knowledge about the use of seasonings that can make meals appetizing and pleasant.

In summary, there is substantial evidence to inidicate that when properly applied, LPDs do not lead to protein energy wasting, even in patients with advanced CKD. Emphasis must be placed on dietary education for patients with CKD to ensure that the diet is adequate and to avoid consumption of foods that increase the accumulation of nitrogenous wastes and which aggravate uremic symptoms. When patients with CKD spontaneously reduce dietary protein, an educational program must be undertaken to plan and implement an appropriate LPD.

ENERGY METABOLISM IN PATIENTS WITH CHRONIC KIDNEY DISEASE

Influence of Energy Metabolism on Protein Turnover

Energy intake influences protein turnover; when the energy intake of patients with CKD was varied from 15 to 45 kcal/kg b.w./day, while their protein intake remained constant (0.60 g protein/kg b.w./day), Bn was more positive with higher levels of energy intake, and the urea nitrogen appearance rate was inversely correlated with energy intake. A decrease in urea appearance means that dietary protein was being used more efficiently to build body protein stores.

Energy Requirements of Patients with Chronic Kidney Disease

The rates of energy expenditure (and hence, energy requirements) at rest and with exercise by patients with uncomplicated CKD are similar to those of healthy subjects. With an energy intake of approximately 35 kcal/kg b.w./day, the levels of serum proteins, anthropometric values, and Bn are maintained even in patients with CKD consuming protein-restricted diets. Note that this recommended level of energy is commonly calculated using the patient's *ideal* body weight (IBW), because *actual* body weight may over- or underestimate energy requirements if the subject is edematous or obese, or malnourished, respectively. In elderly or obese subjects, a lower energy intake (e.g., approximately 30 kcal/kg b.w./day) may be adequate. In addition, given the close relationship between obesity and CKD-related metabolic abnormalities such as inflammation and oxidative stress, it may be reasonable to limit the energy intake to 30 kcal/ kg b.w./day in most, if not all, patients with stage 1–5 CKD who are not on maintenance dialysis. Exercise increases energy requirements. Clearly, the first step in achieving a sufficient energy intake is to schedule counseling sessions with a renal dietician. If changing the intake of conventional foods is unsuccessful in increasing energy intake, then high-energy or low-protein products can be used (as described above and in Chapter 19).

ABNORMALITIES IN GLUCOSE AND LIPID METABOLISM IN CHRONIC KIDNEY DISEASE

Glucose Metabolism

Subjects with uremia exhibit glucose intolerance, with fasting hyperglycemia and hyperinsulinemia, especially when metabolic acidosis complicates CKD. The major metabolic abnormality resides in peripheral tissues; there is decreased glucose uptake by skeletal muscle and adipose tissue, both without and with insulin. In contrast, hepatic glucose production is normal and is appropriately suppressed by insulin. This abnormality occurs after insulin interacts with its receptor via a postreceptor defect, consisting of suppressed phosphatidyl-inositol 3 kinase activity. Several pharmacologic and nutritional interventions, including but not limited to dietary protein restriction, exercise, and the calcium channel blocker, verapamil are shown to improve glucose utilization.

Lipid Metabolism

Hyperlipidemia is found in 20% to 70% of patients with uremia. The predominant abnormality in patients with CKD who are non-nephrotic or in patients receiving hemodialysis therapy is hypertriglyceridemia. There is an increase in very low-density lipoprotein (VLDLs) levels, a decrease in high-density lipoprotein (HDL) cholesterol levels, and normal to below-normal levels of LDLs. This pattern is consistent with a type IV hyperlipoproteinemia. Besides advanced CKD, this abnormal lipoprotein pattern can be aggravated by genetic predisposition, male gender, steroid therapy, and proteinuria.

The mechanism causing hypertriglyceridemia in patients with CKD is mainly defective catabolism of triglyceride-rich lipoproteins. This defect, in turn, is linked to decreased activity of lipoprotein lipase and hepatic triglyceride lipase. The levels of apoprotein C-II, the main activator of lipoprotein lipase, is reportedly decreased in patients with CKD, but metabolic acidosis and hyperinsulinemia also depress lipoprotein lipase activity. Secondary hyperparathyroidism might also contribute to hypertriglyceridemia in CKD. Another factor that aggravates hypertriglyceridemia is increased triglyceride production, which probably reflects insulin resistance. The importance of these abnormalities is that conversion of triglyceride-rich VLDL to LDL is defective, causing accumulation of potentially atherogenic intermediate density lipoproteins (IDL).

Patients with the nephrotic syndrome generally have high plasma levels of total cholesterol consisting of LDL and VLDL cholesterol, normal or low levels of HDL cholesterol, and normal or elevated triglycerides, that is, types IIa, IIb, or V hyperlipoproteinemia pattern. Early in the course of the nephrotic syndrome, VLDL is overproduced and is rapidly catabolized to LDL. However, LDL clearance is often impaired, especially in patients with severe proteinuria. The major factors that increase the risk for atherosclerosis in patients with nephrotic syndrome seem to be hypoalbuminemia and hyperlipidemia, which lead to dysregulation of HMG CoA reductase and 7a-hydroxylase expression.

ASSESSING DIETARY ADEQUACY AND COMPLIANCE

Dietary Adequacy

A key component in designing a successful plan of dietary therapy is a regular assessment of dietary adequacy and compliance. This assessment should not rely solely on indirect measures of dietary adequacy such as changes in serum visceral protein concentrations such as albumin, prealbumin, or transferrin, because there are other factors that influence their serum concentrations including inflammation leading to low values of these serum proteins. Anthropometrics are insensitive to an early change in nutritional status. In short, several indices should be monitored to obtain the most reliable information about nutritional status. Our approach is to monitor serum albumin, serum transferrin, and anthropometric indices of muscle mass *serially* and to interpret the values in comparison with the patient's dietary compliance (see Chapter 18 for more detailed nutritional assessment recommendations).

Monitoring Compliance with the Diet Prescription

Protein Intake

For inpatients, the protein–calorie content of meals can be identified by the dietician, but at the outpatient setting, the amount of protein ingested must be estimated. Fortunately, compliance with a dietary protein prescription can be estimated using a method based on the concept that the waste nitrogen arising from degraded protein is excreted as either urea or nonurea nitrogen (NUN). Because urea is the principal end product of amino acid degradation, the urea appearance rate (or net urea production rate) parallels protein intake. The urea nitrogen appearance rate is measured from the amount of urea excreted in urine plus the urea that is accumulated in body water. NUN excretion (i.e., nitrogen in feces and urinary creatinine, uric acid, amino acids, peptides, and ammonia) does not require measurement, because it does not vary with dietary protein: NUN averages 0.031 g

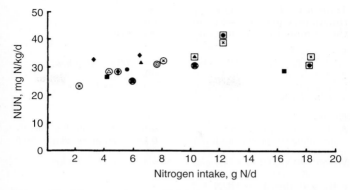

Figure 6-3. Nonurea nitrogen (NUN) losses measured in healthy subjects (*solid triangles, circles,* and *squares*) and patients with chronic kidney disease (CKD) being treated with low-protein diets (LPD) (*solid diamonds, open circles with cross,* and *open triangle*), by hemodialysis (*open circle with solid square* and *open square with solid triangle*) or continuous ambulatory peritoneal dialysis (CAPD) (*open square with cross* and *open square with solid circle*). These results indicate that NUN losses (i.e., nonurea urinary nitrogen plus fecal nitrogen) are relatively constant despite large variations in nitrogen intake and renal function. (From Maroni BJ, Steinman TI, Mitch WE. A method for estimating nitrogen intake in patients with chronic renal failure. Kidney Int 1985;27:58–65, with permission.)

N/kg b.w./day (Fig. 6-3). Thus, if nitrogen balance is assumed to be neutral (i.e., when nitrogen intake equals output and no loss or gain of protein occurs), then nitrogen intake (I_N) equals urea nitrogen appearance (U) plus the estimate of NUN losses or 0.031 g N/kg b.w. (Table 6-1, formula 2). Nitrogen intake can be converted to protein intake by multiplying I_N by 6.25, because protein is 16% nitrogen. In the steady state, when blood urea nitrogen (BUN) and weight are constant, the urea nitrogen appearance (U) rate is measured as the urea nitrogen in a 24-hour urine collection (urinary urea nitrogen [UUN]). In this case, I_N equals UUN plus 0.031 g N/kg b.w. as long as nitrogen balance is zero (Table 6-1, formula 4). If weight is changing because of an increase or decrease in body water, or if BUN is changing, the accumulation of urea should be calculated as shown in Table 6-1.

When the calculated and prescribed values of protein intake are similar, the patient is adhering to the amount of dietary protein prescribed. But if the estimated protein intake is less than prescribed, patients should be sent to the dietician to determine how to increase their protein intake. Conversely, if the estimated intake exceeds that prescribed by more than 20%, the difference might be caused by a superimposed catabolic illness or condition (e.g., gastrointestinal bleeding or metabolic acidosis). Alternately, the patient might need more training to adhere to the dietary prescription. Regardless, the patient should be evaluated

Table 6-1.   Estimating compliance with the dietary protein prescription from the 24-hour urinary urea nitrogen excretion

Formulas
1. $B_N = I_N - U - NUN$, where $NUN = 0.031$ g N/kg b.w.
2. if $B_N = 0$, then $I_N = U + 0.031$ g N/kg b.w.
3. when BUN is unchanging, then $U = UUN$, and
4. $I_N = UUN + 0.031$ g N/kg b.w.

Example
A 40-year-old woman is seen 1 month after instruction in a diet providing 0.6 protein/kg b.w./d (i.e., 60 kg $\times$ 0.6 protein/kg = 36 g protein)
Weight: 60 kg; UUN = 4.1 g/d; NUN = 0.031 g N $\times$ 60 kg = 1.86 g N/d
if $B_N = 0$, then $I_N = UUN + NUN$
= 4.1 + 1.86 = 5.96 g N
= 5.96 g N $\times$ 6.25 g protein/g N
= 37.3 g protein/d

B_N, nitrogen balance (g N/d); BUN, blood urea nitrogen; I_N, nitrogen intake (g N/d); N, nitrogen; NUN, nonurea nitrogen (g N/d); U, urea nitrogen appearance (g N/d); UUN, 24-hour urinary urea nitrogen (g N/d).

for a catabolic condition and referred to the dietician for counseling.

The formula for estimating protein intake can be used for other clinical tasks; for example, if the urea clearance has been measured, the steady state BUN for any prescribed protein intake can be calculated (Table 6-2). This formula is important, because a BUN higher than 60 to 70 mg per dL is associated with uremic symptoms. Secondly, the amount of dietary protein that will achieve this level of BUN can be calculated.

Table 6-2.   Relationship between nitrogen balance, urea nitrogen appearance rate, and steady state blood urea nitrogen*

Dietary Protein (g/d)	I_N-NUN (g N/d)	Steady State BUN (mg/dL)
80	10.6	123
60	7.4	86
40	3.9	49

where

$$BUN = \frac{I_N - g\ N/\text{kg body weight}}{C_{UREA}} \times 100$$

*Calculated for a 70-kg person with a urea clearance of 6 mL/min (8.6 L/d). BUN, blood urea nitrogen; C_{UREA}, urea clearance (L/d); I_N, nitrogen intake (16% of protein intake); N, nitrogen; NUN, nonurea nitrogen, which averages 0.031 g N/kg b.w./d.

Energy Intake

Unlike dietary protein, there is no simple method for estimating the intake of calories (or other components of the diet); dietary diaries or recall are used to assess energy intake of outpatients with CKD, but the accuracy of these methods depends on knowing all foods consumed, the portion size their energy contact, and the number of days each food was eaten. A skilled dietician can derive considerable information using these techniques, and consequently, accuracy is questionable. Moreover, when restricted diets are prescribed, patients quickly learn what foods they should eat, and often they underestimate their actual diet. For this reason, the energy intake derived from dietary records must be interpreted cautiously; we use a 3-day food diary obtained every 3 to 4 months to monitor the energy intake of patients with CKD. If protein intake is calculated and diet records provide a value for the percentage of calories from protein to be calculated, the total amount of dietary calories can be calculated.

The critical issue is to provide both the patient and the family with enough information so that the patient and the individual responsible for preparing the meals will have a clear understanding of the principles of dietary therapy. They must also be trained in meal planning, be knowledgeable about possible choices at restaurants, and be familiar with the protein contents of various foods. With this type of education, the likelihood of achieving adherence and maintaining an adequate nutritional state will be maximized. In addition, dieticians can provide sample menus to learn how to enhance patient satisfaction and to assist with monitoring the patient's nutritional status and dietary compliance. When patients become knowledgeable with the diet, we typically examine them every 3 months. At each visit, we estimate protein intake (to assess hence compliance) from the 24-hour UUN excretion (see Table 6-1). We also estimate caloric intake from food recall or diaries, and we monitor serum albumin, prealbumin and transferrin concentrations, and anthropometrics as suggested by the KDOQI guidelines; we then use these parameters to provide a patient with feedback regarding dietary adequacy and compliance.

PROTEIN REQUIREMENTS OF PREDIALYSIS PATIENTS

Two dietary regimens have been used to treat patients with progressive CKD: (i) a conventional diet that provides approximately 0.6 g protein/kg b.w./day; or (ii) a VLPD that contains approximately 0.3 g protein/kg b.w./day, supplemented with a mixture of EAA or their nitrogen-free ketoanalogs (i.e., keto acids or KA). Keto acids (the nitrogen-free analogues of EAA) are not available in the United States but are used in Europe, Asia, and Latin America. Because energy expenditure (and hence, energy requirements) of patients with CKD are comparable to those of healthy subjects, 30–35 kcal/kg b.w./day is recommended to achieve maximal use of the dietary protein, as described later in this chapter.

In general, the nutritional status of patients treated for prolonged periods with LPD or the VLPD/KA regimen is maintained or improved and uremic symptoms and metabolic complications of chronic renal failure (CRF) (e.g., metabolic acidosis, insulin resistance, and secondary hyperparathyroidism) are reduced. A randomized trial from India also found that the VLPD/KA regimen slowed the loss of kidney function while maintaining an adequate nutritional status. The mechanism of this type of benefit is unknown, but it may be linked to suppression of proteinuria, which decreases the risk for progressive kidney failure and cardiovascular disease.

DIETARY PROTEIN PRESCRIPTION

There are several reasons to limit the dietary protein of patients with CKD: (i) the accumulation of unexcreted waste products is reduced, and uremic symptoms are improved; (ii) the severity of acidosis, secondary hyperparathyroidism, and insulin resistance is reduced; (iii) proteinuria is reduced; and (iv) no evidence exists that feeding an excess of protein increases body protein stores. The effect of reducing dietary protein on the progression of CKD is discussed in Chapter 9.

Generally, we begin dietary protein restriction when patients develop symptoms or complications of uremia, or have edema or poorly controlled hypertension related to salt intake (Chapter 15), and for patients who continue to exhibit progressive renal insufficiency despite control of BP and the use of angiotensin-converting enzyme inhibitors (ACEI). After discussing the goals and methods with the patient, we use the guidelines outlined below and in Table 6-3. Dietary modification does require a substantial commitment, but when properly implemented and monitored, the dietary regimens are safe and nutritionally sound.

Moderate Chronic Renal Failure (Glomerular Filtration Rate 25 to 60 mL/minute)

Dietary therapy for patients with moderate CKD begins with a LPD that provides approximately 0.6 g protein/kg b.w./day, of which approximately two thirds is provided as high–biologic value protein (meat, fish, eggs, etc.; Table 6-3). The advantage of this strategy is that the protein limitation can be achieved using traditional foods. For patients that develop additional symptoms or have problems, we prescribe an essentially vegetarian diet that contains approximately 0.3 g protein/kg b.w./day (approximately 15 to 25 g protein/day) supplemented with a mixture of EAA or KA. These regimens provide the daily requirement of EAA and there is a variety of low-protein, high-calorie food products used to achieve calorie requirements. Examples of calorie-rich products include glucose polymers (Polycose) that can be added to beverages, high-density oral supplements (Suplena), and low-protein breads, pastas, and cookies (see Chapters 18 and 19).

Fortunately, the LPD invariably limits dietary phosphates, as long as milk-based products and high phosphate foods are avoided. This is emphasized because a low-phosphate diet is critical for preventing secondary hyperparathyroidism. The rationale for dietary phosphorus restriction is discussed in more detail in Chapters 3 and 18.

Advanced Chronic Renal Failure (Glomerular Filtration Rate 5 to 25 mL/minute)

The dietary regimens outlined in Table 6-3 are also appropriate for patients with advanced CKD. Proper use of a LPD invariably

Table 6-3. Recommended nutrient intake in patients with chronic kidney disease

Chronic Kidney Disease	Daily Recommendations
Protein*	
GFR (mL/min/1.73m^2)	Amount of protein (g/kg of ideal body weight)
>50	No restriction recommended
25–50	0.6 to 0.75 controlled
<25	0.6 or 0.3 plus supplementation†
Renal transplant recipient	
Early phase or acute rejection	1.3
Stable phase	As CKD
For nephrotic patient	0.8 plus 1 g pf protein/g of proteinuria
Energy	(kcal/kg of ideal body weight)
<60 yrs old	≥35
>60 yrs old	30–35
Carbohydrates	35% of nonprotein calories
Fat	Polyunsaturated to saturated ratio of 2:1
Phosphorus	800–1000 mg
	No restriction in transplant recipient if serum phosphorus is normal
Calcium	Should not exceed 2.5 g (dietary plus calcium based binders)
Potassium	Individualized
Sodium and water	As tolerated, to maintain body weight and blood pressure

*At least 50% of proteins should be of high biological value.
†Mixture of essential amino acids and ketoacids[51].
CKD, chronic kidney disease; GFR, glomerular filtration rate.

leads to fewer uremic symptoms and metabolic complications. Those properties delay the time until dialysis or transplantation is required. Albeit controversial, these diets may also slow the rate at which kidney function is lost (Chapter 9). When CKD is advanced, using the VLPD/EAA or KA regimens has potential advantages. These regimens have a lower nitrogen content, so less waste nitrogen accumulates, and dietary phosphates are reduced; the latter lowers the need for phosphate binders.

Nephrotic Syndrome (Glomerular Filtration Rate less than 60 mL/min)

An LPD reduces proteinuria and can ameliorate hypercholesterolemia in patients with nephrotic syndrome, and because proteinuria is considered an important risk factor for progressive kidney disease and cardiovascular complications, dietary protein restriction can suppress proteinuria in nephrotic patients. Regarding safety, a diet providing 0.8 g protein (plus 1 g protein per g proteinuria) and 35 kcal/kg b.w./day yields neutral Bn in patients with nephrotic syndrome, regardless of the level of renal function (i.e., GFR: 19 to 120 mL per minute). Moreover, long-term studies of LPD (0.45 to 0.8 g protein/kg b.w./day) have been conducted in nephrotic patients, and the results indicate that serum albumin levels either remain stable or increase. Despite these reports, we cannot recommend LPD for patients with extremely high levels of proteinuria (more than 15 g per day) or in patients with catabolic illnesses (e.g., vasculitis and systemic lupus erythematosus), or those receiving catabolic medications (e.g., glucocorticoids).

Until appropriate measurements are available, we recommend that patients with CKD who are infected or who are receiving prednisone should increase dietary protein to the "safe" level of intake (0.75 g protein/kg b.w./day). They should also be monitored by measuring the urea appearance rate regularly; when the urea appearance rate declines, there is evidence that the patient is using amino acids to augment protein stores rather than catabolizing them to form waste products. But if urea appearance rises, a patient is catabolic; in this case, raising dietary protein is very unlikely to reverse the problem. Efforts should be directed at correcting catabolic illnesses.

Role of Phytoestrogens and Vegetable-based Proteins

Evidence from animal experiments and small groups of patients indicates that consumption of soy protein, rich in isoflavones, and of flaxseed, rich in lignans, can prevent progressive CKD. In a randomized cross-over trial of a diet consisting of vegetable proteins compared with animal proteins in a LPD it was found that patients with stage 4 CKD with the vegetarian diet had significantly lower values of serum urea nitrogen and 24-hour creatinine and phosphate excretion rates. The number of patients in this trial was small, and there was no improvement in renal function.

Angiotensin-Converting Enzyme Inhibitors and Low Protein Diets

Agents that inhibit the renin-angiotensin system will reduce proteinuria and slow the progression of CKD. In addition, proteinuria is closely linked to the severity of CKD, yielding an important indication for dietary protein restriction. Combining an ACEI with an LPD will produce an additive response in reducing proteinuria and slowing the progression of kidney disease.

FAT REQUIREMENTS IN CHRONIC KIDNEY DISEASE

Even in healthy individuals, neither an adequate level of dietary fat nor a recommended dietary allowance of fat is established because there is insufficient evidence about what constitutes an inadequate amount of dietary fat. The Food and Nutrition Board of the Institute of Medicine suggests an acceptable range of total fat intake should be 20% to 35% of energy. There is an "Acceptable Macronutrient Distribution Range" (AMDR) based on evidence of the risk for coronary heart disease (CHD) at low intakes of fat and high intakes of carbohydrate and the risks for obesity and its complications (including CHD) at high intakes of fat. An

AMDR for patients with renal disease has not been published so current recommendations are the same as for healthy subjects.

CONCLUSION

In summary, manipulation of the diet remains an integral aspect of the management of patients with CKD who are not on maintenance dialysis. A properly designed diet is both safe and effective. The dietary prescription should be based on each patient's calculated protein and energy requirements. For success, dietary adherence and nutritional adequacy must be monitored regularly, and success with this therapy as with any therapeutic strategy requires motivation. Tangible rewards of nutritional therapy include reduced uremic symptoms and metabolic complications, plus the potential for slowing the progression of CKD. Fortunately, many patients welcome the opportunity to have "control" over their illness.

Selected Readings

Aparicio M, Chauveau P, de Precigout V, et al. Nutrition and outcome on renal replacement therapy of patients with chronic renal failure treated by a supplemented very low-protein diet. J Am Soc Nephrol 2000;11:719–727.

Avesani CM, Draibe SA, Kamimura MA, et al. Resting energy expenditure of chronic kidney disease patients: influence of renal function and subclinical inflammation. Am J Kidney Dis 2004;44:1008–1016.

Beddhu S, Samore MH, Roberts MS, et al. Impact of initiation of dialysis on mortality. J Am Soc Nephrol 2003;14:2305–2312.

Bellizze V, Di Iorio BR, De Nicola L. Very low protein diet supplemented with ketoanalogs improves blood pressure control in chronic kidney disease. Kidney Int 2007;71:245–251.

Di Iorio BR, Minutolo R, De Nicola L, et al. Supplemented very low-protein diet ameliorates unresponsiveness to erythropoietin in chronic renal failure. Kidney Int 2003;64:1822–1828.

Fouque D, Aparicio M. Eleven reasons to control the protein intake of patients with chronic kidney disease. Nat Clin Pract Nephrol 2007;3:383–392.

Gansevoort RT, De Zeeuw D, De Jong PE. Additive antiproteinuric effect of ACE inhibition and a low-protein diet in human renal disease. Nephrol Dial Transplant 1995;10:497–504.

Kaysen GA, Dubin JA, Muller HG, et al. Inflamation and reduced albumin synthesis associated with stable decline in serum albumin in hemodialysis patients. Kidney Int 2004;65:1408–1415.

Maroni BJ, Staffeld C, Young VR, et al. Mechanisms permitting nephritic patients to achieve nitrogen equilibrium with a protein-restricted diet. J Clin Invest 1997;99:2479–2487.

Masud T, Manatunga A, Cotsonis G, et al. The precision of estimating protein intake of patients with chronic renal failure. Kidney Int 2002;62:1750–1756.

Mitch WE, Remuzzi G. Diets for patients with chronic kidney disease, still worth prescribing. J Am Soc Nephrol 2004;15:234–237.

Mitch WE. Malnutrition: a frequent misdiagnosis for hemodialysis patients. J Clin Invest 2002;110:437–439.

Shoji TS, Ishimura E, Nishizawa Y. Body fat measurement in chronic kidney disease: implications in research and clinical practice. Curr Opin Nephrol Hypertens 2007;16:572–576.

Soroka N, Silverberg DS, Greemland M, et al. Comparison of vegetable-based (SOYA) and an animal-based low-protein diet in predialysis chronic renal failure patients. Nephron 1998;79:173–180.

Tranyor JP, Simpson K, Geddes CC, et al. Early initiation of dialysis fails to prolong survival in patients with end-stage renal failure. Nephrol Dial Transplant 2002;13:2125–2132.

Walser M, Mitch WE, Maroni BJ, et al. Should protein be restricted in predialysis patients? Kidney Int 1999;55:771–777.

Nutritional Requirements of Diabetics with Nephropathy

Eberhard Ritz

*"With an excess of fat diabetes begins and from an excess of fat dia-
betics die, formerly of coma, recently of atherosclerosis."*
—Joslin, EP. Atherosclerosis and diabetes. Annals of Clinical Medicine 1927;
5:1061–1079.

WHAT IS DIABETES?

Diabetes is a heterogeneous disease. Traditionally, one distinguishes two major types of diabetes: type 1 diabetes (insulino-
penic), which is usually secondary to the autoimmune destruction
of the insulin-secreting β cells in the pancreas (insulitis) and usually begins at a young age. These patients require insulin treatment within the first year after the onset of diabetes. Type 2
diabetes is usually seen in elderly individuals. Increasingly, however, it is also seen in the obese young. Type 2 diabetes is characterized by insulin resistance that is, to a large extent, genetically
determined. After years or decades, the secretory capacity of the
pancreatic islets is exhausted. The patients respond initially to
weight reduction, oral hypoglycemic agents, or both. As the disease progresses, these patients usually require insulin.

Matters are much more complex than this simple scheme suggests; up to 10% of elderly patients with diabetes have an autoimmune illness (Late Autoimmune Diabetes in Adults [LADA]).
Conversely, 10% to 15% of patients with type 2 diabetes develop
diabetes at a relatively young age as a result of genetic abnormalities of insulin secretion (Maturity Onset Diabetes of the Young
[MODY]) or premature obesity for reasons of lifestyle. The major
health problem in Western populations is currently type 2 diabetes of the adult. It affects approximately up to 10% of the general
population. In some populations, the prevalence is much higher.
For instance, in Saudi women aged 50 years, the prevalence is
no less than 50%. The prevalence increases with advancing age.
Currently, the prevalence of type 2 diabetes is increasing
throughout the Western world and particularly also in rapidly
Westernizing countries, e.g., India and China.

Both type 1 and type 2 diabetes cause similar long-term complications, namely *macrovascular disease* (coronary heart disease
[CHD], cerebrovascular disease, and peripheral arterial disease)
and *microvascular disease* (retinopathy and nephropathy).

THE EPIDEMIOLOGY OF NEPHROPATHY AND END-
STAGE RENAL DISEASE IN DIABETES

Diabetic nephropathy, usually in patients with type 2 diabetes,
recently has become the single most common cause of end-stage
renal disease (ESRD). Currently, more than 50% of patients ad-
mitted to start renal replacement therapy at the University of

Heidelberg have type 2 diabetes. Comparable figures have been reported from the United States, where the incidence of ESRD with diabetes as primary diagnosis has stabilized in recent years at 150 new cases per million population per year according to the United States Renal Data System (USRDS) report 2007 (http://www.USRDS.org). These high rates of diabetic nephropathy not only impose a burden on the health budget but are also associated with immense human suffering as a result of amputation, blindness, heart disease, and kidney disease.

WHY IS THE PREVALENCE OF TYPE 2 DIABETES RISING?

Undoubtedly, a strong genetic predisposition plays an important role, as illustrated by family studies and, more specifically, by twin studies, although the genes that are responsible have not been identified. Despite the strong genetic determination, the risk for developing type 2 diabetes is considerably influenced by intrauterine programming (reflected by birth weight) as well as by lifestyle factors. That lifestyle, particularly the diet, plays an important role as illustrated by observations that indicate that the prevalence of type 2 diabetes is very low in periods of nutritional deprivation, for example, during and after World War II in Europe. Conversely, type 2 diabetes becomes extremely prevalent when indigenous populations adopt a Western lifestyle, for example, Pima Indians, inhabitants of the Pacific island of Nauru, or Australian Aboriginals and particularly the increase in South-East Asia.

The current epidemic of obesity throughout the Western world, particularly in the United States, is certainly a major predisposing factor for type 2 diabetes. Why did the predisposition for such an adverse condition as diabetes not disappear during evolution by natural selection? One very persuasive explanation is provided by the so-called thrifty gene hypothesis. According to this theory, survival in our ancestors was often limited by frequent periods of nutritional deprivation. In that case, insulin resistance and the consecutive storage of energy available in visceral adipose tissue from periods of adequate nutrition provided a survival advantage. Consequently, when individuals whose ancestors had been genetically programmed for survival in a lean environment are today exposed to an environment with excessive calorie supply and physical inactivity, this persisting metabolic program causes insulin resistance, central obesity, dyslipidemia, and hypertension. This constellation has been called *metabolic syndrome* or *syndrome X* and is thought to be the forerunner of type 2 diabetes. This subject is covered in more detail in Chapter 16.

Several observations suggest that lifestyle modification still provides major benefit even once type 2 diabetes has developed. Australian investigators sent diabetic Australian aborigines back into the desert to adopt the lifestyle of their ancestors as hunters and gatherers. Within several weeks, glycemia and dyslipidemia were reversed. The salutary effects of dietary restriction and physical exercise have been known for several millennia. Wise ancient Indians advised individuals whose (glycosuric) urine attracted flies to visit on foot at least 100 villages—a therapy that involved physical exercise and weight reduction.

Table 7-1. Optimal glycemic control for individuals with diabetes according to the recommendations of the American Diabetes Association

	Goal	Action Suggested
Preprandial glucose (mg/dL)*	80–120	<80 or >140
Bedtime glucose (mg/dL)*	100–140	<100 or >160
HbA1c (%)	<7	>8

*Whole blood values.
From Sheard NF, Nathaniel GC. The role of nutrition therapy in the management of diabetes mellitus. Nutr Clin Care 2000;6:334–348, with permission.

THE ROLE OF NUTRITION THERAPY IN THE MANAGEMENT OF DIABETES MELLITUS

Nutrition therapy is not only one of the most challenging aspects of diabetes care but is also an essential component of successful diabetes management. Current thinking about nutrition and diabetes is reviewed in the recent statements of Franz et al. and Sheard in the nutrition recommendations of the American Diabetes Association (ADA). The interested reader is referred to these excellent in-depth reviews.

The goals of nutrition therapy in terms of optimal glycemic control are summarized in Table 7-1. One major goal is to achieve and maintain near-normal glucose concentrations. A second goal is to manage dyslipidemia, particularly in view of the excessive cardiovascular risk of the patient with diabetes, a risk comparable to that of the survivor of an acute myocardial infarction. Recognition of this risk has prompted a marked downward revision of acceptable low-density lipoprotein (LDL) cholesterol concentrations in the Third Report of the National Cholesterol Education Program. Table 7-2 summarizes the recommended lipid concentrations for a patient with diabetes.

Table 7-2. Goals for treating plasma lipid disorders in diabetic patients according to the third report of the national cholesterol education program (NCEP)

- Diabetes is a CHD risk equivalent
- Patients with CHD or CHD risk equivalents have an LDL cholesterol goal of <100 mg/dL
- In diabetic patients with high triglycerides (≥200 mg/dL) the sum of LDL + VLDL (equivalent to total cholesterol–HDL cholesterol) is a secondary target. The goal value is <130 mg/dL
- A low HDL (<40 mg/dL) should receive clinical attention; currently, insufficient evidence exists to specify a goal of therapy

From Executive Summary of the Third Report of the National Cholesterol Education Program (NCEP). Expert panel on detection, evaluation, and treatment of high blood cholesterol in adults (Adult Treatment Panel III). JAMA 2001;285:2486–2497, with permission.
CHD, coronary heart disease; HDL, high-density lipoproteins; LDL, low-density lipoproteins; VLDL, very low-density lipoproteins.

Table 7-3.   History of dietary recommendations for diabetes mellitus

Year	Carbohydrate (%kcal)	Protein (%kcal)	Fat (%kcal)
1921	20	10	70
1950	40	20	40
1971	45	20	35
1986	Up to 60	12–20	<30
1994	Variable*	10–20	Variable†

*Based on nutritional assessment and treatment goals.
†Less than 10% from saturated fats.
From Sheard NF, Nathaniel GC. The role of nutrition therapy in the management of diabetes mellitus. Nutr Clin Care 2000;6:334–348, with permission.

Another goal is to control or even reverse obesity in type 2 diabetics through lifestyle modifications that include caloric restriction and physical exercise. Clinical data strongly support the potential for moderate weight loss to reduce the risk for developing diabetes. The benefit from loss of weight is improved control of glycemia, of dyslipidemia, and of blood pressure; these interventions often become less effective, however, as the disease progresses.

The dietary recommendations regarding the relative proportions of carbohydrates, protein, and fat have changed with greater insights into the pathologic mechanisms. Table 7-3 shows that the recommended relative contribution of calories from carbohydrates has progressively increased, whereas the recommended proportion of fat has progressively decreased. The currently accepted recommendations can be summarized as follows. There has been a recent trend, however, to reduce carbohydrate intake compared with previous recommendations and to increase the proportion of unsaturated fat.

CARBOHYDRATE

In contrast to previous opinion, the total amount of carbohydrate in a diet rather than the type of carbohydrate is what is important in controlling postprandial glucose levels. Individuals with diabetes should reduce their intake of low molecular weight sugars (mono- and disaccharides) to the same extent as, but no more than, individuals without diabetes. The general philosophy is that patients with diabetes should eat the same prudent diet that is recommended for the general population. The problem is to adjust the insulin dose, or oral hypoglycemic agents, to dietary carbohydrates, taking into account the effectiveness of insulin (i.e., insulin sensitivity). Although carbohydrates provoke differing glycemic responses, evidence of a long-term benefit is still insufficient to recommend the use of low glycemic index diets as a primary strategy in dietary advice.

FAT

In patients with type 1 diabetes, hyperlipidemia and, to a major extent, hypertriglyceridemia can be reversed by tight glycemic control. In contrast, in patient with type 2 diabetes dyslipidemia had usually been present even before the onset of diabetes. Although somewhat improved by adequate glycemic control, it usually persists despite dietetic measures. The difficulties with lipid control are aggravated with the onset of renal disease and proteinuria, particularly at nephrotic levels of proteinuria. Specifically in individuals with diabetes and elevated LDL cholesterol, decreasing saturated fat intake to less than 7% of total calories is recommended. In individuals with pronounced hyperglycemia, weight reduction and decreasing intake of sucrose, total carbohydrates, and alcohol are recommended; carbohydrates should be exchanged for more monounsaturated fat (olive oil or canola oil) in the diet. Specific recommendations have been made for patients with chronic kidney disease. Apart from dietary measures, administration of statins is strongly advocated by all recent guidelines.

PROTEIN

The recommended dietary allowance (RDA) for protein in the general population is 0.8 g/kg b.w., or approximately 10% of total calories. The usual protein intake in Europe and in the United States is far greater than RDA. The nutritional requirement for protein in the patient with well-controlled diabetes is not different from that recommended for the general population. However, in hyperglycemic individuals, protein synthesis is decreased and protein breakdown is increased, thus leading to a negative nitrogen balance. During periods of hyperglycemia or weight loss, somewhat higher protein intakes may improve nitrogen balance, but this theory is not proved. The influence of reduced dietary protein intake on the progression of chronic kidney disease (CKD), especially diabetic nephropathy, is discussed in detail in Chapter 9.

The impressive changes of dietary recommendations to diabetic patients with time and today's more liberal approach have been nicely summarized by Sheard and Nathaniel (Table 7-3).

SODIUM CHLORIDE

Blood pressure in diabetic individuals tends to be sodium sensitive. It is wise to follow the recommendation of the Joint National Committee on Prevention, Detection, Evaluation and Treatment of High Blood Pressure for individuals with hypertension and lower the sodium chloride intake to 6 g per day; the importance of reducing dietary sodium intake has been illustrated by recent studies, which show that reduced sodium intake lowers blood pressure and that sodium intake even predicts cardiovascular mortality. Whether the interesting experimental results showing that in diabetic rats high salt intake reduced proximal tubular reabsorption thus reducing glomerular hyperfiltration via the tubulo-glomerular feedback have clinical implications is not clear. The salient features of the nutritional recommendations by the ADA for individuals with diabetes mellitus are summarized in Table 7-4.

**Table 7-4.   Nutritional recommendations
of the American Diabetes Association**

General recommendations
- Moderate caloric restriction (250–500 calories less than average daily intake) for individuals with type 2 diabetes
- Increase in physical activity

Protein
- 10%–20% of daily caloric intake (both animal and vegetable sources)
- 0.8 g/kg b.w./day in patients with overt nephropathy
- Once GFR decreases, further restriction to 0.6 g/kg b.w./day (in our view controversial because of the risk of malnutrition)

Total fat
- <10% of calories from saturated fats (<7% in individuals with high LDL cholesterol)
- <10% of calories from polyunsaturated fats
- 10%–15% of calories from monounsaturated fats
- Limitation of dietary cholesterol to <300 mg daily (<200 mg daily in individuals with high LDL cholesterol) can be handled somewhat more liberally when patients are treated with statins
- Two to three servings of fish to provide dietary $n3$ polyunsaturated fat can be recommended

Carbohydrates and sweeteners
- Carbohydrates from whole grains, fruits, vegetables, and low-fat milk should be included
- Regarding the glycemic effects of carbohydrates, the total amount is more important than the source or type
- Avoid excessive simple sugars
- Sucrose, if used, must be substituted for, not simply added to, other carbohydrates
- Moderate consumption of fructose-sweetened food is allowed
- Calories from all nutritive sweeteners must be accounted for in the meal plan

Fiber
- Daily consumption of 20–35 g dietary fiber from both soluble and insoluble fibers is recommended

Sodium chloride
- 6–7.5 g/day (approx. 100–130 mmol/day) in individuals without hypertension
- <6 g/d (<100 mmol/day) in individuals with mild to moderate hypertension
- <5 g/d (<85 mmol/day) in individuals with hypertension and nephropathy (difficult to achieve because of the high proportion of "hidden salt" in commercial food items)

Alcohol
- No more than two drinks/day for men and one drink/day for women
- To reduce the risk of hypoglycemia, alcohol should be consumed with food

Vitamins and minerals
- Generally no need for additional vitamin and mineral supplementation for the majority of individuals with diabetes

From American Diabetes Association. Nutrition principles and recommendations in diabetes. Diabetes Care 2004;27:S36–S46, with permission.
GFR, glomerular filtration rate; LDL, low-density lipoproteins.

Alcohol

Several studies documented that moderate alcohol consumption reduced the incidence of type 2 diabetes, and a recent observational study found even less risk of end-stage kidney disease with moderate use of alcohol. Moderate use of alcohol should not be completely discouraged, but an eye must be kept on the sugar content of the beverages and the risk of hypoglycemia in patients on glucose-lowering agents must be considered.

Vitamin D

Vitamin D deficiency increases the risk of onset of type 1 and type 2 diabetes, and there is some evidence that vitamin D and calcium insufficiency negatively influences glycemic control and that supplementation with both nutrients may be beneficial in optimizing glucose control. The pleiotropic effect of Vitamin D on insulin sensitivity is a subject of further studies.

WHAT ARE THE NUTRITIONAL REQUIREMENTS OF PATIENTS WITH DIABETES AND NEPHROPATHY?

To answer this question one has to address several different issues:

- Do dietary factors contribute to the development or progression of diabetic nephropathy?
- Does the presence of advanced diabetic nephropathy necessitate changes in the management of patients with diabetes?
- Does renal replacement therapy have an effect on the management of patients with diabetes?

In this context, it is helpful to first describe the natural history of diabetic nephropathy, because the interventions depend on the stage of nephropathy. At the time of diagnosis, when the patient is markedly hyperglycemic, kidney function is usually increased (renal hyperfunction), as shown in Table 7-5. This abnormality is ameliorated but not normalized during the so-called phase of clinical latency. The first indication of kidney damage is the appearance of albumin ("microalbuminuria") in the urine at concentrations that are not detected by routine measurements of urine protein but can be detected using sensitive techniques (Elisa, Radioimmunoassay [RIA], specific dipsticks). With the increase of urinary albumin excretion, blood pressure also increases. This stage is a window of opportunity, because kidney function is still normal, but the high-risk patient can be identified and given specific therapy, primarily administration of angiotensin-converting enzyme (ACE) inhibitors or angiotensin receptor blockers (pharmacologic blockade of the renin angiotensin aldestrone system [RAAS]). After several years, frank proteinuria supervenes. From this time it used to take an average of only 7 years before patients were in ESRD requiring renal replacement therapy. Modern interventions, particularly more aggressive blood pressure lowering and blockade of the RAAS, have extended this period, particularly if begun very early in the course of diabetes. With increasing frequency deviations from the above scheme are observed, particularly reduced glomerular filtration rates without albuminuria in the presence of small kidneys presumable as a consequence of vascular disease.

Table 7-5. The stages of diabetic nephropathy

Stage	Glomerular Filtration	Albuminuria	Blood Pressure	Time Course (years after diagnosis)
Renal hyperfunction	Elevated	Absent	Normal	At diagnosis
Clinical latency	High/normal	Absent		
Microalbuminuria (incipient nephropathy)	Within the normal range	20–200 µg/min (30–300 mg/day)	Rising within or above the normal range	5–15
Macroalbuminuria or persisting proteinuria (overt nephropathy)	Decreasing	200 µg/min (300 mg/day)	Increased	10–15
Renal failure	Diminished	Massive	Increased	15–30

Table 7-6. Factors that increase the risk of developing or progression of diabetic nephropathy

	Importance for Development of Diabetic Nephropathy	Importance for progression of Diabetic Nephropathy
Hypertension	↑↑↑	↑↑↑↑↑
High protein intake	↑↑	↑↑
Dyslipidemia?	↑	↑↑
Hyperglycemia	↑↑↑↑↑	↑↑↑
Proteinuria	N/A	↑↑↑↑
Smoking	↑↑↑↑	↑↑↑

Do Dietary Factors Contribute to the Development and Progression of Diabetic Nephropathy?

Development of Diabetic Nephropathy

As shown in Table 7-6, apart from genetic predisposition and nonmodifiable factors such as gender (higher risk in men than in premenopausal women) and ethnicity (higher risk in Blacks, Hispanics, and Asians than in other ethnic groups), several modifiable factors increase the risk that individuals with type 1 and type 2 diabetes will develop diabetic nephropathy.

THE ROLE OF HYPERGLYCEMIA

Diabetic nephropathy cannot develop in the absence of hyperglycemia. An important risk factor is the quality of glycemic control, as documented in type 1 diabetes by the DCCT (Diabetes Control and Complications Trial) and in type 2 diabetes by the Kumamoto study in Japan and the UK-PDS study in the United Kingdom. Notably, no safe cutoff value exists for blood glucose concentration (Table 7-7). Glycemic control is reflected by the level of hemo-

Table 7-7. Effect of intensified insulin treatment on development (primary prevention) and progression (secondary prevention) of nephropathy in Japanese type 2 diabetic patients

	Percent of Patients after 6 years		
	Conventional Insulin Treatment ($n = 55$)	Intensified Insulin Treatment ($n = 55$)	p
Primary prevention (development)	28%	7.7%	.03
Secondary prevention (progression)	32%	11.5%	.04

From Ohkubo Y, Kishikawa H, Araki E. Intensive insulin therapy prevents the progression of diabetic microvascular complications in Japanese patients with non-insulin-dependent diabetes mellitus: a randomized prospective 6-year study. Diabetes Res 1995;28:103–117, with permission.)

globin A1c, that is, the proportion of hemoglobin molecules that have undergone postribosomal modification by glycation. The normal value is about 6.1% (depending on the method used). The risk of diabetic nephropathy (and retinopathy) rises with increasing levels of hemoglobin A1c. The hemoglobin A1c value is superior to spot measurements of blood glucose, because it reflects the level of glycemia in the past 4 to 6 weeks; that is, it is the integral of glucose concentrations (preprandial and postprandial) over time. In advanced CKD, particularly in patients on erythropoietin (EPO) and on iron therapy, the erythrocyte half-life is altered, and glycated albumin is more reliable than $HbA1_c$.

THE ROLE OF HYPERTENSION

Another important risk factor is blood pressure. At least in type 2 diabetes, the presence of hypertension before the onset of diabetes clearly determines the ultimate risk for developing diabetic nephropathy. Recent evidence indicates that lowering blood pressure reduces the risk for developing diabetic nephropathy in type 2 diabetes. Furthermore, the evidence is overwhelming that lowering blood pressure is effective in attenuating the rate of progression in established diabetic nephropathy. Hypertension is strongly modified by body weight and salt intake, two aspects that have obvious implications for the dietary management of patients.

Blood pressure is influenced by salt intake, as shown in the recent DASH study (Dietary Approach to Stop Hypertension). Reducing sodium intake from 144 ± 58 mmol per day to 67 ± 46 mmol per day by eating a diet rich in vegetables, fruits, and low-fat dairy products reduced systolic blood pressure by 7.1 mm Hg in normotensive individuals and no less than 11.5 mm Hg in hypertensive individuals. The salt dependency of blood pressure is particularly pronounced in individuals with diabetes. Studies have shown that blood pressure is "salt sensitive," that is, increased by more than 3 mm Hg when salt intake was increased from 20 to 200 mmol per day, in no less than 43% of patients with type 1 diabetes, regardless of the presence or absence of microalbuminuria. There are several potential reasons for this finding. One reason is that insulin is an antinatriuretic hormone and acutely lowers sodium excretion. Second, in the presence of hyperglycemia, increased amounts of glucose and sodium are reabsorbed in the proximal tubule via the glucose–sodium cotransporter. As a result, exchangeable sodium and extracellular fluid volume tend to be higher in patients with diabetes than in healthy individuals. Salt sensitivity of blood pressure and volume expansion is even more pronounced once patients have developed kidney disease and ESRD. Conversely, dietary sodium restriction, administration of diuretics, or both are particularly effective in reducing the blood pressure of patients with diabetes and the benefit is particularly pronounced if the RAAS is blocked by ACE inhibitors and/or angiotensin receptor blockers.

In a recent prospective study, high sodium intake also predicted mortality and risk for CHD, independent of other cardiovascular factors, including blood pressure. The cardiovascular risk is extremely high in the patient with diabetes. These considerations provide a further rationale to recommend reducing dietary salt intake in patients with diabetes.

Patients with type 2 diabetes tend to be obese. In obese individuals without diabetes, particularly individuals with visceral obesity, blood pressure is sodium sensitive as well; in several small clinical trials, even moderate weight loss diminished salt sensitivity. This observation is less surprising in view of recent molecular evidence, which indicates that adipose tissue is not only a storehouse of energy but is also an active endocrine organ, with a complete local renin-angiotensin system and the capacity to synthesize endocrine factors, including estrogens, leptin, adiponectin, and others. When motivating patients to lose weight, it is important to emphasize that complete normalization of body weight is not necessary to achieve at least some benefits against hypertension. Even a reduction by several kilograms can lead to a marked decrease in blood pressure. The obesity subject is discussed in more detail in Chapter 16.

The Joint National Committee on Prevention, Detection, Evaluation, and Treatment of High Blood Pressure (JNC7) and its European counterpart (2007 ESH-ESC Practice Guidelines for the Management of Arterial Hypertension) as well as the ADA recommend an average of 6 g sodium chloride per day, that is, approximately 100 mmol per day. Patients should be instructed that this goal may be achieved by reducing the consumption of cured meat, canned food, salted varieties of bread, hard cheese, and seafood. Obviously, meals should be prepared without adding salt, and soups are a notorious source of salt. The great difficulty is that almost 80% of the salt consumed is contained already in the commercial food items the patient consumes. Measuring sodium excretion occasionally in 24-hour urine collections is prudent.

THE ROLE OF DIETARY INTAKE OF PROTEIN

That high protein intake increases the progression risk in different animal models of kidney damage is well known. Conversely, restricting protein intake reduces hyperfiltration and intraglomular pressure. As a result, the increase of proteinuria, glomerulosclerosis, and hypertension is lessened, and progression is slowed.

In patients with diabetes who do not have nephropathy, only fragmentary evidence exists that high dietary protein intake increases the risk for developing microalbuminuria. In one important cross-sectional study (EURODIAB study), 2696 patients with type 1 diabetes in 16 European countries were examined. It was noted that in individuals whose protein consumption was more than 20% of total energy intake, the albumin excretion rates were higher, particularly in individuals with hypertension and poor metabolic control. This association was found specifically for animal protein; no association was found for vegetable protein. In animal experiments, manipulation of dietary protein intake was particularly effective early in the course of progressive CKD. Therefore, recommending a reduction of protein consumption to less than 20% of total energy intake (as proposed by the EURODIAB investigators) would seem prudent. This advice is also in line with the recommendations of the ADA. Whether a more drastic reduction of dietary protein is effective when kidney function is already markedly impaired is quite controversial not to the least because of the risk of malnutrition. Long-term adherence to dietary restriction of protein is notoriously poor. This is one more argument against waiting until the patient is in advanced kidney failure and for educating him from the very beginning of diabetes to stick to a prudent diet, i.e., a protein intake of 0.8 g/kg b.w./day, emphasizing substitution of vegetable protein for protein from animal sources. An added benefit of this policy is that the consumption of total fat and saturated fat will also be reduced.

THE HYPOTHETICAL ROLE OF DYSLIPIDEMIA

A potential risk factor for CKD and its progression is dyslipidemia. This risk has been well documented in cross-sectional and longitudinal association studies, in which dyslipidemia was found to be a potent predictor of progressive loss of kidney function. Furthermore, a large body of experimental evidence in different models of renal damage suggests that a high intake of fat (in particular, oxidized fat) aggravates progression of kidney disease, whereas dietary restriction of fat (or lowering of fat by antilipidemic agents) attenuates progression. Controlled evidence for such a relationship is missing, however.

The renal benefit of lipid lowering by dietary measures (and by administering lipid lowering medication) has not been definitely proven, but a strong rationale for it exists because of the excessive atherosclerosis risk among patients with diabetes. Recent recommendations of the National Cholesterol Education Program (Table 7-2), including the stringent goals for LDL cholesterol, can usually be achieved safely and economically only with a combination of dietary measures and lipid-lowering agents, particularly statins. Whether the so-called pleiotropic effects of these agents also play significant role, apart from their lipid-lowering effects, is currently unclear.

What practical dietary recommendations should be given to the patient with diabetes and incipient nephropathy? Patients with diabetes should follow a prudent diet and, in principle, follow the recommendations outlined in Table 7-4.

Progression of Diabetic Nephropathy

The factors involved in the progression of established diabetic nephropathy differ from the factors operative in the development of diabetic nephropathy, not in principle, but with respect to their relative importance, as summarized in Table 7-6.

THE ROLE OF HYPERTENSION

An overwhelming body of evidence documents that the single most important factor that determines progression of established diabetic nephropathy is hypertension. Blood pressure rises when the patient develops microalbuminuria. In particular, the usual decrease of blood pressure during nighttime is attenuated or even reversed. In recent years, the fact that conventional levels of "normotension" are not good enough for the patient with diabetes and CKD has become apparent. Several national committees propose a target blood pressure less than or equal to 125/75 mm Hg in patients with diabetes who have proteinuria, at least in the absence of coronary heart or cerebrovascular disease. Because of disturbed autoregulation, diabetic patients, particularly in the presence of autonomic polyneuropathy, are particularly prone to develop hypotensive episodes. It is presumably for this reason that in the Irbesartan Diabetic Nephropathy Trial population with high comorbid condition profile, the mortality was substantially higher, if the achieved systolic blood pressure was below 120 mm Hg. Although it is uncertain whether the relationship is causal, caution against excessive blood pressure lowering is prudent. The 125/75 mm Hg blood pressure target can usually be reached only if one administers more than one class of antihypertensive agents; ACE inhibitors or angiotensin receptor blockers are the medication of first choice. Nevertheless, dietary salt restriction remains a very important component of antihypertensive management in patients with CKD with diabetic nephropathy. Although diuretics must usually be administered in addition to restricting salt intake, the side effects of diuretic treatment, particularly hypokalemia and hypomagnesemia, are reduced if the patient is on a low salt intake. Blood pressure control with antihypertensive agents is markedly facilitated by a low-salt diet, so that less antihypertensive medication is required. With the exception of calcium channel blockers, the blood pressure-lowering effect of all antihypertensive agents is increased by low-salt intake and reversal of hypervolemia. Notably, diuretics, particularly in patients with hypokalemia, may cause or aggravate insulin resistance and dyslipidemia. It is also important that only the concentration of free diuretic in the tubular fluid, and not the total concentration (also comprising protein bound diuretic) is able to inhibit tubular sodium uptake; as a result the dose-effect relationship is shifted to the right, i.e., higher doses are required in the proteinuric diabetic patient.

THE ROLE OF PROTEINURIA

In the past, optimal renal protection was assumed to have been achieved when blood pressure was lowered to the target level, i.e., less than or equal to 125/75 mm Hg (see preceding text). More recently, in addition to lowering blood pressure, reducing proteinuria has become a second important therapeutic goal. Proteinuria can be considered a "nephrotoxin." Several studies in patients with diabetic and nondiabetic CKD have shown that long-term preservation of kidney function was greatest in those patients in whom the most pronounced reduction of proteinuria could be achieved. For this reason, when administering ACE inhibitors or angiotensin receptor blockers (ARBs), urinary protein excretion should be monitored. When the reduction of proteinuria is not satisfactory, i.e., <1 g/day, escalating the dose of the ACE inhibitor or ARB is recommended, even when target blood pressure has been reached. Notably, several studies have shown that reduction of proteinuria by ACE inhibitors was amplified by a low protein intake. One further approach is the use of ACE inhibitors plus ARBs and also the administration of aldosterone receptor blockers in patients with "aldosterone escape" (i.e., those patients with a secondary increase in the level of serum or urinary aldosterone occurring after the initial decrease in aldosterone production that follows administration of ACE inhibitors or ARBs).

THE ROLE OF DIETARY PROTEIN INTAKE

The Modification of Diet in Renal Disease (MDRD) study, which enrolled exclusively patients without diabetes, showed a slight delay in dialysis dependency when patients with advanced CKD were given a very low-protein diet (0.58 g/kg b.w./day), but the benefit was not impressive and certainly was much smaller than the benefit derived from aggressive lowering of blood pressure. The results of this controlled trial are in striking contrast to those of a few uncontrolled studies that had shown marked benefit from protein restriction. A meta-analysis showed that the effect of protein restriction was greater in 11 nonrandomized studies comprising 2248 patients than in 13 randomized studies comprising 1919 patients. Others concluded that "the benefit of a low-protein diet on slowing the progression of renal failure is negligible and that the delay of dialysis for a few months, i.e., short-lasting freedom from dialysis, is not cost-effective, particularly since it may lead to poor nutritional status."

Specific information is available on the effect of protein restriction in patients with diabetes. In a prospective parallel group study, 20 patients with type 1 and manifest nephropathy were given a low-protein (0.6 g/kg b.w./day) diet with 500 to 1000 mg phosphorus and 2000 mg of sodium. The control group of 15 patients received 1 g protein/kg b.w./day and the same amount of phosphorus and sodium. The glomerular filtration rate (GFR) was measured using the iothalamate clearance. Iothalamate clearance decreased by 3.1 mL/minute/month with the low-protein diet and by 12.1 mL/minute/month in the control diet group. Although the difference between groups was statistically significant ($p = 0.02$), large interindividual differences were observed.

In a cross-over study, patients with type 1 diabetes and overt nephropathy were switched from a normal protein diet (1.13 g/kg b.w./day) to a low-protein diet (0.67 g/kg b.w./day). As shown in Figure 7-1, the rate of loss of GFR, measured by the radiochelate method, was markedly attenuated when patients were on the low-protein diet, and this change was associated with a decrease in albuminuria. The study is confounded, however, by lower blood pressure with low-protein diet, the possibility of carryover effects, and nonstandardized concurrent treatment.

Almost all studies showed that albuminuria (a surrogate marker of glomerular damage) decreases with a low-protein diet, but the effect on GFR is not entirely consistent. To this result must be added the fact that a decrease in muscle strength, an increase in fat mass, and reduced whole body leucine oxidation were observed when patients with type 1 diabetes and early nephropathy were given 0.6 g protein/kg b.w./day. This finding illustrates the potential danger of malnutrition and is of particular concern because malnutrition is a potent predictor of cardiovascular death in patients with ure-

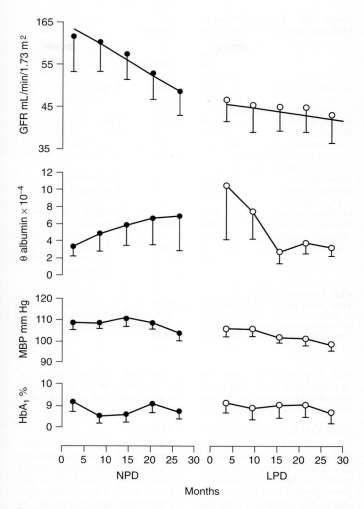

Figure 7-1. Changes in glomerular filtration rate (GFR), fractional clearance of albumin (calculated as clearance [UV/P] of albumin divided by the GFR), mean blood pressure, and glycosylated haemoglobin (HbA1) in 19 proteinuric insulin-dependent diabetic patients on normal protein diets (NPD) (*closed circles*) and low-protein diets (LPD) (*open circles*). (From Walker JD, Dodds RA, Murrells TJ, et al. Restriction of dietary protein and progression of renal failure in diabetic nephropathy. Lancet 1989;2:1411–1415, with permission.)

**Table 7-8.   Two different types of
malnutrition in chronic kidney disease**

	Type 1 "Uremia-Induced"	Type 2 "Cytokine-Driven"
Comorbidity (for example, chronic heart failure)	Low association	High association
Serum albumin	Normal/low	Low
Presence of inflammatory markers (high levels of CRP and cytokines)	No	Yes
Food intake	Low	Low/normal
Resting energy expenditure	Normal	Elevated
Oxidative stress	Increased	Markedly increased
Protein catabolism	Decreased	Increased
Optimal treatment strategy	Dialysis/ nutritional support	First priority elimination of the sources of chronic inflammation

CRP, C-reactive protein.
From Stenvinkel P, Heimburger O, Lindholm B, et al. Are there two types of malnutrition in chronic renal failure? Evidence for relationships between malnutrition, inflammation and atherosclerosis (MIA syndrome). Nephrol Dial Transplant 2000;15:953–960, with permission.

mia. The issue is more complex, however, because indices of malnutrition may additionally be attributable to a state of microinflammation with increased expression of inflammatory cytokines, as illustrated in Table 7-8.

THE ROLE OF GLYCEMIC CONTROL

Although blood pressure control is of overwhelming importance, the rate of progression is also determined to a minor degree by the quality of glycemic control. Hemoglobin A1c concentrations have been shown to correlate with the rate of loss of GFR at any given level of blood pressure and is presumably a factor contributing to the excessive frequency of cardiovascular events. In the diabetic patient with preterminal/terminal uremia, good glycemic control is also important for another reason; because cells shrink in a hyperosmolar milieu, hyperglycemia causes translocation of potassium from the intracellular to the extracellular compartment as part of a homeostatic effort to hold intracellular solute content constant. Therefore, hyperglycemia predisposes the patient to hyperkalemia. In patients with impaired kidney function, the amount of glucose lost in the urine (glucosuria) is limited, so glycemic decompensation may cause excessive hyperglycemia and predispose patients to hyperosmolar coma. Finally, catabolism and impaired infection control are common in patients with poor glycemic control. One important measure against catabolism

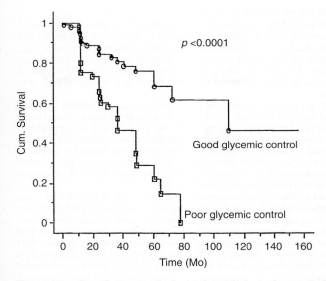

Figure 7-2. Cumulative survival with hemodialysis therapy in Taiwanese patients with type2 diabetes having good glycemic control (HbA1c 5% to 10%) and poor glycemic control (HbA1c > 10%) in the 6 months preceding dialysis. (From Wu MS, Yu CC, Yang CW, et al. Poor predialysis glycemic control is a predictor of mortality in type II diabetic patients on maintenance hemodialysis. Nephrol Dial Transplant 1997;12:2105–2110, with permission.)

is to immediately put the patient on insulin rather than to waste time with oral hypoglycemic agents.

As shown in Figure 7-2, Chinese authors documented that patients with type 2 diabetes who were treated with dialysis had substantially poorer survival when glycemic control was poor in the 6 months preceding the start of dialysis. In patients with diabetes who were undergoing dialysis, several other trials showed higher mortality in patients with higher HbA1c levels than in patients with good blood glucose control, albeit this is observed only in patients with HbA1c levels higher than 10.

Does Presence of Advanced Diabetic Nephropathy Necessitate Changes in a Patient's Dietary Management?

In the patient with advanced diabetic nephropathy, the most important components of medical management are:

- Maintaining glycemic control
- Maintaining blood pressure control
- Monitoring progression
- Controlling dyslipidemia
- Avoiding malnutrition

Maintaining Glycemic Control

When the GFR is reduced, the half-life of insulin is prolonged, because the renal and the extrarenal clearances of insulin are diminished. This relation holds for both endogenous insulin (e.g., released by sulfonylureas) and exogenous insulin (i.e., insulin injection). As a result, when the dosage of insulin is not adjusted, the patient with advanced CKD is at risk of developing hypoglycemia.

The propensity to develop hypoglycemia is modulated by additional factors. Patients with impaired kidney function tend to be anorectic. Inadequate dietary intake predisposes to hypoglycemia. According to experimental studies anorexogenic factors are excreted in normal urine, and such factors presumably accumulate in patients with advanced CKD. Furthermore, the plasma concentration of leptin, an adipocyte hormone that reduces appetite, is increased in advanced CKD.

Most sulfonylurea compounds (or their active metabolites) accumulate in CKD, with the exception of gliquidone and glimepiride. This accumulation is particularly pronounced for glibenclamid, which may cause prolonged episodes of hypoglycemia and necessitate prolonged infusion of large quantities of glucose. Most of the newer oral antihyperglycemic agents, for example, glinides and thiazolidiones, do not accumulate in CKD, even in advanced stages.

Conversely, the action of insulin is impaired in advanced CKD. Because of aggravated insulin resistance, the patient with diabetes and advanced CKD is prone to develop hyperglycemia. Insulin resistance is caused by low-molecular-weight, water-soluble substances that are removed by dialysis (vide infra). In the individual patient, the net effect of these opposing tendencies, i.e., to develop hypoglycemia on the one hand or hyperglycemia on the other hand, cannot be safely predicted. Consequently, strict monitoring of glycemia is necessary in the CKD patient with diabetes.

Because of the risks associated with oral hypoglycemic agents, and to avoid protein catabolism, it is wise to be more liberal about the decision to begin insulin therapy. The use of insulin is indispensable in the patient with intercurrent disease, particularly in the case of infection or surgical intervention. One important factor that may render glycemic control particularly difficult is gastroparesis, the disturbance in gastric emptying as a result of autonomic polyneuropathy. Delayed transfer of food from the stomach to the intestine may make dietary management difficult. After the patient with diabetic gastroparesis has eaten, up to several hours may be required for the glucose derived from food items to enter the circulation.

When managing glycemia in patients with diabetes and advanced nephropathy, one must be aware that HbA1$_c$ levels may be artifactually increased and reflect not only glycation but also carbamylation of hemoglobin. If the patient is receiving EPO, younger erythrocytes are in the circulation and HbA1c concentrations will decrease, even though glycemic control is unchanged. This artifact results from the fact that such young erythrocytes are exposed to a hyperglycemic milieu for shorter periods of time. The measurement of glycosylated albumin is a more reliable alternative.

Table 7-9. Adverse effects of common antihypertensive drugs in the diabetic patient

Betablocker	Decreased glucose tolerance
(Nonspecific > β_1-selective)	"Masking" of the symptoms of hypoglycemia delayed recovery from hypoglycemia dyslipidemia
Diuretics	Dyslipidemia
Thiazides > furosemide	Hyperglycemia via insulin resistance and diminished glucosuria
ACE inhibitors/Ang II receptor blockers	Hyperkalemia
	Increase in serum creatinine (in patients with hypovolemia, renal artery stenosis)
α receptor blocker	Orthostatic hypotension, congestive heart failure

Maintaining Blood Pressure Control

As stated in the preceding text, dietary salt restriction, use of diuretics, or both are the cornerstone of blood pressure control. However, one has to be aware that antihypertensive agents may influence the control of glycemia and lipidemia (Table 7-9).

A physician who recommends salt restriction and administers diuretics must also be aware that hypovolemia is undesirable. This complication can be recognized from the constellation of hypokalemia, metabolic alkalosis (elevated serum bicarbonate concentration), increased uric acid concentration, and a tendency for an acute rise of serum urea and creatinine concentrations. The patient also tends to have orthostatic hypotension.

Hypovolemia is particularly undesirable in patients with diabetes and left ventricular hypertrophy (because a stiff left ventricle requires a higher filling pressure) or in the patient with diabetes and autonomic polyneuropathy, who is not able to achieve appropriate vasoconstriction when blood pressure decreases.

Monitoring Progression

Accurately measuring the rate of GFR loss requires the use of marker substances that are not available in clinical practice. Usually physicians rely on serum creatinine or endogenous creatinine clearance. In individuals with low muscle mass, particularly elderly, wasted, diabetic women, the serum creatinine concentration may grossly underestimate GFR. The explanation is that creatinine is chiefly derived from conversion of creatine to creatinine in muscle, and a wasted individual with a low muscle mass will produce less creatinine.

After ingestion of cooked meat, serum creatinine level increases transiently, because prolonged cooking can increase the production of creatinine from creatine in muscle. Serum creatinine (SCR) levels tend to decrease when patients are given meat-free diets. A good index of GFR is the endogenous creatinine clearance (CCR), which requires a 24-hour urine collection. Because 24-hour urine collections for measurement of CCR are tedious and error-prone, algorithms have been proposed to assess GFR; for example, the Cockroft–Gault formula:

Ccr = (140 − age) (wt in kg)/72 × SCR (mg/100 mL)

or the modified MDRD formula for (estimated) eGFR based on serum creatinine (standardized measurement according to Cleveland clinic protocol) and patient age and gender:

eGFR = 175 × (standardized S-crea) − 1.154 × (age) − 0.203 × 0.742
(for females)

The rate of urinary protein excretion is an important surrogate marker to monitor the progression of diabetic nephropathy. Monitoring proteinuria enables assessing the effect of therapeutic interventions to retard progression, for example, blood pressure lowering and glycemic control.

Controlling Dyslipidemia

Patients with advanced diabetic nephropathy tend to have more dyslipidemia. This condition is the combined result of CKD yielding hypertriglyceridemia and accumulation of incompletely catabolized lipoprotein particles (e.g., intermediate-density lipoproteins [IDL]) and chylomicrons. Severe proteinuria aggravates dyslipidemia through mechanisms analogous to the ones operative in the nephrotic syndrome.

In principle, hypertriglyceridemia would respond well to fibrates. Most fibrates, with the exception of gemfibrozil, accumulate in patients with advanced CKD, exposing them to the risk of muscle necrosis (rhabdomyolysis). Statins do not accumulate in CKD.

An important clinical observation is that medications that reduce proteinuria (e.g., ACE inhibitors) also tend to improve dyslipidemia, so that blood pressure control by ACE inhibitors (or ARBs) can have clinically important benefits for the lipid status.

Avoiding Protein Energy Wasting of Kidney Disease

The main issue in the patient with advanced diabetic nephropathy is avoiding malnutrition and wasting. For any given degree of CKD, patients with diabetes tend to be more wasted than patients without diabetes. One important reason for this observation is that insulin is an anabolic hormone, so the absence of, or the resistance to, its effects diminishes synthesis of muscle protein and predisposes individuals to loss of muscle. Important confounding factors are anorexia (common in advanced CKD), gastroparesis, and catabolism during intercurrent illness or surgery and, particularly, during long periods of fasting (often during ill-advised efforts to reduce weight). Experimental studies showed that breakdown of muscle protein in the fasting state is considerably greater in uremic animals than in nonuremic animals. Consequently, the combination of uremia and diabetes is particularly disadvantageous. The risk of a negative protein balance is further aggravated by high-grade proteinuria.

Against this background, it is problematic to advise low-protein diets to patients with advanced diabetic nephropathy to retard progression. Such diets are not safe unless calorie intake is strictly maintained (patients tend to eat less rather than to eat less protein when they are not properly instructed and monitored). The occurrence of catabolism can be recognized by monitoring serum urea concentrations and urinary urea excretion rates, but the simple clinical examination of inspecting the patient and assessing his muscle mass is usually sufficient. Anthropometric measurements are rarely required for this purpose.

Biochemical markers such as serum albumin concentration and concentrations of complement factors may be misleading in CKD. Notably, many patients with uremia have signs of "microinflammation," including increased concentrations of C-reactive protein (CRP) and serum amyloid A protein (SAA). As shown in Table 7-8, a simple list of variables has been proposed to differentiate between malnutrition caused by uremia per se and malnutrition resulting from microinflammation (see Chapters 6 and 16).

There is consensus that renal replacement therapy, either continuous ambulatory peritoneal dialysis (CAPD) or hemodialysis, should be started earlier in the patient with diabetes than in nondiabetic patients with uremia. Timely start of dialysis is often necessary not because of symptoms of uremia but because of fluid overload, vomiting because of gastroparesis, recurrent episodes of left ventricular dysfunction with pulmonary edema, or wasting. In patients with stage 4 and 5 CKD not yet on maintenance dialysis, the most important task is to avoid insidious protein energy wasting.

Does Renal Replacement Therapy Affect Dietary Management of the Diabetic Patient?

Hemodialysis has the beneficial effect of removing substances that interfere with the action of insulin, so that sensitivity to endogenous or exogenous insulin increases. As a consequence, patients tend to be less hyperglycemic. Conversely, hemodialysis removes hypothetical anorexigenic substances, so that appetite increases and patients gain weight, with an increase in lean body mass. This increase may cause glycemic control to deteriorate. The net effect is difficult to predict, and monitoring of glycemia and of HbA1$_c$ concentrations is necessary. There is no further documented benefit for lowering Hba1$_c$ below 8% in patients with ESRD.

Dialysates most often contain glucose in concentrations ranging from 100 to 200 mg per dL. Particularly the anuric patient is at risk of hyperglycemia because spillover of glucose into the urine is no longer taking place. In this case, glucose concentrations increase to very high levels, causing hypervolemia, thirst, and hyperkalemia. Another consequence of hemodialysis is loss of amino acids, so the protein requirement is higher; a dietary intake of 1.2 g/kg b.w./day is therefore commonly recommended (see Chapter 11).

For patients treated with CAPD, the dialysate in the abdominal cavity contains glucose in concentrations ranging from 1500 to 4000 mg/dL. This high concentration is used to osmotically remove excess fluids from the patient (see Chapter 12). The net uptake of glucose is 100 g/day and more. Because of these excess calories, obesity is common among patients treated with CAPD. Theoretically CAPD may offset one problem, because insulin can be administered intraperitoneally, thus imitating the natural delivery of insulin into the portal circulation. This mode of adminis-tration of insulin is not consistently used, however, and most pa-tients are on subcutaneous insulin. The earlier CAPD fluids contained advanced glycation end (AGE) products produced dur-ing the sterilization process, but this problem has been circum-vented with novel sterilization and bag handling techniques.

For the patient with diabetes who has successfully received a combined pancreas and kidney transplant, reversing diabetes and restoring normal insulin secretion does not pose specific die-tetic problems, with the exception of the advice that patients should avoid major weight gain. The patient with diabetes who has received a kidney graft has several hazards such as higher infection rates and a higher cardiovascular morbidity and mortal-ity in the long run. The patient without diabetes who is treated with steroids and calcineurin inhibitors (e.g., cyclosporin A or tacrolimus) has a long-term risk of developing type 2 diabetes that is as high as 30%. Major culprits are presumably genetic predisposition, weight gain, use of steroids, and, specifically in the case of tacrolimus, selective disturbance of insulin secretion. The latter effect is dose dependent (see Chapter 13).

Selected Readings

American Diabetes Association. Nutrition principles and recommen-dations in diabetes. Diabetes Care 2004;27:S36–S46.

Cosio FG, Hickson LJ, Griffin MD, et al. Patient survival and cardio-vascular risk after kidney transplantation: the challenge of diabe-tes. Am J Transplant 2008;8:593–599.

DCCT Research Group. The effect of intensive treatment of diabetes on the development and progression of long-term complications in insulin-dependent diabetes mellitus. N Engl J Med 1993;329: 977–986.

Diabetes Prevention Program Research Group. Reduction in the inci-dence of type 2 diabetes with lifestyle intervention or metformin. N Engl J Med 2003;346:393–403.

Executive Summary of the Third Report of the National Cholesterol Education Program (NCEP). Expert panel on detection, evaluation, and treatment of high blood cholesterol in adults (Adult Treatment Panel III). JAMA 2001;285:2486–2497.

Franz MJ, Bantle JP, Beebe CA, et al. Evidence-based nutrition prin-ciples and recommendations for the treatment and prevention of diabetes and related complications (technical review). Diabetes Care 2002;25:148–198.

Inaba M, Okuno S, Kumeda Y, et al. Glycated albumin is a better glycemic indicator than glycated hemoglobin values in hemodi-alysis patients with diabetes: effect of anemia and erythropoietin injection. J Am Soc Nephrol 2007;18:896–903.

Ohkubo Y, Kishikawa H, Araki E. Intensive insulin therapy prevents the progression of diabetic microvascular complications in Japa-nese patients with non-insulin-dependent diabetes mellitus: a ran-domized prospective 6-year study. Diabetes Res 1995;28:103–117.

Ritz E, Orth SR. Nephropathy in patients with type 2 diabetes melli-tus. N Engl J Med 1999;341:1127–1133.

Ruggenenti P, Schieppati A, Remuzzi G. Progression, remission, regression of chronic renal diseases. Lancet 2001;357:1601–1608.

Sacks FM, Svetkey LP, Vollmer WM, et al. Effects on blood pressure of reduced dietary sodium and the Dietary Approaches to Stop Hypertension (DASH) diet. N Engl J Med 2001;344:3–10.

Sato A, Hayashi K, Naruse M, et al. Effectiveness of aldosterone blockade in patients with diabetic nephropathy. Hypertension 2003;41:64–68.

Sheard NF, Nathaniel GC. The role of nutrition therapy in the management of diabetes mellitus. Nutr Clin Care 2000;6:334–348.

Stevens LA, Coresh J, Greene T, et al. Assessing kidney function—measured and estimated glomerular filtration rate. N Engl J Med 2006;354:2473–2483.

Toeller M, Buyken A, Heitkamp G, et al, EURODIAB IDDM Complications Study Group. Protein intake and urinary albumin excretion rates in the EURODIAB IDDM complications study. Diabetologia 1997;40:1219–1226.

UK Prospective Diabetes Study (UKPDS) Group. Intensive blood-glucose control with sulphonylureas or insulin compared with conventional treatment and risk of complications in patients with type 2 diabetes (UKPDS 33). Lancet 1998;352:837–853.

Wu MS, Yu CC, Yang CW, et al. Poor pre-dialysis glycemic control is a predictor of mortality in type II diabetic patients on maintenance hemodialysis. Nephrol Dial Transplant 1997;12:2105–2110.

Nephrotic Syndrome: Nutritional Consequences and Dietary Management

Jane Y. Yeun, Michel Zakari, and George A. Kaysen

Nephrotic syndrome results from urinary loss of albumin and other plasma proteins and is characterized by hypoalbuminemia, hyperlipidemia, and edema. Quantifying the loss of tissue protein is more difficult than measuring the urinary loss of albumin and other plasma proteins. However, marked muscle wasting (sometimes obscured by edema) occurs in patients with continuous proteinuria. In addition, micronutrients such as vitamin D, iron, and zinc are bound to plasma proteins that are lost, so depletion syndromes can occur when proteinuria is massive and continuous. Lipid metabolism is abnormal in the nephrotic syndrome resulting in hyperlipidemia and potentially, accelerated atherosclerosis and renal failure.

The major rationales for modifying a patient's diet, then, are to blunt manifestations of the syndrome (such as edema and hyperlipidemia), to replace nutrients lost in the urine, and to reduce risks for progressive kidney disease and atherosclerosis. It should be mentioned that specific allergens in food may cause kidney disease in some patients, and dietary modification might be curative.

DIETARY PROTEIN

Metabolic abnormalities in nephrotic syndrome include depletion of plasma and tissue protein pools. Nephrotic syndrome in this case, resembles protein–calorie malnutrition (i.e., kwashiorkor) because in both cases, the plasma albumin concentration is reduced, plasma volume is expanded, and albumin pools shift from the extravascular to the vascular compartment. In protein–calorie malnutrition, providing the needed protein and calories will correct all of the manifestations of malnutrition. This is not the case in patients with the nephrotic syndrome.

In patients with nephrotic syndrome, there are several causes of hypoalbuminemia: (i) albumin loss in the urine; (ii) an inappropriate increase in the fractional catabolic rate of albumin; and (iii) an insufficient increase in the synthesis rate of albumin to replace the loss. Placing patients with nephrotic syndrome on a high protein diet might seem reasonable in light of the massive urinary protein and amino acid losses. However, while average values for urinary protein losses are approximately 6 to 8 g per day (the amount contained in a hen's egg), simply increasing dietary protein is of little benefit. This strategy is not recommended because dietary protein and, specifically, certain amino acids in the diet, increase glomerular permselectivity, i.e., an increase in the defect in the filtration barrier of the glomerular cap-

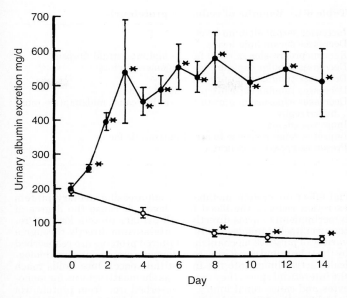

Figure 8-1. The effect of dietary protein augmentation on urinary albumin excretion (UAE) in rats with nephrotic syndrome. Nephrotic syndrome was induced by injection of anti-FX 1A antibody to produce passive Heymann nephritis. Twenty-eight rats were initially fed a diet containing 8.5% protein as sodium caseinate. On day 0, 15 animals had dietary protein increased to 40% casein (*solid circles*), and 13 animals remained on the 8.5% casein diet (*open circles*). Urinary albumin excretion increased significantly in the animals fed a high-protein diet by the second day and remained significantly greater thereafter, whereas urinary albumin excretion decreased in the low-protein diet by day 8. *$p < 0.05$ versus time 0.

illary when compared with low-protein diets; filtration barrier defects result in increased urinary protein losses (Fig. 8-1). This increase in permselectivity increases urinary protein loss and results in a net decrease in plasma protein mass despite any increase in albumin synthesis because of augmentation of dietary protein. Indeed, high protein diets likely contribute to loss of kidney function.

Conversely, dietary protein restriction in contrast, has several benefits in patients with chronic kidney disease (CKD) with nephrotic syndrome. There is reduced urinary protein excretion and plasma fibrinogen levels, decreased protein degradation and amino acid oxidation with improvement or achievement in neutral nitrogen balance, and a potential salutary effect on progressive loss of kidney function.

Reducing urinary protein excretion, regardless of how it is achieved, is desirable for several reasons. In addition to its benefi-

Table 8-1.   Benefits of reducing proteinuria

Increases serum albumin levels
Decreases serum lipid levels
Retards progression of renal failure and interstitial fibrosis
Decreases tubular exposure to complement factors
Decreases tubular exposure to iron
Decreases tubular exposure to oxidized lipids
Decreases exposure to growth factors that cause maladaptive renal
   hypertrophy
Improves edema
Improves renal response to atrial natriuretic factor
Preserves growth in children

cial effect on protein metabolism, suppressing urinary protein excretion reduces the blood lipid levels, because the degree of hyperlipidemia varies directly with urinary protein losses. Proteinuria itself damages the renal interstitium directly through a variety of putative mechanisms. Filtered proteins are reabsorbed by the tubule and carry iron, complement components, and biologically active lipids into the interstitial space. Once lipids reach the interstitial space, they may act as chemoattractants for monocytes and cause renal injury. Reabsorbed iron from proteinuria is biologically active and may act as an oxidant to injure the kidney. In addition, diets that are high in protein also are high in acid content, leading to acidosis with increased ammoniagenesis by the kidney. The accelerated rates of renal ammonia production also may lead to renal injury. The reduction in urinary protein excretion that follows the initiation of a low-protein diet can have a potentially salutary effect on progressive renal injury through any or all of these mechanisms (Table 8-1).

Several studies have suggested that the composition of proteins in the diet may be as important as its absolute nitrogen content. In experimental studies in rats, dietary augmentation of certain amino acids causes a prompt increase in urinary albumin excretion (UAE), whereas branched-chain amino acid supplementation does not affect proteinuria. Studies in animal models of nephrotic syndrome and in humans with CKD also suggest that specific types of dietary proteins may be particularly important. When patients with nephrotic syndrome were fed a vegetarian soy diet, urinary protein excretion decreased, as did blood lipid levels. In rats with puromycin-induced nephrotic syndrome, not only did a 20% soy protein diet lower proteinuria and blood lipid levels, but it also improved the creatinine clearance and decreased glomerular sclerosis while reducing the level of proinflammatory cytokines in the kidney. Because the soy protein diet was low in fat (28% of calories) and protein (0.71 g per kg ideal body weight), distinguishing whether the beneficial effects of a soy-based diet in patients with nephrotic syndrome from a special amino acid composition alone or from the lower fat and protein content is difficult. Studies of nephrotic rats suggested, however, that much of the benefit of a soy-based diet derives from a direct effect of soy proteins on the kidney (possibly through reducing the degree of nitrotyrosine formation), rather than through changes in hepatic lipid metabolism. Curiously, urinary protein excretion differed only slightly when diets containing 1.1 g were compared with those containing 0.7 g soy protein/kg/day.

More recent animal studies suggest that a flaxseed-based protein diet may offer even more benefit than soy protein. In a study of the effects of 20% casein, 20% soy protein, or 20% flaxseed meal in a rat model of diabetic nephropathy using the obese spontaneously hypertensive rat model, flaxseed meal reduced proteinuria and glomerular and tubulointerstitial injury more than a casein- or soy protein–based diet; creatinine clearance and plasma creatinine levels did not differ. The common pathway for the beneficial effects of plant-protein diets may be the phytoestrogens that are present in soybeans as isoflavones and in flaxseed as lignans. These compounds are estrogen-like but how they affect the kidney is unknown. Plant-protein diets are high in polyunsaturated lipids, including α-linolenic acid in flaxseed. Polyunsaturated fats can improve the lipid profile and may reduce kidney injury. However, mechanisms for these responses are unknown.

In nephrotic patients, concomitant use of an angiotensin-converting enzyme (ACE) inhibitor with a high-protein diet (1.3 to 1.6 g protein/kg/day) prevented the diet-induced increase in urinary protein excretion. Serum protein and albumin levels increased significantly in eight patients after they crossed over to the high-protein diet with ACE inhibitor, compared with results with a mildly protein-restricted diet (0.8 g per day). The use of ACE inhibitor or angiotensin receptor blocker (ARB) in patients with normal to moderately restricted protein intake (0.8 g per day), in contrast, lowered levels of proteinuria, triglycerides, total cholesterol, and low-density lipoprotein (LDL) cholesterol. Recent data suggest that more complete blockade of the renin-angiotensin-aldosterone system (RAAS) with a combination of ACE inhibitor and ARB or addition of aldosterone inhibitor to the ACE inhibitor or ARB regimen is even more effective in reducing proteinuria. Unfortunately, hyperkalemia may develop. Whether protein restriction in addition to RAAS blockade offers further benefit is debated.

MICROALBUMINURIA

Although the focus of this chapter is on patients with nephrotic proteinuria, a much larger numbers of patients have low levels of urinary albumin loss (i.e., microalbuminuria). Microalbuminuria is found in hypertensive and diabetic subjects and predicts progression of kidney disease and cardiovascular risk in both populations. Microalbuminuria also increases the risk of cardiovascular disease even among patients who are not hypertensive or diabetic. The risk for developing urinary albumin excretion (UAE) in hypertensive diabetic subjects is related to the fraction of total calorie intake that is composed of dietary protein. Restriction of protein intake reduces UAE in both noninsulin-dependent and insulin-dependent diabetic subjects. The type of protein consumed also has an effect on UAE in diabetic subjects, suggesting

Table 8-2.   Dietary recommendations in nephrotic syndrome

Calorie	35 kcal/kg/day
Protein	0.8–1.0 g/kg/day Soy and vegetarian proteins may be more beneficial than "high-quality protein"
Fat	<30% of total calories Cholesterol <200 mg/d Higher proportion of polyunsaturated fatty acids (10% of energy) Fish oil may be beneficial for IgA nephropathy (12 g/d)
Minerals	<2 g Na Iron only when clearly iron deficient Calcium, if vitamin D deficient (2 g/day)
Vitamins	1,25-$(OH)_2$-vitamin D, if vitamin D deficient

IgA, immunoglobulin A.

that either the amino acid composition or the lipid composition of the food ingested contributes to the effect of a protein-rich meal.

Recommendations

Because urinary protein excretion varies from day to day in individual patients, we recommend collecting 3 separate 24-hour urine specimens, with simultaneous measurements of serum albumin and protein, to establish baseline values. Patients are then placed on a 35-kcal per kg diet that contains 0.8 to 1.0 g protein per kg and is restricted to 2 g of sodium. We then monitor 24-hour urinary urea excretion every 2 to 3 months to ensure that patients are not eating more (or less) protein than recommended. The goal is to decrease proteinuria without reducing serum albumin and protein concentration. This goal is usually attainable when dietary protein intake is restricted to these levels (Table 8-2).

Dietary protein intake can be estimated from nitrogen excretion measured in the steady state. The steady-state nitrogen excretion (previously abbreviated as the protein catabolic rate or PCR) is principally determined by the urea nitrogen excretion. Therefore, if total body urea pools are constant (i.e., the blood urea nitrogen [BUN] and weight are stable), then the amount of protein ingested can be estimated from the formula:

Protein intake = [0.031 gN/kg/day]body weight in kilograms/0.16 + [24-hour urine urea nitrogen excretion/0.16] g/day + 24-hour urine protein excretion g/day (see Chapter 6)

If the estimated protein intake by this method varies from the amount of protein prescribed for the diet, the patient should be referred to the nutritionist/dietician.

Although "high-quality" protein (meat and dairy products) contain a higher fraction of essential amino acids (EAA), vegetarian diets based on soy protein are more effective in reducing urinary

Table 8-3.   Proatherogenic factors in nephrotic syndrome

High cholesterol	Increased low-density lipoprotein
	Increased very low-density lipoprotein
	Increased intermediate-density lipoprotein
	Normal to low high-density lipoprotein
Altered high-density lipoprotein structure	
High lipoprotein(a)	
High triglycerides	
Increased fibrinogen	

protein loss, increasing serum protein levels, correcting hyper-lipidemia, and reducing renal inflammation and fibrosis. Consequently, we recommend soy-based protein in the diet. A plant-based diet may be even more useful in preventing the development of diabetic kidney disease, in ameliorating the progression of diabetic nephropathy, and in preventing obesity-related kidney diseases. An ACE inhibitor and/or ARB should be used concomitantly to reduce urinary protein losses.

LIPIDS

Several lipid and biochemical abnormalities occur in nephrotic syndrome (Table 8-3). In the patient without nephrosis, the same abnormalities are associated with accelerated atherosclerosis. Although it is not documented that nephrotic patients are definitively at increased risk for developing accelerated atherosclerosis, this is most likely the case and hence, suggests therapy.

One hallmark of nephrotic syndrome is hyperlipidemia, characterized by high serum levels of total cholesterol and triglycerides, mostly in the LDL, very–low-density lipoprotein (VLDL), and intermediate-density lipoprotein (IDL) fractions. Clearances of triglycerides, VLDL, and IDL are decreased because of (i) reduced lipoprotein lipase (the enzyme responsible for the metabolism of lipoproteins) on the vascular endothelium in the setting of hypoalbuminemia; and (ii) a proteinuria-induced alteration in the structure of the lipoproteins. Thus, reducing proteinuria would be expected to reduce the levels of these lipoproteins, independently of the effect on albumin concentration. LDL synthesis is increased but does not correlate with serum albumin levels, suggesting that LDL synthesis is not driven by a general increase in protein synthesis in the liver. The high-density lipoprotein (HDL) cholesterol levels are either unaffected or are reduced, leading to an increased ratio of LDL/HDL cholesterol. In addition, maturation of HDL is impaired through alterations in apolipoprotein levels, resulting in smaller HDL moieties that contain more oxidized lipids and are more atherogenic. Similar changes in HDL structure are present even at low levels of albuminuria but can worsen with progressive proteinuria.

Plasma lipoprotein(a) [Lp(a)] levels also are increased in patients with nephrotic syndrome. The concentration of plasma

Lp(a) is genetically determined in patients without kidney disease and largely depends on the specific isoform of the apolipoprotein(a) moiety synthesized by the liver. In patients with nephrotic syndrome, plasma Lp(a) levels are increased, including different isoforms plus higher plasma fibrinogen levels, because of increased hepatic synthesis. The increased levels of both proteins are associated with atherosclerosis. As with lipids, the plasma Lp(a) and fibrinogen levels decrease when the degree of proteinuria abates.

In experimental animals with kidney disease, elevated lipid levels alone can induce severe and progressive renal injury, and reducing plasma lipid levels favorably alters the course of the renal damage. The effect of hyperlipidemia on the progression of CKD in humans is much less certain. But the dyslipidemia associated with the nephrotic syndrome should predispose to cardiovascular disease even if they change CKD progression only minimally. Therefore, it should be treated. In addition, there is evidence that disordered lipid metabolism can initiate or cause progressive kidney disease. Hereditary lecithin cholesterol acyl transferase (LCAT) deficiency may be linked to progressive mesangial and glomerular sclerosis. Patients with lipoprotein glomerulopathy, presumably from an inherited abnormality in apolipoprotein E, develop nephrotic syndrome, progressive CKD, and glomerular lipoprotein thrombi. All elements of the metabolic syndrome, hypercholesterolemia, hypertriglyceridemia, and low HDL cholesterol level function as independent risk factors for the progression of kidney disease in diabetic patients; the same factors represent risk factors for developing microalbuminuria. Several small observational clinical studies reveal that treating nephrotic patients with a cholesterol-lowering agent (a 3-hydroxy-3-methyl-glutaryl-coenzyme A [HMG CoA] reductase inhibitor or statin] can reduce urinary protein excretion along with increasing serum albumin levels; there was no benefit on serum creatinine levels. For example, 43 nephrotic patients randomly assigned to therapy with or without fluvastatin were examined. After 1 year, there was a significant decrease in total cholesterol, LDL, and triglyceride levels associated with fluvastatin therapy. With fluvastatin, urinary protein excretion decreased, serum albumin levels increased, and creatinine clearance was higher. There also was improvement in the kidney biopsy with less interstitial fibrosis and significantly less fat but no difference in the degree of glomerular sclerosis. Another strategy is to use apheresis to selectively remove LDL and Lp(a) levels. This was associated with an increase in serum albumin and reduced proteinuria. Even though comparisons were prospective, only small numbers of patients were studied, and the testing was not randomly assigned or blinded. The studies were also too brief for a meaningful assessment of the effects of treating hyperlipidemia on ultimate renal outcome (death or dialysis). Still, a reduction in urinary protein excretion is a reasonable surrogate for an improved outcome, and apparently reducing lipoproteins does reduce proteinuria. Finally, another strategy would be to reduce lipid peroxidation; this is suggested by the finding of high glomerular levels of lipid peroxidation products in patients with congenital nephrotic syndrome of the Finnish type. These levels were associated with down-regulation of antioxidant systems in the kidney. In conclusion, reversing changes in plasma lipid levels and their biochemical composition can help nephrotic patients to reduce the risk for cardiovascular disease and potentially to retard the progression of renal injury. Consequently, efforts should be made to reduce high plasma lipid levels, both by nutritional and by pharmacologic means, in patients with the nephrotic syndrome. Protein restriction and supplementation with vegetarian proteins can improve the plasma lipid profile in both animal models and humans with the nephrotic syndrome. These results suggest that patients with the nephrotic syndrome and an elevated LDL cholesterol and reduced HDL cholesterol should be treated to improve plasma lipids. There is insufficient evidence to provide lipid-lowering drugs to patients with nephrotic syndrome and a normal lipid profile.

As with varying protein intake, the types of lipids ingested may be important because lipids include compounds such as prostaglandins (PGs) and leukotrienes (important regulators of vascular resistance). Polyunsaturated fatty acids (PUFAs), which are not synthesized by mammals but are available only via dietary means, are metabolized to PGs and leukotrienes. For this reason, supplementing the diet with specific PUFAs could change the levels and activity of important vasoactive compounds. Another source of specific lipids is those derived from marine sources and hence is rich in ω-3 PUFAs (e.g., eicosapentaenoic acid). In contrast, vegetable oils are rich in ω-6 PUFAs and are metabolized to produce other lipids (e.g., arachidonic acid). The metabolism and function of different classes of lipids are complicated and depend not only on enzyme activities but also the dietary composition of lipids because they are the precursors of vasoactive lipids. For this reason, dietary plans should include the impact of lipids provided. For example, dietary addition of specific PUFAs can alter the course of renal injury and reduce blood lipid levels in experimental animals. But in human studies, benefits and results have not been so easily demonstrated. Compared with results of a vegetarian soy diet, there was no additional beneficial effect on either proteinuria or blood lipid levels in nephrotic patients who were treated by adding low doses of fish oil (5 g per day) to the vegetarian soy diet,. Higher doses of fish oil (15 g per day) added to an unrestricted diet led to a decrease in plasma levels of total triglycerides and LDL triglycerides along with an increase in LDL-cholesterol levels. This is relevant because fish oil showed early promise in reducing progression and proteinuria in patients with IgA nephropathy. Unfortunately, subsequent studies have had more equivocal results. Possibly, varying fatty acid composition in fish oil preparations and an improved influence on dose might improve treatment outcomes. Finally, young children with congenital or persistent nephrotic syndrome may be at risk for developing essential fatty acid deficiency. This occurs because there are losses of albumin-bound fatty acids with the nephrotic syndrome.

Recommendations

Dietary fat restriction can at least partially reduce blood lipid levels in patients with nephrotic syndrome. Diets low in fat (<30% of total calories) and cholesterol (<200 mg per day) but rich in polyunsaturated fatty acids and in linoleic acid (10% of energy) can reduce blood lipid levels (Table 8-2).

If serum total cholesterol remains high (>200 mg/dL) despite restriction of dietary lipids plus attempts to minimize urinary protein excretion, then statin therapy should be instituted. In addition to lowering blood lipid levels, statins may reduce cardiovascular events and proteinuria while retarding progressive renal injury. Providing a supplement of high-dose fish oil of at least 12 g per day may be beneficial for patients with IgA nephropathy (Table 8-2).

ANTIOXIDANTS

Experimentally, the nephrotic syndrome can be associated with an imbalance in oxidation-reduction, resulting in oxidative stress and activation of cytokines and mediators of inflammation. Oxidative stress in turn is implicated in the development and acceleration of cardiovascular disease it may contribute to progressive renal injury. Specifically, oxidative stress increases with oxidized lipoproteins, which can cause atherosclerosis and possibly progressive kidney disease via direct damage glycation to glomeruli and the interstitium. Glucose can oxidize proteins via the Amadori reaction or through reactions with advanced glycation end products (AGEs). In nondiabetic patients, AGEs are derived from exogenous sources such as foods cooked at high temperatures (e.g., the browning of barbecued or broiled meats) and possibly during oxidative stress and the lipid peroxidation. Experimentally, rats fed a diet low in AGEs had less proteinuria and suppressed loss of kidney function plus reduced interstitial fibrosis and macrophage infiltration in the kidneys as well as lower levels of monocyte chemoattractant protein-1, oxidative stress markers and glomerular basement membrane glycation. In patients with the nephrotic syndrome, the utility of dietary restriction of AGEs is not known. In nephrotic patients, antioxidant levels of selenium, vitamin E, vitamin C, and L-carnitine are normal to low; the significance of these levels is unknown. Interestingly, albumin has powerful antioxidant properties, likely related to an ability to scavenge free oxygen radicals. Therefore, a low serum albumin level because of the nephrotic syndrome could contribute to problems caused by oxidative stress. This is relevant because proteinuria is associated with altered endothelial function and decreased vascular reactivity, possibly because of increased oxidative stress and decreased production of endothelial derived nitric oxide. Moreover, reducing lipid levels or administering dietary antioxidants (selenium, vitamin E, and L-carnitine) can reduce proteinuria and albumin levels in animal studies. To date, these benefits have not been demonstrated in nephrotic patients.

Recommendations

Because benefits have not been proven in humans, supplementation with antioxidants such as selenium, vitamin E, vitamin C, and L-carnitine is not recommended. But the finding that albumin has antioxidant properties suggests that strategies for reducing proteinuria in nephrotic syndrome could prove to be beneficial.

SALT AND WATER

Edema formation is one of the most bothersome symptoms of the nephrotic syndrome. It results from pathologic retention of salt and water. The classic model of this edema formation includes a lower plasma albumin concentration as the stimulus causing fluid shift from plasma to the interstitium because albumin losses cause the difference between the interstitial and plasma oncotic pressures. Ultimately, there is a contraction of the plasma volume. Edema occurs when the amount of fluid entering the interstitium exceeds maximal lymph flow, further decreasing circulatory volume. Contraction of the plasma volume activates the RAAS causing sodium retention by the kidney. Contraction of the plasma volume also stimulates vasopressin release causing water retention and hyponatremia. The understanding of the mechanism of edema formation in nephrotic syndrome has changed recently. It has been shown that a low oncotic pressure is a less common mechanism for edema formation, occurring only when serum albumin is <1.5 to 2.0 g/dL. Dietary sodium restriction and strategies for correcting hypoalbuminemia is important in managing edema in nephrotic patients. The second and more important mechanism causing edema formation is a reduction in the ability of nephrotic patients to excrete a sodium load even when there is plasma volume expansion or administration of atrial natriuretic peptide (ANP). Experimentally, the problem appears to be intrinsic to the nephrotic kidney rather than changes in circulating blood volume. The reduced ability of the proteinuric kidney to excrete sodium leads to salt retention and edema. Consequently, the effective plasma volume may not be reduced. Restriction of dietary sodium chloride plus diuretics is effective in treating edema because the defect is in the kidney. In nephrotic patients, a low protein diet may increase the production of natriuretic peptide, which is frequently low. Whether the response of natriuretic peptide translates into a direct effect on avid renal sodium and water retention is undecided. Excess dietary sodium may contribute directly to renal injury via stimulation of intraglomerular capillary pressure, transforming growth factor-β (TGF-β) levels, and reactive oxygen species in the kidney. Amelioration of any of the above proposed mechanisms through dietary sodium restriction can reduce the proteinuria of hypertensive patients and diabetic patients with microalbuminuria.

Recommendations

A low-sodium (less than 2 g per day) diet is recommended. Patients with hyponatremia should be restricted to less than 1 L of fluid per day. Concomitant diuretic use is usually necessary.

VITAMIN D

Reduced levels of total and ionized calcium levels in plasma are common in nephrotic patients, while parathyroid hormone (PTH) levels are often elevated. Vitamin D−binding protein, a member of the albumin supergene family, is lost in the urine of patients with nephrotic syndrome and may contribute to the loss of vitamin D metabolites. Whether the synthesis of vitamin D–binding protein increases in response to urinary losses or is modulated by changes in dietary protein is unknown. Plasma levels of 25-hydroxyvitamin D [25(OH)D] and 1,25-dihydroxyvitamin D [1,25(OH)$_2$D] are reduced and correlate inversely with the degree of urinary albumin excretion, but only 25(OH)D levels correlate directly with plasma albumin concentration. A reasonable mechanism for the low 25(OH)D levels may be through urinary loss of vitamin D-binding protein, as levels may rise promptly with clinical remission of nephrotic syndrome. However, patients may continue to have low 1,25(OH)$_2$D levels even after remission of the nephrotic syndrome. Animal data suggest that 1,25(OH)$_2$D deficiency in the nephrotic syndrome may be multifactorial. Administering 25(OH)D$_3$ orally to nephrotic rats increased serum 1,25(OH)$_2$D levels, suggesting a lack of substrate as the underlying mechanism. Furthermore, a decrease in 1-α-hydroxylase activity and a blunted response of cyclic AMP to PTH were found in the kidney, perhaps because of impaired proximal tubular function.

Hypovitaminosis D may have important clinical implications because recent evaluations of patients undergoing dialysis and CKD patients indicate there is an inverse association between 25(OH)D levels and cardiovascular risk. Interpretation of such data is complicated, however, by the measurements being made because total 1,25(OH)$_2$D can be reduced while the plasma level of "free" or unbound vitamin D is normal. The evidence for a functional insufficiency of vitamin D in nephrotic patients is that serum PTH levels are often increased in relation to ionized calcium and vitamin D levels. Hypovitaminosis D and hypocalcemia can cause rickets when severe and reduce bone density in milder cases, especially in children who may receive treatment with high dose glucocorticoids. Fortunately, oral calcium and vitamin D supplements for children can ameliorate the decrease in bone density.

Recommendations

If the serum calcium level is low in a nephrotic patient, the plasma levels of 25(OH)D, 1,25(OH)$_2$D, and intact PTH should be measured. The patient with a low level of 1,25(OH)$_2$D should have it supplemented. If the 25(OH)D level is low, the patient should be treated with United States Pharmacopoeia (USP) vitamin D because 25(OH)D is not available commercially. In addition, these patients should receive oral calcium supplements provided serum phosphorus levels are normal. Based on the reports that vitamin D deficiency is associated with increased mortality, a level of 25(OH)D <47 nM should prompt treatment with vitamin D supplementation. If plasma-intact PTH level is high despite normal vitamin D levels, treatment should be initiated with 1,25(OH)$_2$D and calcium. An alternative approach is to treat all nephrotic patients receiving high-dose steroids with oral vitamin D and calcium supplements. The response to 500 units of oral vitamin D may not be optimal, however, and plasma levels should be monitored. It is also important to maintain the dietary calcium intake at 1200–1500 mg per day.

IRON

Urinary losses of iron and transferrin are increased by the nephrotic syndrome, but anemia in these patients is more likely to result from decreased erythropoietin rather than iron deficiency. For this reason, iron supplements are recommended only when there is unequivocal iron deficiency. This is recommended because filtered transferrin releases iron in the renal tubule especially when the urine pH is below 6 and inorganic iron can contribute to renal injury and interstitial fibrosis by generating oxygen free radicals. The cause for erythropoietin deficiency in nephrotic patients is thought to be marked urinary losses of erythropoietin, although decreased synthesis of erythropoietin can also occur.

Recommendations

Anemia associated with the nephrotic syndrome should prompt measurement of iron stores, and iron should not be administered unless absolute iron deficiency is documented. Concomitant erythropoietin administration may be necessary to correct the anemia. Because erythropoietin is excreted in the urine, the dose required for correcting anemia may be high. Additional information is needed to define the safety and efficacy of iron and erythropoietin-stimulating agents in nephrotic patients with normal renal function and anemia.

ZINC AND COPPER

The most important circulating zinc-binding protein is albumin, so losses of urinary zinc can be substantial in nephrotic patients. Zinc deficiency, however, probably arises from both reduced absorption and urinary losses of zinc. The effect of proteinuria on zinc metabolism has been largely ignored, and the extent to which zinc depletion plays a role in the clinical manifestations of nephrotic syndrome is not known.

Copper, like iron, is bound to circulating ceruloplasmin, and hence, the urinary copper losses correlate with proteinuria. Results from studies of animals or humans suggest that copper metabolism is normal in patients who do not express ceruloplasmin, suggesting that ceruloplasmin may not be essential for copper transport or metabolism. Unfortunately, this complicates recommendations for therapy because urinary loss of ceruloplasmin may cause a decrease in blood copper levels; the clinical importance of this loss is unknown.

Recommendations

If zinc deficiency is documented, oral replacement is indicated.

CONCLUSION

In summary, the loss of protein in the urine of patients with nephrotic syndrome could directly or indirectly cause abnormalities in nutritional status, acceleration of atherosclerosis, and progressive renal injury. There also can be losses of several ions, trace elements, and vitamins. Because a high protein diet increases urinary protein losses, maneuvers including dietary

Table 8-4.   Beneficial effects of dietary restrictions on the expression of nephrotic syndrome

Type of Restriction	Effects
Protein	Reduces proteinuria
	Increases serum albumin levels
	Decreases hyperfiltration
	Decreases tubular exposure to complement, iron, other toxins
	Retards the rate of progression of renal disease
Lipid	Decreases tubular exposure to oxidized lipids
	Decreases risk for atherosclerosis
	Retards the rate of progression of renal disease
Sodium	Reduces edema
	Optimizes diuretic effect
	Reduces proteinuria
	Improves blood pressure control
	May retard the progression of renal disease
Water	Corrects hyponatremia

manipulation and other methods of decreasing urinary protein losses are critical for the management of nephrotic CKD patients. We recommend a mild restriction of dietary protein to 0.8–1.0 g/kg/day plus the addition of a soy vegetarian diet. As in all manipulations of the diet, compliance should be monitored by frequent measurements of urinary urea nitrogen and an estimation of protein intake. There also should be restriction of fat intake to <30% of calories along with an increase in the proportion of polyunsaturated fatty acids. Unless contraindicated, ACE inhibitors, ARBs, or both, are mainstays of therapy. The patient should be instructed in how to achieve dietary sodium restriction because salt restriction and diuretic use are crucial for the treatment of edema. There may be additional benefit from the use of aldosterone antagonists in ameliorating the proteinuria and interstitial fibrosis. Trace elements and vitamins are frequently lost in the urine, but the contribution of these losses to the clinical manifestations of nephrotic syndrome is not established. There are potentially harmful effects of replacing ions and vitamins (e.g., iron), so we do not recommend routine supplementation with iron and vitamins. However, if a specific deficit is documented, it should be replaced. Supplements of calcium and vitamin D are reasonable for patients receiving repeated courses of high-dose glucocorticoids to counteract loss of bone density.

The principal effects of dietary manipulation in nephrotic syndrome are summarized in Table 8-4. These concepts are particularly important for pediatric patients because growth in children with steroid-resistant nephrotic syndrome seems to depend on the preservation of kidney function, the cumulative dose of steroids, and the severity of hypoalbuminemia.

Nonvegetarian High-quality Protein

DAY 1

Breakfast

2 waffles, plain (4 tbsp fat-free Cool Whip, 1/2 cup frozen
strawberries)
1/2 cup low-fat yogurt, plain
6 oz apple juice

Lunch

1 chicken-salad sandwich (2 oz chicken salad, 1 tbsp
mayonnaise, 2 slices whole wheat bread)
1 cup romaine lettuce, shredded (2 tbsp oil-and-vinegar
dressing)
1 blueberry muffin
1 cup 1% milk

Dinner

3 oz. lean roast beef (cooked with 1/8 tsp salt)
1/2 cup mashed potatoes (1 tsp margarine)
1/2 cup broccoli, seasoned
2 dinner rolls (2 tsp margarine)
1 orange
1 cup tea/coffee (2 tsp sugar)

DAY 2

Breakfast

1/4 cup Egg Beaters (1 tsp vegetable oil)
1 cup oatmeal (2 tsp sugar)
1 slice whole wheat toast (1 tsp jelly)
1 cup 1% milk

Lunch

1 tuna sandwich (2 oz tuna, 1 tsp mayonnaise, 2 slices whole
wheat bread)
4 carrot sticks
1 apple
4 graham crackers
1 cup tea/coffee (2 tsp sugar)

Dinner

3 oz baked chicken, seasoned (cooked with 1/8 tsp salt)
1/2 cup rice
1/2 cup boiled cabbage
1/2 cup corn
1/12 angel-food cake
6 oz grape juice

Strict Vegetarian Soy Diet

DAY 1

Breakfast

2 oz tofu scramble
1 cup oatmeal (2 tsp sugar)
1/2 English muffin (2 tsp jelly)
1 medium orange
1 cup soy milk

Lunch

1 tempeh burger (soy product, 1/4 cup tempeh, 1 hamburger bun, 1 tbsp mayonnaise)
1/2 cup baked beans, homemade (1/2 tsp salt)
1/2 cup applesauce
1 cup grape juice

Dinner

8 oz soy spaghetti
2 oz soy cheese
4 oz fruit salad
1 medium baked potato (1 tbsp margarine)
Tea/coffee (nondairy creamer, 2 tsp sugar)

DAY 2

Breakfast

1/2 cup soy sausage
2 pancakes (4 tbsp syrup)
1/2 cup applesauce
6 oz orange juice

Lunch

3 oz soy bologna (2 slices whole wheat bread, 1 tbsp mayonnaise)
1/2 cup corn
1/2 cup carrot/raisin salad (2 tsp mayonnaise, 1 tsp sour cream substitute)

Dinner

6 oz tofu stir-fry
1 cup mixed vegetables (1/2 cup broccoli, 1/2 cup cauliflower, 1 tsp oil, 1/8 tsp salt)
1/2 cup stewed potatoes (1/8 tsp salt)
1 cup soy milk
2 oatmeal raisin cookies

Soy Products

Breakfast

Soy milk (8 oz)
Protein = 7 g
Fat = 5 g
Na = 40 mg
Carbohydrate = 5 g
Tempeh (soy bacon)
Soy sausage (per serving)
Protein = 9 g
Fat = 0 g
Na = 240 mg
Carbohydrate = 8 g
Soy pancake mix
Tofu scramble

Lunch

Soy bologna (per serving)
Protein = 14 g
Fat = 0 g
Na = 335 mg
Carbohydrate = 8 g

Dinner

Tofu stir fry (3 oz.)
Protein = 5 g
Fat = 1 g
Na = 70 mg
Carbohydrate = 19 g

Selected Readings

Azadbakht L, Atabak S, Esmaillzadeh A. Soy protein intake, cardiore-
   nal indices, and C-reactive protein in type 2 diabetes with nephropathy. Diabetes Care 2008;31:648–654.

Bak M, Serdaroglu E, Guclu R. Prophylactic calcium and vitamin D
   treatments in steroid-treated children with nephrotic syndrome.
   Pediatr Nephrol 2006;21:350–354.

Bovio G, Piazza V, Ronchi A, et al. Trace element levels in adult
   patients with proteinuria. Minerva Gastroenterol Dietol 2007;53:
   329–336.

Castellino P, Cataliotti A. Changes of protein kinetics in nephrotic
   patients. Curr Opin Clin Nutr Metab Care 2002;5:51–54.

Chauveau P, Combe C, Rigalleau V, et al. Restricted protein diet is
   associated with decrease in proteinuria: consequences on the progression of renal failure. J Renal Nutr 2007;17:250–257.

De Mello VDF, Zelmanovitz T, Perassolo MS, et al. Withdrawal of
   red meat from the usual diet reduces albuminuria and improves
   serum fatty acid profile in type 2 diabetes patients with macroalbuminuria. Am J Clin Nutr 2006;83:1032–1038.

Dusol B, Iovanna C, Raccah D, et al. A randomized trial of low-protein
   diet in type 1 and type 2 diabetes mellitus patients with incipient
   and overt nephropathy. J Renal Nutr 2005;15:398–406.

Feng JX, Hou FF, Liang M, et al. Restricted intake of dietary advanced glycation end products retards renal progression in the remnant kidney model. Kidney Int 2007;71:901–911.

Kim SW, Frokiaer J, Nielsen S. Pathogenesis of oedema in nephrotic
   syndrome: role of epithelial sodium channel. Nephrology 2007;
   12(Suppl 3):S8–S10.

Kronenberg F. Dyslipidemia and nephrotic syndrome: recent ad-
   vances. J Ren Nutr 2005;15:195–203.

Nakao N. Yoshimura A, Morita H, et al. Combination treatment of
   angiotensin-II receptor blocker and angiotensin-converting enzyme
   inhibitor in non-diabetic renal disease (COOPERATE): a randomized controlled trial. Lancet 2003;361:117–124.

Newman JW, Kaysen GA, Hammock BD, et al. Proteinuria increases
   oxylipid concentrations in VLDL and HDL but not LDL particles
   in the rat. J Lipid Res 2007;48:1792–1800.

Remuzzi G, Benigni A, Remuzzi A. Mechanism of progression and
   regression of renal lesions of chronic nephropathies and diabetes.
   J Clin Invest 2006;116:288–296.

Teixeira SR, Tappenden KA, Carson LA, et al. Isolated soy protein
   consumption reduces urinary albumin excretion and improves the
   serum lipid profile in men with type 2 diabetes mellitus and
   nephropathy. J Nutr 2004;134:1874–1880.

Vaziri ND. Erythropoietin and transferrin metabolism in nephrotic
   syndrome. Am J Kidney Dis 2001;38:1–8.

9

Nutritional Intervention in Progressive Chronic Kidney Disease

Denis Fouque and Fitsum Guebre-Egziabher

Lipids and carbohydrates are completely processed or stored in the body so protein and its nitrogen derivatives are the most important food-derived compounds handled by the kidney. At equilibrium, every gram of nitrogen from the diet is absorbed and rapidly eliminated into the urine. This property allows easy monitoring of protein intake by measuring excreted nitrogen (or urea) in urine. In healthy adults, increasing protein intake is associated with a concomitant increase in nitrogen output, whereas a diet with inadequate protein is associated with a markedly reduced urinary urea nitrogen output. This adaptive ability is limited because the body has obligatory daily nitrogen losses that are not influenced by protein intake, for example, nitrogen losses in feces, perspiration, hair, and nails. In patients with kidney disease, this loss has been estimated to be approximately 0.031 mg nitrogen per kg of body weight.

Protein requirements are estimated by standard methods, such as nitrogen balance or labeled *amino acid turnover*. These methods can characterize body nitrogen metabolism and the optimal level of protein intake for healthy adults and patients with chronic kidney disease (CKD). From these data, safe diets are devised for patients with varying levels of kidney disease.

Protein intake influences the degree of proteinuria (Fig. 9-1). Because proteinuria has been identified as one of the most important and independent risk factors for CKD progression, every attempt to lower proteinuria to minimal levels seems worthwhile. We will address the potential influence of protein intake on kidney function, the optimal dietary protein for patients with CKD who have various levels of kidney function, the ways to monitor such diets, the potential side effects, and the results of large clinical trials and meta-analyses of low-protein dietary interventions on the course of CKD.

PROTEIN METABOLISM AND KIDNEY DISEASE

Overnutrition is associated with altered renal hemodynamics, particularly when there is a high level of protein or amino acid intake. Whether lipids or carbohydrates directly affect kidney function or disease is unclear, but there is ample evidence that a high protein intake will acutely increase glomerular filtration rate (GFR) and urinary albumin excretion. With long-term dietary restriction, protein intake also influences the degree of glomerulosclerosis. By contrast, reducing the protein load may stop or even induce remission in the progression of experimental renal scarring. Several mechanisms or compounds have been proposed to explain these alterations, including glucagon, insulin, insulin-

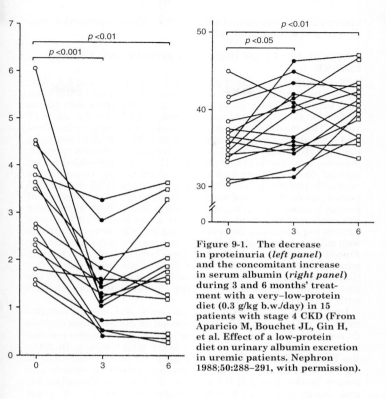

Figure 9-1. The decrease in proteinuria (*left panel*) and the concomitant increase in serum albumin (*right panel*) during 3 and 6 months' treatment with a very–low-protein diet (0.3 g/kg b.w./day) in 15 patients with stage 4 CKD (From Aparicio M, Bouchet JL, Gin H, et al. Effect of a low-protein diet on urinary albumin excretion in uremic patients. Nephron 1988;50:288–291, with permission).

like growth factor-1, angiotension II, prostaglandins, and kinins. Sodium retention may also be associated with protein-induced hyperfiltration via activity of the proximal, sodium–amino acid cotransporter. Protein restriction ablates hemodynamic changes related to 5/6 nephrectomy because it reduces glomerular pressure and flow.

Glomerular protein trafficking induces hypermetabolism and oxidant stress, while a low-protein diet (LPD) reduces oxygen consumption and malondialdehyde production. The nature of protein absorbed may also influence the renal response because the GFR of vegetarians is reportedly lower than that of omnivores. When rats with CKD were fed casein or soy proteins, proteinuria and histologic renal damage were always more severe compared with results in rats fed protein of animal origin.

Levels of growth factors and profibrotic agents, such as transforming growth factor (TGF)-beta, fibronectin, and plasminogen activator inhibitor-1 (PAI-1) are modulated by an LPD, resulting in reduced proteinuria and kidney injury. Finally, albuminuria per se possesses pathogenic effects promoting tubulointerstitial scar and apoptosis, and LPD can independently decrease glomerular capillary pressure and albuminuria, adding a protective anti-fibrotic and antiapoptotic effect.

OPTIMAL LEVEL OF DIETARY PROTEIN AND ENERGY INTAKE

A Western diet contains approximately 1.4 g protein/kg b.w./day; women have a daily protein intake that is 35% to 50% lower than men because of their lower body weight, and aging also affects protein intake; it is spontaneously reduced 15% by the age of 70 years. The mean optimal protein intake, according to the Food and Agriculture Organization (FAO) in 1985, is 0.50 g protein/kg b.w./day. To ensure that 97.5% of individuals maintain nitrogen balance, two standard deviations of the mean are added for an optimal daily intake to 0.75 g protein/kg b.w./day. To correct for vegetable protein (less absorption by a factor of 10%), the optimal protein intake was raised to 0.8 g protein/kg b.w./day. More recent research using sophisticated measurements of protein turnover has confirmed these values. There is a Gaussian distribution of protein requirements, however, explaining why some patients do well with protein intakes below the average recommended values. Finally, the protein requirements have been estimated in healthy adults or in patients with kidney disease who were receiving a controlled energy intake of at least 35 kcal/kg b.w./day, and the diet may not be applicable to healthy adults or patients with CKD with a reduced energy intake.

Interestingly, the basal metabolic rate and energy requirements in patients with CKD who are not on maintenance dialysis do not differ from those in healthy adults, and nitrogen balance is obtained when a protein intake is 0.6 g/kg b.w./day. In 2000, the Kidney Disease Outcomes Quality Initiatives (K/DOQI) of the National Kidney Foundation recommended that protein and energy intake should be 0.6 g protein/kg b.w./day (Guideline 24) and energy intake, 35 kcal/kg b.w./day for patients <60 years with CKD and 30 to 35 kcal/kg b.w./day for patients >60 with CKD (Guideline 25). These recommendations change when maintanence dialysis treatment is initiated. However, there are spontaneous reductions in energy and protein intake when kidney function decreases leading to intake values as low as 21 kcal and 0.85 g protein/kg b.w./day in patients with stage 3 CKD (estimated GFR <30 mL per minute). Notably, for an equal amount of protein, a diet with 70% of protein from vegetable sources enables a greater amount of calories to be consumed than a diet consisting of 70% of its protein from animal sources. Because energy intake may decrease when kidney function falls, a defect in protein metabolism may occur with an inadequate dietary energy intake. Obviously, patients with CKD will need instruction in methods for achieving an optimal, moderately low protein intake and adequate energy intake.

METABOLIC CONSEQUENCES OF REDUCED PROTEIN INTAKE IN CHRONIC KIDNEY DISEASE

Nature of Protein Restricted Diets

Healthy adults or patients with CKD have been shown to adapt to a dietary protein intake as low as 0.3 g protein/kg b.w./day, if energy and essential amino acid (EAA) requirements are met. To avoid nutritional deficits, supplements of EAA or ketoacids (KA) of amino acids have been suggested; the ketoacids are synthesized into the corresponding EAAs. Without these supplements, intakes as low as 0.6 g protein/kg b.w./day can be safely used if at least 50% of the protein is of high biologic value (e.g., principally from animal sources) and energy intake meets the recommended goal (i.e., 35 kcal/kg b.w./day for patients younger than 65 years and 30 to 35 kcal/kg b.w./day for those >65 years). If lower levels of protein intake are prescribed, supplements (EAA or KA) should be considered to avoid inducing an EAA deficit. The potential benefits are that low dietary protein intake can slow the progression of CKD and alleviate uremic symptoms and postpone the start of maintenance dialysis or prolong survival when dialysis opportunities are limited.

Adaptation to Protein Metabolism

An adaptive response (i.e., a decrease in whole body leucine flux and oxidation) occurs in patients with stage 3 to 4 CKD who had a 40% reduction in their dietary protein intake (i.e., from 1.1 to 0.7 g/kg/day) during a period of 3 months; body composition is maintained. This adaptive response was also observed with a more restricted protein intake (0.35 g/kg/day supplemented with KA) treated over an extended period of 16 months. The adaptation has also been observed in patients with CKD with nephrotic syndrome when their protein intake was reduced from 1.85 to 1.0 g protein/kg/day. The LPD was even more beneficial in nephrotic patients with CKD who were tested while their intake was reduced from 1.20 to 0.66 g protein/kg/day; amino acid metabolism improved, and there was strong reduction in proteinuria leading to increased serum albumin concentrations. Thus, with adequate energy supply, patients with CKD correctly adapt their protein metabolism.

Glucose Metabolism

Insulin resistance is common during the course of CKD, and glycemic control can improve with attention to nutrition. After 3 months of an LPD, insulin sensitivity improved and there was reduced fasting serum insulin or daily insulin needs and blood glucose values and endogenous glucose production. The mechanisms for these benefits are unclear, but the results are encouraging.

Control of Chronic Kidney Disease—Mineral and Bone Disorders

Because proteins of animal origin are strongly associated with phosphates (1 g protein approximately contains 13 mg of phosphorus), limiting dietary protein intake reduces the phosphate intake and hence the amount that must be excreted. With calcium salts of KA as a supplement, there also is extra calcium. Both low phosphate intake and calcium supplements reduce serum parathormone (PTH) levels and improve renal osteodystrophy, and this has been shown during 12 months of an LPD supplemented with KA. Given the recent reports regarding the adverse effects of excessive calcium intake in patients with advanced

CKD, use of calcium containing KA supplements must be used with caution.

Improvement in Lipid Profile

The reduced protein intake of animal origin (e.g., meat and dairy products) generally entails a decrease in saturated lipids, leading to an improvement in the overall serum lipid profile. For example, reducing protein intake for 3 months from 1.1 to 0.7 g/kg/day resulted in an increase in serum lipoprotein AI and in the Apo-AI/Apo-B ratio, changes considered to reduce the cardiovascular risk in general population. Likewise, a 6-month LPD regimen improved decreased red cell malondialdehyde and increasing polyunsaturated fatty acids, particularly C22:4 and C22:5, thereby limiting oxidative stress.

Reduction in Proteinuria and Amelioration of Kidney Injury

Lowering dietary protein intake induces a decrease in proteinuria (see Fig. 9-1). Because proteinuria is now identified as an independent risk factor for progression of CKD, every attempt to reverse proteinuria is worthwhile. Whether reducing protein intake will protect the kidney from progressive injury in humans is less clear. First, experimental studies used diets with extreme differences in protein intake. Obviously, the clinical use of these diets does not permit this much variation. Second, protein in food is associated with other factors such as phosphorus, sodium, energy, and water that could affect kidney function. Third, a single intervention can be studied experimentally, but in clinical practice, patients generally receive several nephroprotective interventions that may mask the true effect of the diet as a single intervention. Besides angiotensin-converting enzyme (ACE) inhibitors, AT1 receptor blockers, or both, an LPD might confer additional protection against progression of kidney disease and may potentuially postpone end-stage renal disease (ESRD).

Hypocaloric Risk

Without adequate counseling, too few calories may be contained in the protein-restricted diet. With adequate supervision, however, energy intakes are usually greater than 30 kcal/kg/day, and body composition is unchanged during long-term LPD therapy. However, clinical trials have led to the conclusion that even at fairly low energy intake, long-term nutritional status, as measured by dual-energy x-ray absorptiometry (DEXA) or anthropometry, does not reveal significant changes. Furthermore, patients treated with LPD for years had a survival rate during maintenance dialysis similar to that achieved by other therapies.

MONITORING NUTRITIONAL INTAKE

Protein intake can be estimated from two sources: (i) intake from dietary reports; and (ii) output from urinary urea excretion in patients without ESRD, or protein nitrogen appearance (PNA), formerly called protein catabolic rate (PCR). Two formulas are routinely used to assess nitrogen (N) and thus protein intake in CKD:

Table 9-1.   Estimation of dietary protein intake based on a daily urinary nitrogen appearance in a stable, 80-kg adult patient prescribed with a 0.6 g protein/kg/day diet

Patient's UNA = 5.2 g/day and protein is 16% nitrogen
(Nitrogen intake × 6.25 protein intake)

Eq 1:   UNA + 0.031 × 80 kg = 5.2 + 2.48 = 7.68 g N
        DPI = 7.68 g × 6.25 = 48 g; thus, DPI/kg = 48 g/80 kg
        = 0.60 g/kg b.w./day

Or

Eq 2:   1.2 × UNA + 1.74 = 6.24 + 1.74 = 7.98 g N
        DPI = 7.98 × 6.25 = 49.9 g; thus, DPI /kg = 49.9/80
        = 0.62 g/kg b.w./day

Protein intake <20% more than prescribed intake, is considered acceptable (i.e., a UNA = 6.3 g per day for this patient).
DPI, dietary protein intake; UNA, urinary nitrogen appearance.
From Masud T, Manatunga A, Cotsonis G, et al. The precision of estimating protein intake of patients with chronic renal failure. Kidney Int 2002;62: 1750–1756, with permission.

Eq 1:   N intake (g/day) = UNA (g/day) + 0.031 × b.w. (kg)
Eq 2:   N intake (g/day) = 1.20 × UNA (g/day) + 1.74
where b.w. is the patient's edema-free body weight (Table 9-1).

Adherence to an LPD is defined by an intake equal to ±20% of prescribed intake. In well-controlled studies, protein intake tends to be greater than the prescribed amount by 10% to 20%, with 40% to 70% of patients meeting the required intakes. Thus, repeated efforts are needed to support the nutritional care of patients with CKD.

Energy expenditure can be reliably assessed through indirect calorimetry, the Harris–Benedict formula, or physical activity questionnaires. The optimal energy intake is 35 kcal/kg/day and 30 to 35 kcal/kg/day in patients older than 60 years, but energy intake can only be deduced from dietary interviews or records. We estimate that at least four interviews are necessary to ensure an understanding by the patient of the goals and requirements of an LPD and an optimal energy intake as well as how an adequate home food record should be kept. The K/DOQI guidelines recommend that at least one dietetic interview be performed every 3 to 4 months. A general system for patient follow-up is proposed in Table 9-2.

EVIDENCE FOR AN OPTIMAL PROTEIN INTAKE FOR PATIENTS WITH PROGRESSIVE CHRONIC KIDNEY DISEASE

Numerous trials have tried to assess the relationship between the level of protein intake and the potential deleterious or protective effects on the kidney. Some concessions have to be made when interpreting the findings of these trials.

Table 9-2. Nutritional follow-up and dietary counseling in patients with chronic kidney disease before end-stage renal disease

Time Span	To Do	Result
Every month for 4 months; then every 3–4 months	Dietary interview	Develop a care plan; tailor diet to patient taste and economic situation
	Home 3-day food record	Record energy intake; verify adequate understanding of diet and adherence from urinary urea
	24-hour urinary urea	Estimate protein intake
Every 3 months	Body weight, anthropometry (optional), subjective global assessment (optional) Serum albumin, serum prealbumin, serum cholesterol C-reactive protein	

If GFR is <15 mL/minute, the nutritional survey should be more frequent, particularly if a superimposed disease occurs; consider starting dialysis treatment if follow-up does not show improvement in nutritional status or laboratory markers.

Assessing Kidney Tissue Damage and Estimating Kidney Function

A major caveat for quantifying renal damage in humans is that repeated histologic analyses are not available. In addition, serial measures of kidney function over time are difficult because of the interaction between kidney function markers (e.g., serum creatinine, 1/serum creatinine, urinary creatinine clearance, or formula-derived creatinine clearance) and protein intake. Indeed, variations in dietary protein intake with changes in creatine and creatinine intake can interfere with estimates of kidney function. Serum creatinine and creatinine clearance can also be affected by several medications, such as cimetidine, interfering with tubular excretion of creatinine. Third, and more importantly, a large change in dietary protein index (DPI) can acutely change GFR. Reducing DPI may initially lower GFR by 10% to 20% until a new equilibrium is reached. Consequently, a delay of 3 to 4 months is mandatory before an effect of protein intake on changes in GFR can be identified as a benefit on progression of kidney failure.

Methodological Caveats

An important aspect of clinical research relies on the methodological quality, design, and reports of trials. Several criteria now exist for rating trials, generating evidence, and producing clinical guidance: evidence level A is obtained from the best-quality, large, randomized, and controlled trials (RCT) and meta-analyses (grades 1 or 2). Evidence level B is from prospective controlled clinical trials (CCT) (grade 3), and evidence level C, the lowest ranking, is information acquired from retrospective trials, case reports, or expert opinion (grades 4 and 5). We extensively searched the literature published since 1974 and excluded more than 50 low-quality studies (too small in size or uncontrolled), leaving only nine randomized, controlled trials and four meta-analyses that are suitable for evaluating the influence on dietary protein and changes in kidney function.

Results of Major Randomized Clinical Trials and Meta-analyses

Randomized Clinical Trials

Rosman et al. studied the influence of protein restriction in 247 patients over 2 or 4 years. Protein intake was 0.90 to 0.95 g/kg/day in patients whose GFR was between 60 and 30 mL/minute and was reduced to 0.70 to 0.80 g/kg/day in patients whose GFR was between 30 and 10 mL/minute; protein intake for the control groups was not restricted. After 2 years of the restricted diets, the loss of GFR was significantly slowed. Patients with polycystic kidney disease did not improve with a restricted diet. After 4 years, a marked improvement in survival was observed in patients treated with the more restricted protein intake (survival without proceeding to dialysis was 60% for the dietary protein-restricted group but only 30% for the dietary protein unrestricted patients, $p < 0.025$). Adherence to the LPDs was very good after a short period of training and was sustained over time. Notably, dietary protein restriction did not cause malnutrition.

Ihle et al. studied 72 patients with advanced kidney disease for 18 months. The patients were randomized to a protein-unrestricted control diet or 0.4 g protein/kg/day. Actual protein intake, estimated from urinary urea, was 0.8 or 0.6 g/kg/day. The GFR (^{51}Cr-ethylenediaminetetra-acetate [^{51}Cr-EDTA]) decreased only in the control group eating unrestricted diets. There was no decrease in the GFR of the LPD group. The number of patients who started dialysis during the trial was significantly greater in patients with an uncontrolled diet ($p < 0.005$). Body composition varied, with a loss of body weight in the LPD group but no change in other anthropometric measures or in serum albumin levels occurred in either group. No food records were published, so an insufficient energy intake cannot be ruled out to explain the weight loss in those eating the LPD. The authors concluded that moderate reduction in protein intake exerts a beneficial effect.

Williams et al. studied the three different interventions in 95 patients with stage 4–5 CKD over 18 months. Patients were randomly assigned to receive a diet of 0.6 g protein/kg/day and 800 mg phosphate (LPD group), a diet of 1000 mg phosphate/day plus phosphate binders but no specific dietary protein restriction (low-phosphate group), or a diet with no protein or phosphate restriction. Dietary adherence, estimated both by urinary urea output and diet recalls, averaged 0.7, 1.02, and 1.14 g protein/kg b.w./day and 815, 1000, and 1400 mg phosphorus per day, respectively. Slight weight losses were observed in the protein- and phosphate-restricted groups (-1.3 and -1.65 kg for the LPD and low-phosphate group, respectively). No difference was observed in any of the three groups in the rate of decrease in creatinine clearance over time. Death or the commencement of dialysis therapy did not differ among the three groups. Both the small size of the study and the GFR estimation by creatinine clearance greatly limit the value of this study.

The Northern Italian Cooperative Study Group carried out a randomized controlled study of 456 patients with GFRs <60 mL/minute during 2 years of follow-up. Patients were prescribed 1 g/kg/day (control group) or 0.6 g/kg/day (LPD), and both diets provided at least 30 kcal/kg/day. The main outcome tested was "renal survival," defined as beginning dialysis or doubling of the serum creatinine. The control group ate 0.90 g protein/kg/day, and the low-protein group ate 0.78 g/kg/day with a large overlap between groups. Only a borderline difference existed between control and LPD groups, with slightly fewer patients in the LPD group reaching a renal endpoint ($p = 0.059$).

Malvy et al. examined a diet with more severe protein restriction (0.3 g protein/kg/day) plus a supplement of KAs (Ketosteril [Fresenius Kabi, Bad Homburg, Germany], 0.17 g/kg/day) and compared results from patients eating 0.65 g protein/kg/day. Fifty patients with severe kidney disease (creatinine clearance ≤20 mL/minute) were followed until dialysis or until creatinine clearance was <5 mL/minute/1.73 m^2. Renal survival between diets did not differ, but the small number of patients prevents any valid conclusions. For patients with the most advanced disease at inclusion (GFR of 15 mL/minute/1.73 m^2), the "half-life" for renal death was 9 months in those prescribed 0.65 g protein/kg/day; it was 21 months in those treated with the most restricted diet. There was a loss of 2.7 kg over 3 years in the group assigned to the very–low-protein diet; the loss was equally from fat and lean body mass; no weight loss or body composition change occurred with those assigned to the 0.65 g protein/kg diet.

Mirescu et al. assessed a more severe protein restriction (0.3 g protein/kg/day) diet supplemented with ketoacids (Ketosteril, 1 capsule/5 kg/b.w./day) and compared results with those from patients assigned to 0.60 g protein/kg/day; 53 nondiabetic patients with stage IV CKD with moderate proteinuria were studied. The supplemented, very–low-protein diet (SVLPD) was associated with an increase in serum bicarbonate and serum calcium and a reduction in blood urea nitrogen (BUN) and serum phosphate. Although there was no change in kidney function over time (estimated GFR), after 48 weeks, there were significantly fewer patients entering dialysis in the SVLPD group (4%) compared with the LPD group (27%) ($p = 0.01$).

Cianciaruso et al. reported a larger study (423 patients with stage 4–5 CKD) who received either a 0.8 or a 0.55 g protein/kg/day diet for 18 months. Actual protein intakes estimated from urinary nitrogen were 0.92 versus 0.72 g protein/kg/day, respectively. There were 9 renal deaths in the 212 patients in the dietary protein restricted group versus 13 in the 211 patients assigned to the 0.8 g/kg/day group (p = NS). Most metabolic parameters and/or medications were improved with the lower protein intake group.

The MDRD study tested the effects of low protein intake and strict blood pressure control on the progression of kidney disease in more than 800 patients separated into two groups: Study A, GFR: 25 to 55 mL/minute/1.73 m^2 of body surface area and Study B, GFR: 13 to 24 mL/minute/1.73 m^2 of body surface area. In Study A, patients received 1 g protein/kg/day or more and were treated to a mean blood pressure of 105 mm Hg. The low-protein patients received 0.6 g protein/kg/day and a mean blood pressure of 92 mm Hg. In Study B, patients received 0.6 g protein/kg/day or 0.3 g protein/kg/day, plus a KA supplement and were treated to blood pressure goals comparable to those in Study A. The loss of GFR was estimated by the slope of ^{125}I-iothalamate clearance was measured over 2 years. The mean follow-up was only 2.2 years, and actual protein intakes were 1.11 g protein/kg/day versus 0.73 g protein/kg/day in Study A (n = 585), and 0.69 versus 0.46 g protein/kg/day in Study B (n = 255). No difference was observed in GFR decline between groups in Study A. There was a somewhat faster decline in GFR in the group prescribed the 0.60 g protein/ kg b.w./day diet as compared with the 0.46 g/kg/ day plus KA group of Study B (p = 0.07).

At first glance, these results were disappointing, but some caveats should be emphasized. During the first 4 months in Study A, a sharp decrease in GFR was observed in the group with the more restricted protein intake (0.73 g/kg/day). This difference was attributed to the physiologic reduction in glomerular hemodynamics that follows protein restriction. Subsequently, there was a slower decrease in GFR compared with results from the group eating the higher protein intake (1.11 g/kg/day). If the initial hemodynamic effect is eliminated, (i.e., from 4 months after the start until 3 years), the slope of GFR decrease was significantly lower in the patients assigned to more restricted protein group; renal survival also improved (p = 0.009). Secondly, the actual rate of progression of renal failure was lower than expected from the pilot study, and patients were randomly treated with ACE inhibitors (subsequently shown to influence progression of CKD). These factors increase the number of patients needed to test the study outcomes. For example, in the Diabetes Control and Complications Trial of the effects of strict blood glucose control, no renal benefit was detected at 2 years, but a protection from microalbuminuria or proteinuria was observed only after 4 years in patients with strict blood glucose control.

Secondary analyses of the MDRD, although less robust, are of interest. When the outcome of patients was analyzed according to actual protein intake, there was a strong relation between actual protein intake and the decline in GFR (p = 0.011) or the number of renal deaths (p = 0.001). Indeed, for every reduction of 0.2 g protein/kg/day of intake, a 1.15 mL/minute/year reduction was observed in GFR decline and a 49% reduction in renal death. These analyses support the conclusion that there is a moderate beneficial effect of reduced protein intakes in patients with CKD.

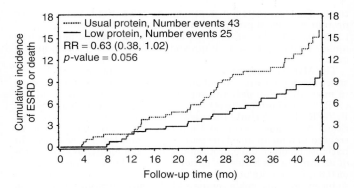

Figure 9-2.   Occurrence of renal failure or death in Study A of the Modification of Diet in Renal Disease Study including a 10-month additional follow-up after completion of the study (p = 0.056 between the two levels of protein intake). (From Levey AS, Greene T, Beck GJ, et al. Dietary protein restriction and the progression of chronic renal disease: what have all of the results of the MDRD study shown? Modification of Diet in Renal Disease Study Group. J Am Soc Nephrol 1999;10:2426–2439, with permission).

Meta-analyses

To clarify issues about trial design and numbers of patients, a series of meta-analyses have been performed. The criterion analyzed was renal death (i.e., the occurrence of death, the need to start dialysis, or a GFR decrease during the course of the study). Literature published since 1974 was examined, and to reduce biases and for robustness of conclusions, only randomized controlled trials were included in the final analysis. Results of "renal deaths" appear in Figure 9-2. The odds ratios (i.e., a treatment effect estimate between treated and control group) and the overall pooled analysis from the selected trials are shown in Figure 9-3. Among more than 1400 patients (753 in LPD groups and 741 in control or larger protein intake groups), a 39% reduction in renal death (p <0.006) was seen for patients consuming a lower protein diet. When using a meta-analysis to address the effect of LPDs on GFR, Kasiske et al. reported that in more than 1900 patients, a beneficial effect for patients with lower protein intake spared 0.53 mL/minute/year of GFR (p <0.05). The number needed to treat (NNT) among patients with an LPD to prevent 1 renal death per year was estimated to be 18, a number that compares favorably with the well-accepted mortality reductions that is observed with treatment with statin drugs in the 4S trial (NNT = 30) and the WOSCOPS study (NNT = 111).

The case for protein restriction in patients with diabetes is somewhat less clear. Indeed, most clinical trials are of shorter duration, during which renal death cannot be taken into account. Furthermore, they address surrogate criteria such as reductions in microalbuminuria, proteinuria, and creatinine clearance. In

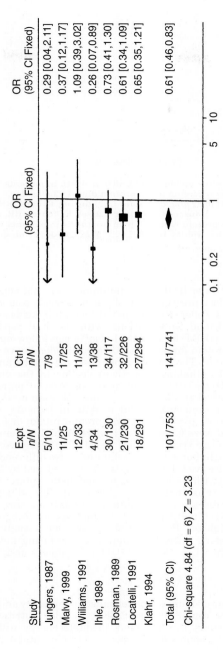

Study	Expt *n*/*N*	Ctrl *n*/*N*	OR (95% CI Fixed)	OR (95% CI Fixed)
Jungers, 1987	5/10	7/9		0.29 [0.04,2.11]
Malvy, 1999	11/25	17/25		0.37 [0.12,1.17]
Wiiliams, 1991	12/33	11/32		1.09 [0.39,3.02]
Ihle, 1989	4/34	13/38		0.26 [0.07,0.89]
Rosman, 1989	30/130	34/117		0.73 [0.41,1.30]
Locatelli, 1991	21/230	32/226		0.61 [0.34,1.09]
Klahr, 1994	18/291	27/294		0.65 [0.35,1.21]
Total (95% CI)	101/753	141/741		0.61 [0.46,0.83]

Chi-square 4.84 (df = 6) Z = 3.23

Figure 9-3.   Meta-analysis of the results of low-protein diets in patients with CKD. A *square* denotes the odds ratio (treatment/control) for each trial, and the *diamond* indicates the overall results of the seven trials combined. 95% confidence intervals are represented by *horizontal lines*. Overall "common" odds ratio = 0.61 (95% CI: 0.46, 0.83), *p* = 0.006. (From Fouque D, Laville M, Boissel JP. Low protein diets for chronic kidney disease in non diabetic adults. Cochrane Database Syst Rev 2006;(2):CD001892, with permission).

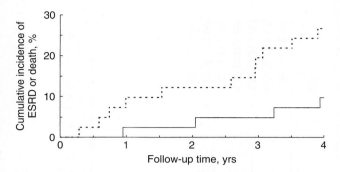

Figure 9-4. **Cumulative incidence of ESRD or death in patients with type 1 diabetes receiving usual protein diet (1.02 g/kg/day, *dashed line*) or LPD (0.89 g/kg/day, *solid line*) during 4 years; p = 0.042, log rank (From Hansen HP, Tauber–Lassen E, Jensen BR, et al. Effect of dietary protein restriction on prognosis in patients with diabetic nephropathy. Kidney Int 2002;62:220–228, with permission).**

addition, in many older trials, ACE inhibitors were not equally distributed, and blood pressure control was not strictly comparable between groups. Zeller et al. compared 1 g protein/kg/day versus 0.6 g protein/kg/day in 36 patients with insulin-dependent diabetes mellitus (IDDM) for at least 1 year (mean follow-up, 35 months). Actual protein intake was 1.08 g protein/kg/day versus 0.72 g protein/kg/day. The investigators observed a substantial reduction in GFR (iothalamate method) decline in the group treated with a LPD ($p < 0.02$) but only in the subgroup of patients with a GFR greater than 45 mL per minute. Hansen et al. reported the longest randomized trial to date in patients with IDDM. Patients were given their usual protein intake or 0.6 g protein/kg/day and were followed for 4 years. Actual protein intake during the entire trial duration was 1.02 g/kg/day versus 0.89 g/kg/day, a slight but significant difference. No difference in proteinuria was observed, but renal death was reduced by 36% in patients treated with moderately restricted dietary protein, as seen in Figure 9-4. Cox analysis was performed after adjusting for cardiovascular disease, and the difference was even more significant ($p = 0.01$). Finally, in the meta-analysis of a subgroup of patients with diabetes, Pedrini et al. showed that a combined criterion of increasing microalbuminuria and reducing kidney function was improved by 44% ($p < 0.001$) in subjects assigned to a LPD.

CONCLUSION

Patients with impaired kidney function must have dietary adjustments to avoid the complications of CKD. Regular nutritional surveys are mandatory to verify that adequate energy will be provided and to recommend changes in protein intake that evolves during different stages of kidney disease. There is convincing evidence that during CKD stages 3 and 4 (i.e., for a GFR between 60 and 15 mL/minute), protein intake should be reduced from a typical Western diet to 0.6 to 0.8 g/kg/day. The diet must be tailored to meet individual requirements, adherence, and body composition by regular support and education of nutritional principals and dietary advice.

Selected Readings

Bernhard J, Beaufrere B, Laville M, et al. Adaptive response to a low-protein diet in predialysis chronic renal failure patients. J Am Soc Nephrol 2001;12:1249–1254.

Cianciaruso B, Pota A, Pisani A, et al. Metabolic effects of two low protein diets in chronic kidney disease stage 4–5: a randomized controlled trial. Nephrol Dial Transplant 2008;23:636–644.

de Zeeuw D, Remuzzi G, Parving HH, et al. Proteinuria, a target for renoprotection in patients with type 2 diabetic nephropathy: lessons from RENAAL. Kidney Int 2004;65:2309–2320.

Fouque D, Laville M, Boissel JP, et al. Controlled low protein diets in chronic renal insufficiency: meta-analysis. Br Med J 1992;304: 216–220.

Fouque D, Laville M, Boissel JP. Low protein diets for chronic kidney disease in non diabetic adults. Cochrane Database Syst Rev 2006; (2):CD001892.

Gansevoort RT, de Zeeuw D, de Jong PE. Additive antiproteinuric effect of ACE inhibition and a low-protein diet in human renal disease. Nephrol Dial Transplant 1995;10:497–504.

Goodship TH, Mitch WE, Hoerr RA, et al. Adaptation to low-protein diets in renal failure: leucine turnover and nitrogen balance. J Am Soc Nephrol 1990;1:66–75.

Ikizler TA, Greene JH, Wingard RL, et al. Spontaneous dietary protein intake during progression of chronic renal failure. J Am Soc Nephrol 1995;6:1386–1391.

Kasiske BL, Lakatua JD, Ma JZ, et al. A meta-analysis of the effects of dietary protein restriction on the rate of decline in renal function. Am J Kidney Dis 1998;31:954–961.

Klahr S, Levey AS, Beck GJ, et al. Modification of Diet in Renal Disease Study Group. The effects of dietary protein restriction and blood-pressure control on the progression of chronic renal disease. N Engl J Med 1994;330:877–884.

Kopple JD, Greene T, Chumlea WC, et al. Relationship between nutritional status and the glomerular filtration rate: results from the MDRD study. Kidney Int 2000;57:1688–1703.

Levey AS, Greene T, Beck GJ, et al. Dietary protein restriction and the progression of chronic renal disease: what have all of the results of the MDRD study shown? Modification of Diet in Renal Disease Study Group. J Am Soc Nephrol 1999;10:2426–2439.

Masud T, Manatunga A, Cotsonis G, et al. The precision of estimating protein intake of patients with chronic renal failure. Kidney Int 2002;62:1750–1756.

Peters H, Border WA, Noble NA. Angiotensin II blockade and low-protein diet produce additive therapeutic effects in experimental glomerulonephritis. Kidney Int 2000;57:1493–1501.

Peuchant E, Delmas-Beauvieux MC, Dubourg L, et al. Antioxidant effects of a supplemented very low protein diet in chronic renal failure. Free Radic Biol Med 1997;22:313–320.

Rand WM, Pellett PL, Young VR. Meta-analysis of nitrogen balance studies for estimating protein requirements in healthy adults. Am J Clin Nutr 2003;77:109–127.

Rigalleau V, Blanchetier V, Combe C, et al. A low-protein diet improves insulin sensitivity of endogenous glucose production in pre-dialytic uremic patients. Am J Clin Nutr 1997;65:1512–1516.

Vendrely B, Chauveau P, Barthe N, et al. Nutrition in hemodialysis patients previously on a supplemented very low protein diet. Kidney Int 2003;63:1491–1498.

Trace Elements and Vitamins

Joel D. Kopple

TRACE ELEMENTS

Overview

The body burden and tissue concentrations of many trace elements are altered in chronic kidney disease (CKD) and kidney failure. Various factors contribute to these alterations: many trace elements are excreted primarily by the kidney, and with renal failure they may accumulate. Secondly, elements such as iron, zinc, and copper, which are protein bound, may be lost in excessive quantities with urinary protein losses as in the nephrotic syndrome. Excessive uptake or losses of trace elements may also occur during dialysis therapy depending on their relative concentrations in plasma and dialysate and the degree of binding to protein or red cells. Hemodialysis of copper, strontium, zinc, and lead should be minimal because they are largely bound to plasma proteins or red cells. Table 10-1 shows commonly recognized abnormalities in trace elements in patients with chronic renal failure.

Hemodialysis or hemodiafiltration (MHD) may remove some trace elements if the dialysate concentrations are sufficiently low (e.g., bromide, iodine, lithium, rubidium, cesium, and zinc). Because many trace elements are bound avidly to serum proteins, they may be taken up by blood against a concentration gradient when present in even small quantities in dialysate. In fact, therapeutic doses of trace elements may be administered through dialysis, as has been done for zinc. These observations provide part of the rationale for the intensive purification of dialysate used for maintenance dialysis patients. Besides changes in removal, inhalation could result in increased intake of certain trace elements as may occur in people exposed to certain industrial processes, fertilizers, insecticides, herbicides, or burning of fossil fuels.

Protein-energy wasting can be associated with lowered serum concentrations of proteins that bind trace elements to decrease the serum levels of elements including zinc, manganese, and nickel. Occupational exposure or pica can increase the burden of some trace elements. The effect of the altered dietary intake of the patient with CKD on body pools of trace elements is unknown. Oral and, for maintenance dialysis patients, intravenous iron supplements are commonly provided for patients with renal failure.

Assessment of the trace element burden in patients with renal failure is often difficult because the serum concentrations of binding proteins may be decreased, thereby lowering serum trace element levels, or the binding characteristics of these proteins may be altered in renal failure as well. Also, red cell concentrations of trace elements may not reflect levels in other tissues. In general,

Table 10-1. Commonly recognized abnormalities in trace elements and vitamins in patients with chronic renal failure*

Micronutrient	Effect of Chronic Renal Failure†
Zinc	Serum‡↓-N; RBC↑; leukocyte↓ in CRF and HD; N in CPD
Selenium	Serum↓ in CRF, HD, and CPD
Iron	Serum↓-N; tissue↓ in CRF, HD, and CPD
Aluminum	Serum N-↑ in CRF; serum and tissue↑ in HD and CPD
Copper	Serum N-↑ in CRF and HD, N in CPD; RBC↓-N
Thiamin	Serum↓-N in CRF, HD, and CPD
Riboflavin	Serum↓-N in CRF, HD, and CPD
Pyridoxine	Serum↓-N in CRF, HD, and CPD; RBC↓ in CRF and HD
Cobalamin	Serum↑ in CRF; serum N in HD and CPD
Folic acid	Serum↓-N and RBC N-↑ in CRF, HD, and CPD
Ascorbic acid	Serum↓-N in CRF, HD, and CPD
Vitamin A	Serum↑ in CRF, HD, and CPD
Vitamin E	Serum↓-N-↑ in CRF, HD, and CPD; RBC↓ in HD and CPD

*Refers to persons with CRF who are not receiving trace element or vitamin supplements.
†Serum levels of many trace elements and vitamins may be reduced in the nephrotic syndrome because of increased urinary losses and low serum levels of binding proteins.
‡Values ascribed to serum refer to serum or plasma.
↓, decreased compared to normal values; ↑, increased compared with normal values; CPD, chronic peritoneal dialysis; CRF, chronic renal failure; HD, maintenance hemodialysis;.
N, not different from normal values; RBC, erythrocytes.

supplements of trace elements should be undertaken with caution, because impaired urinary excretion and the poor dialysance of trace elements, because of protein binding, increases the risk of overdosage. Dietary requirements for trace elements have not been defined for patients with CKD because of the difficulties in conducting the studies to determine nutritional requirements plus the problems of identifying sensitive and reliable methods of determining deficiency of trace elements.

Iron

Iron deficiency is common, particularly in patients receiving hemodialysis (Table 10-2). Because intestinal iron absorption can be impaired, because there are often blood losses from the intestinal tract and from blood drawing, and because blood may be sequestered in the hemodialyzer, iron deficiency is occurs frequently. Also, iron may bind to the dialyzer membrane while the erythropoietin-induced rise in hemoglobin concentrations may deplete the body's iron supply. Not only do iron requirements increase during the time between initiation of erythropoietin therapy and

Table 10-2.   Factors leading to iron deficiency in patients with chronic renal failure or patients receiving maintenance dialysis

- Increased demand for iron during erythropoiesis stimulated by rhEPO
- Decreased iron uptake by intestinal mucosal cells
- Gastrointestinal tract blood loss which may be clinically apparent or occult
- Massive proteinuria
- Blood retention in hemodialyzer and blood lines at end of hemodialysis
- Blood drawing for testing
- Accidental blood loss from vascular access tubing, grafts, and fistulae
- Menstruation

rhEPO, recombinant human erythropoietin.

the rise in hemoglobin but also higher serum iron levels are associated with a greater response to erythropoietin. Some researchers recommend that, in general, patients undergoing MHD or chronic peritoneal dialysis (CPD) should maintain serum transferrin saturation (TSAT) at 30% to 50% and serum ferritin at about 400 to 800 ng/mL.

Although some patients receiving maintenance dialysis can maintain these iron values with oral iron supplements, many patients will require parenteral iron therapy. Oral ferrous sulfate, 300 mg three times per day, one-half hour after meals should be tried, but some patients will develop anorexia, nausea, constipation, or abdominal pain; these individuals sometimes will tolerate other iron compound, including ferrous fumarate, gluconate, or lactate. The levels sought include TSAT at 30% to 50% and serum ferritin levels of 400 to 800 ng/mL, and if these are not achieved with oral iron, the patient can be treated with intravenous iron (intramuscular injections cause pain and staining of skin, so intravenous iron, given as ferrous gluconate, ferrous sucrose, or iron dextran is generally the preferred method of administration). Iron dextran has a slightly greater risk of anaphylactic reactions, from 0.6% to 0.7%, and 31 deaths have been reported from anaphylactic reactions to iron dextran between 1976 and 1996 in the United States. Consequently, many physicians prefer to use other iron salts. Although rare, iron overload can be treated by simply halting intake or by removal using deferoxamine (see below) or by injections of erythropoietin along with repeated phlebotomy. Recommendations for iron therapy in patients receiving erythropoietin treatment are given in Chapter 11.

Aluminum

In patients with stage 5 CKD or those receiving maintenance dialysis, increased aluminum has been implicated as a cause of a progressive dementia syndrome (particularly in patients receiving MHD), osteomalacia, weakness of the proximal muscles of the limbs, impaired immune function, and anemia. Although contamination of dialysate with aluminum previously was the major source of aluminum toxicity, current methods of water treatment have removed virtually all aluminum from the dialysates. Instead, ingestion of aluminum binders of phosphate is probably the major cause of the excess burden of aluminum, and aluminum binders are now used sparingly if at all. Increased body burden and toxicity of iron or aluminum in patients receiving MHD or CAPD may be reduced simply by eliminating intake or by infusion of deferoxamine (a dialyzable chelator of divalent cations). Care must be taken with the latter method because deferoxamine can promote loss of iron as well as certain serious infections, particularly mucormycosis.

Zinc

Although the zinc content of most tissues is normal in patients with chronic renal failure (CRF), serum and hair zinc levels are reported to be low, but red cell zinc content is increased. Some reports indicate that dysgeusia (poor food intake) reduced peripheral nerve conduction velocities, abnormal serum cholesterol levels, low sperm counts, and impaired sexual function, and helper/suppressor T-cell (CD4/CD8) ratios may be improved in patients undergoing CKD and MHD by giving zinc supplements. Other studies have not confirmed these findings. Zinc deficiency in non-CKD persons is manifested by Beau lines (transverse horizontal grooves in the fingernails), discolored nail plates, paronychia, and impaired growth in children. Intestinal absorption of zinc is not affected by administration of 1,25-dihydroxycholecalciferol.

The dietary requirement for zinc in CKD and patients with end-stage kidney disease (ESKD), especially in patients receiving MHD, is unclear. In nondialyzed patients with CKD, the fractional urinary excretion of zinc is increased. But with a reduced glomerular filtration rate (GFR), urinary zinc excretion is decreased. There is the potential for fecal losses of zinc, and this can increase the dietary zinc to rise above the recommended dietary allowance (RDA). The problem in estimating zinc needs is compounded because the dietary zinc intake of many patients with CKD and patients undergoing MHD and CAPD is below the RDA for normal adults (i.e., 15 mg/day). It is probably both safe and clinically indicated to ensure that patients receiving CKD and MHD ingest this level of zinc. Unfortunately, zinc does not appear to be commercially available as a single supplement but can be found in some multivitamin preparations.

Selenium

Selenium is necessary for the selenium-dependent, glutathione peroxidases, and it participates in the defense against oxidative damage of tissues, an important problem for patients with renal failure. Selenium is largely protein-bound and binds to sulfur-containing amino acids as selenomethionine and selenocysteine.

The finding of low values of serum or plasma selenium in patients undergoing dialysis and in patients with CKD suggests there is a need for a supplement. Generally, these patients have low plasma or serum selenium levels; red cell selenium levels in patients with ESKD are conflicting. Impaired gastrointestinal absorption of selenium and selenium losses during dialysis are suggested as reasons for low serum selenium levels. Indeed, low selenium values can contribute to the reduced plasma glutathione reductase activity found for patients undergoing MHD. Whether these abnormalities cause clinical disorders in patients with CKD and/or patients undergoing MHD or CAPD is unknown. Selenium deficiency in adults without CKD can cause Keshan disease, which is associated with a cardiomyopathy. Interestingly, patients undergoing MHD who develop a cardiomyopathy have lower plasma and platelet selenium levels and low glutathione peroxidase activity as compared with patients undergoing MHD without cardiomyopathy. Low selenium levels in patients receiving MHD are associated with a decrease in the red cell and platelet half-lives plus an altered thyroid status. Selenium deficiency and toxicity syndromes have not been identified in patients with CKD or ESKD, so routine selenium supplementation is not recommended.

Copper
Many years ago, an epidemic of copper toxicity occurred because copper was being leached from dialysis equipment. Currently, patients with CKD and patients undergoing MHD are reported to have normal serum levels of copper and ceruloplasmin (although inflammation will elevate ceruloplasmin because it is an acute phase reactant). Nutritional deficiency of copper is rare or absent in patients with CKD or patients undergoing MHD, unless there is an enteropathy or a requirement for total parenteral nutrition that does not contain copper.

Other Trace Elements
Plasma or tissue levels of other trace elements reported to be altered by CKD or dialysis are shown in Table 10-3. Notably, the evidence for clinical nutritional deficiencies or excesses of these elements in patients with CKD or patients undergoing MHD is very limited and almost certainly occurs uncommonly.

VITAMINS
Overview
Individuals with CKD and particularly the patient receiving MHD who do not receive vitamin supplements will have a high incidence of vitamin deficiencies. Table 10-1 shows commonly recognized abnormalities in vitamins in patients with chronic renal failure. Deficiencies are because of several factors: first, 1,25-dihydroxycholecalciferol production by the diseased kidney is impaired; and second, vitamin intake is often decreased in patients with CKD and patients receiving MHD and CAPD because of anorexia and reduced food intake. Intercurrent illnesses, frequently present in patients with CKD and patients undergoing MHD also impair food intake. Many foods that are high in water-soluble vitamins are often restricted because of the elevated protein and potassium content of such foods. Specifically, diets prescribed for nondialyzed patients with CKD and patients undergoing MHD frequently contain less than the recommended daily allowances for certain water-soluble vitamins. For example,

Table 10-3. Summary of serum, plasma, or tissue concentrations of other trace elements in patients with chronic renal failure and patients undergoing maintenance dialysis and their possible clinical consequences

	CRF	HD	CPD	Dialysis Induced	Clinical Consequences*
Bromine	N	↓	↓	Yes	Altered sleep
Cadmium	Kidney↓ liver↑ Serum N-↑	Kidney↓ liver↑ Serum N-↑	N Serum N-↑		Growth retardation, hypertension, ↓ serum PTH
Chromium	N	↑	↑	Yes	Carcinogenic
Cobalt	N	↑	↑	?	?
Lead	↑	↑	↓-N	No	Hypertension, gastrointestinal and neurological diseases
Manganese	↓	↓-N	↓-N	No	Anemia, impaired glucose tolerance
Molybdenum	N	↑	?	?	Arthropathy
Nickel	↑	↑-N↓	?	Yes	Degeneration of heart muscle
Rubidium	N	↑-N↓	N	Yes	Depression, central nervous system disturbances
Silicon	↑	↑	↑	Yes	↑ serum Si protects against Al toxicity
Strontium	↑	↑↓	↑-↓	?	Osteomalacia
Tin	↓	?	?	?	
Vanadium	N	↑	?	No	Bone disease, hypoglycemia

*Adverse clinical effects that have been observed in the general population.
↓, decreased compared with normal; ↑, increased compared with normal; ?, unknown; CPD, chronic peritoneal dialysis; CRF, chronic renal failure; HD, maintenance hemodialysis; N, not different from normal; PTH, parathyroid hor

Table 10-4. Recommended daily supplemental vitamins for persons with chronic kidney disease and those undergoing maintenance hemodialysis or chronic peritoneal dialysis[*,†]

Vitamin	Stage 3–5 CKD[‡]	Maintenance Hemodialysis	Chronic Peritoneal Dialysis
Thiamine (mg/day)	1.2	1.2	1.2
Riboflavin (mg/day)	1.3	1.3	1.3
Pantothenic Acid (mg/day)	5	5	5
Niacin (mg/day)	16	16	16
Pyridoxine HCl (mg/day)[§]	5	10	10
Vitamin B_{12} (mcg/day)	2.4	2.4	2.4
Vitamin C (mg/day)	90	90	90
Folic Acid (mg/day)	1	1	1
Vitamin A	No addition	No addition	No addition
Vitamin D	See text	See text	See text
Vitamin E (mg/day)	15	15	15
Vitamin K	None	None	None

[*]These quantities are recommended in addition to the patient's daily intake of vitamins from foods ingested.

[†]The proposed supplemental daily vitamin intakes are based on the recommended daily requirements for normal adults. Because the recommended daily allowances may vary according to gender and age group in adults, the highest recommended level for nonpregnant, nonlactating adults was selected. Exceptions are made to this policy when evidence indicates that patients with CKD or patients receiving maintenance dialysis have an increased need or a decreased tolerance for a given vitamin.

[‡]CKD: patients with chronic kidney disease who are not receiving dialysis treatments.

[§]10 mg of pyridoxine HCl is 8.21 mg of free pyridoxine.

low levels of thiamine and, in some patients, thiamine and pyridoxine occur in patients with CKD who are prescribed low protein diets. Third, CKD appears to alter the absorption, metabolism, or activity of some vitamins. Animal studies indicate that intestinal absorption of riboflavin, folate, and vitamin D_3 are impaired in renal failure. In addition, the metabolism of folate and pyridoxine can be abnormal in patients with CKD. Fourth, certain medicines interfere with the intestinal absorption, metabolism, or actions of vitamins. Fifth, water-soluble vitamins are removed by dialysis, and the high-flux/high-efficiency hemodialysis procedures can remove great quantities of these water-soluble vitamins.

Vitamin deficiencies have also been observed for 1,25-dihydroxycholecalciferol, folic acid, vitamin B_6 (pyridoxine), vitamin C, and, to a lesser extent, other water-soluble vitamins. Because a substantial proportion of patients with stage 4 or 5 CKD and especially patients undergoing MHD appear to develop laboratory evidence for one or more vitamin deficiencies, a supplemental intake of multivitamins is recommended (Table 10-4). It is recommended that this multivitamin supplement be given in addition to the vitamins that are ingested with foods.

Vitamin B$_1$ (Thiamine)

Decreased plasma or red blood cell levels of thiamine have been reported in patients undergoing MHD who were not receiving vitamin supplements (not every study has confirmed this requirement). But there are syndromes in patients undergoing MHD that are suggestive of dementia or beriberi heart disease that have been found to improve when the patients were given large doses of thiamin. Because both syndromes can occur in patients undergoing MHD from other causes, an extensive investigation of the abnormality is required. Nonetheless, to essentially remove the possibility that symptomatic thiamine deficiency will occur in patients with stage 3–5 CKD or in patients undergoing MHD, a multivitamin supplement providing the recommended daily dose of thiamine is recommended (Table 10-4).

Vitamin B$_6$ (Pyridoxine HCl)

Many have found an abnormally high prevalence of low concentrations of vitamin B$_6$ in the plasma and red blood cell in subjects with advanced CKD or those undergoing MHD or CAPD. Activation coefficients of erythrocyte transaminase enzymes (i.e., the activity of the enzyme divided into the activity of the same enzyme after the vitamin B$_6$ cofactor pyridoxal-5-phosphate is added to the assay) are commonly elevated in patients undergoing MHD who are not receiving supplemental vitamin B$_6$. This is evidence that the subjects are deficient in vitamin B$_6$. Improvement in the activation coefficient during hemodialysis can occur, suggesting there might be an inhibitor of vitamin B6 in uremic sera that is removed by dialysis. Low stimulation ratios in mixed lymphocyte cultures are also reported in these patients undergoing MHD, and pyridoxine hydrochloride supplements can improve several parameters including lymphoblast formation. These observations suggest that vitamin B$_6$ deficiency, which is known to cause abnormal immunologic function, may be an important cause of the altered immune response in patients with stage 5 CKD or patients undergoing MHD. Interestingly, serum glutamate-oxaloacetate transaminase activity is also reduced in patients with renal failure, apparently related to vitamin B$_6$ activity, possibly from a uremic inhibitor in serum.

Treatment with large doses of folic acid and/or pyridoxine HCl (and sometimes with vitamin B$_{12}$) has been used to treat elevated plasma homocysteine levels. This is done because plasma homocysteine is increased in nondialyzed patients with CKD as well as patients receiving MHD and CAPD and renal transplant recipients. In addition, a high plasma homocysteine in the general population is a risk factor for adverse cardiovascular events including thrombosis of vascular access sites such as the arteriovenous fistulae. In patients undergoing MHD, the relation of an elevated plasma homocysteine to adverse outcome is less clear. A reverse risk factor pattern is thought to be related to the association of protein-energy wasting and/or inflammation to a low or normal plasma homocysteine level. Unfortunately, clinical trials in both the general population and in patients with CKD or patients undergoing MHD (i.e., the Veterans Administration HOST Study) have failed to show a survival benefit of vitamin treatment of hyperhomocysteinemic subjects, even though plasma or serum homocysteine levels were observed to decrease with the vitamin supplement. In the HOST study, over 2000 patients with stage 4, 5 CKD and patients undergoing MHD with hyperhomocysteinemia were randomized in a double-blind fashion to treatment with large doses of folic acid, pyridoxine HCl, and vitamin B_{12} or to placebo. The treatment group displayed a significant fall in serum homocysteine levels, but there was no reduction in cardiovascular or overall mortality. In clinical trials of subjects in the general population, adverse effects of megavitamin treatment of hyperhomocysteinemic patients occur occasionally. Consequently, treatment of hyperhomocysteinemia with large doses of pyridoxine HCl, folic acid (see below), or vitamin B_{12} is no longer recommended.

Plasma oxalate levels are elevated in patients with renal failure. The increase in plasma oxalate appears to be largely because of impaired urinary excretion. However, large doses of vitamin C (ascorbic acid), a precursor of oxalate, can increase oxalate production (see the subsequent text). Glyoxylate, a metabolic precursor of oxalate, may also be transaminated to form glycine, and this reaction is catalyzed by vitamin B_6. Vitamin B_6 deficiency also can increase urinary oxalate excretion in rats with experimental renal insufficiency as well as in normal adults. In patients with CKD, treatment with large doses of pyridoxine HCl can decrease plasma oxalate levels but not to normal values. Five milligrams per day of pyridoxine hydrochloride seems to produce a normal red cell erythrocyte glutamate-pyruvate transaminase activation index in nondialyzed, clinically stable patients with stage 5 CKD, and 10 mg per day of pyridoxine hydrochloride normalized this index in stable patients undergoing MHD as well as in nondialyzed patients with CRF with superimposed infections.

Vitamin C

In patients undergoing MHD, there are substantial losses of vitamin C into the dialysate. Hence, low plasma and leukocyte ascorbic acid concentrations can occur in patients receiving MHD who are not receiving supplemental vitamin C. Clinical signs suggestive of mild scurvy have been described in several patients undergoing MHD who have very low plasma ascorbic acid concentrations. Administration of ascorbic acid orally or into the dialysate can prevent negative vitamin C balance during hemodialysis.

Folate

Blood folate concentrations have been reported to be decreased in some patients undergoing MHD who did not take folic acid supplements. In addition, several investigators found hypersegmentation of polymorphonuclear leukocytes in such patients and reported that these abnormalities decreased with administration of folate supplements. In addition, the reticulocyte count and hematocrit can rise when patients undergoing MHD are given folic acid supplements. We have observed that serum folate concentrations are normal in virtually all patients undergoing MHD who received 1.0 mg per day of supplemental folic acid. Dietary folic acid requirements do increase in patients with stage 4 or 5

CKD when they commence erythropoietin therapy and undergo a major rise in their hemoglobin levels.

Folate also can improve abnormal vascular enthothelial function, a risk for factor for atherosclerosis risk in patients with ESKD. Folinic acid is reported to improve endothelium dependent-vasodilation in the forearm in patients with ESKD. As has been observed in the general population, the patient receiving MHD who is emotionally depressed can also have lower serum folate and red blood cell folate levels and lower serum cobalamin concentrations than nondepressed patients undergoing MHD. The response of depressed patient to the vitamin supplements is not established.

Vitamin B_{12}

Deficiency of vitamin B_{12} is uncommon in patients with CKD because the daily requirement for this vitamin is so small (e.g., 2.4 mcg/day for normal, nonpregnant, nonlactating adults). In addition, body stores of this vitamin are great, and little is removed during hemodialysis because vitamin B_{12} is protein-bound and hence, poorly dialyzed. There is a report of low serum vitamin B_{12} concentrations in 19 of 60 patients undergoing MHD; the serum vitamin B_{12} concentrations tended to fall progressively over months of dialysis treatment. More interestingly, serum vitamin B_{12} levels were directly correlated with nerve conduction velocities, which improved with ingestion of large quantities of vitamin B_{12}. Low serum vitamin B_{12} levels were also found in four patients receiving hemodialysis even though only one had an intestinal absorption defect for vitamin B_{12}. In these subjects, the hematocrit improved after receiving vitamin B_{12} injections. The explanation for these two discrepant reports of low serum vitamin B_{12} levels in patients undergoing MHD is not known, but it is important to recognize that the average age of maintenance dialysis patients is similar to the age at which pernicious anemia is most likely to occur.

Other Water-Soluble Vitamins

Despite the water solubility of riboflavin, thiamine, pantothenic acid, and biotin, plasma concentrations of these vitamins are usually not decreased in Patients undergoing MHD. It is possible that losses of these vitamins into hemodialysate are offset by their lack of urinary excretion. Low plasma niacin concentrations have been reported in some patients undergoing MHD, but other reports have not confirmed these findings in patients receiving 7.5 mg per day of supplemental nicotinic acid.

Fat-Soluble Vitamins

Serum retinol-binding protein and vitamin A are increased in patients with CRF, and an increase in liver vitamin A content may occur. Even relatively small supplements of vitamin A, i.e., 7500 to 15,000 IU/day (about 1500 to 3000 retinal equivalents or micrograms per day), are reported to be associated with bone toxicity and hypercalcemia in some individuals. In contrast, vitamin K deficiency is uncommon unless the patients do not eat foods containing vitamin K or are receiving antibiotics that suppress intestinal bacteria. In such patients, supplemental vitamin K is required to prevent deficiency of this vitamin.

Normal, low, and increased plasma or red cell vitamin E (alpha-tocopherol) levels have been described in nondialyzed patients with CKD or patients undergoing MHD. Vitamin E deficiency can cause oxidative injury to tissues, and several studies have indicated that administration of 1200 IU of vitamin E (all-racemic alpha-tocopherol acetate) to patients undergoing MHD may decrease oxidative stress. This conclusion was reached after formal testing that included measurements of the oxidative stress that is induced by 100 mg of iron sucrose. The antioxidant effect can be enhanced by administration of a combination of vitamin E and vitamin C. Treatment with vitamin E (α-tocopherol) is also reported to reduce progression of carotid artery stenosis in patients undergoing MHD. For example, there can be significantly less intima-media thickness in the common carotid artery, and there is an associated increase in brachial artery flow-mediated dilatation in patients with CKD who were treated with the HMGCoA reductase inhibitor, pravastatin. The latter was obtained when vitamin E and homocysteine reduction therapy were added over a period of 2 years. Conversely, in the general population, randomized, prospective placebo controlled clinical trials indicate that vitamins E, C, beta carotene, or combinations of these compounds do not significantly reduce total adverse cardiovascular events or cancer. Indeed, in the HOPE and HOPE-TOO trial, a moderate dose of vitamin E (400 IU), as compared with placebo, was associated with an increased risk of heart failure and hospitalization for heart failure. The reasons why discrepant responses occur in patients with advanced CKD (and patients undergoing MHD) compared with the general population is not known. It has been suggested that the greater oxidant stress of patients with CKD may enable them to benefit from vitamin E therapy.

Is There a Need for Routine Vitamin Supplements?

Some investigators suggest that patients undergoing MHD who do not receive vitamin supplementation can avoid developing signs of water-soluble vitamin deficiencies for months. These results suggest that vitamin supplements should not be prescribed routinely to patients receiving maintenance dialysis. This conclusion is supported by findings indicating the maintenance of normal plasma or blood cell levels of vitamins in patients undergoing MHD even though they did not receive supplements for periods of less than 1 year. Still, levels of water-soluble vitamins can fall to borderline low levels in several patients.

In patients undergoing CAPD, dietary intake of several vitamins, including vitamin A, vitamin C, vitamin B_1 (thiamine), vitamin B_6, vitamin B_{12}, and nicotinamide, is often lower than the recommended allowances for normal adults. Patients undergoing CAPD who are not receiving supplements can have a high incidence of low or normal plasma folate levels, low vitamin B_1, and low vitamin B_6 and vitamin C. Reduced plasma vitamin E has been reported in 13% of patients undergoing CAPD, whereas others found increased plasma vitamin E levels.

Overall, a low intake of several vitamins is still common in patients with renal failure, and many reports continue to show that substantial numbers of these patients show evidence for vitamin deficiencies. Because the water-soluble vitamin supplements are generally safe, I believe it is wise to recommend them routinely until these issues are more completely resolved. What is missing? The nutritional requirements for most vitamins are not well defined for patients with renal failure. Besides the vitamins present in foods, the following daily supplements of vitamins will prevent or correct vitamin deficiency: pyridoxine hydrochloride, 5 mg in nondialyzed patients with stage 3–5 CKD and 10 mg for patients receiving MHD or CAPD; folic acid, 1.0 mg; and for all other water-soluble vitamins, I recommend the daily allowance for normal nonpregnant, nonlactating adults. Because the recommended daily allowances may vary according to gender and age group in adults, the highest recommended level for nonpregnant, nonlactating adults should be selected. Based on the disappointing results arising from the treatment of hyperhomocysteinemia in patients with CKD and patients undergoing MHD, the large doses of vitamins B_6, vitamin B_{12}, and folic acid are not recommended. Of course, this negative recommendation does not apply to individuals who have the genetic forms of hyperhomocysteinemia, because this problem can be associated with severely elevated plasma homocysteine concentrations that might be treated with vitamins.

A supplement of vitamin C should be limited to only 60 mg per day (the recommended daily allowance) because ascorbic acid can be metabolized to oxalate. Large oral or intravenous doses of ascorbic acid have been associated with an increase in plasma oxalate and the risk of deposition on tissue of renal failure patients. Oxalate is highly insoluble. The concern about high plasma oxalate concentrations could lead to precipitation in the kidney, possibly causing further impairment in renal function in the nondialyzed patient with renal insufficiency.

Supplemental vitamin A is not recommended because serum levels are increased, and there is a high risk of vitamin A toxicity with even small supplements. Although some studies indicate that vitamin E supplements in patients undergoing MHD may be beneficial, it is still not certain that vitamin E supplements are necessary. Indeed, there are negative or adverse results resulting with vitamin E supplementation in the general population. Additional vitamin K is not needed unless the patient is not eating and receives antibiotics that suppress intestinal bacteria that synthesize vitamin K. Recommendations for vitamin D intake are given in Chapter 3.

Selected Readings

Anderson TJ, Sun YH, Hubacek J, et al. Effects of folinic acid on forearm blood flow in patients with end-stage renal disease. Nephrol Dial Transplant. 2006;21:1927–1933.

Antoniou LD, Shalhoub RJ, Sudhakar T, et al. Reversal of uremic impotence by zinc. Lancet 1977;2:895.

Blomfield J, McPherson J, George CRP. Active uptake of copper and zinc during hemodialysis. Br Med J 1969;2:141.

Blomfield J. Dialysis and lead absorption. Lancet 1973;2:666.

Boelaert JR, de Locht M, Van Cutsem J, et al. Mucormycosis during deferoxamine therapy as a siderophore-mediated infection—in vitro and in vivo animal studies. J Clin Invest 1993;91:1979.

Bovio G, Piazza V, Ronchi A, et al. Trace element levels in adult patients with proteinuria. Minerva Gastroenterol Dietol 2007;53: 329–336.

Cannata JB, Briggs JD, Junor BJR, et al. Aluminum hydroxide intake: real risk of aluminum toxicity. Br Med J 1983;286:1937.

Cartwright GE, Gubler CJ, Wintrobe MM. Studies on copper metabolism in the nephrotic syndrome. J Clin Invest 1954;33:685.

Chazot C, Kopple JD. Vitamin metabolism and requirements in renal disease and renal failure. In: Kopple JD, Massry SG, eds. Nutritional Management of Renal Disease. 2nd Ed, Baltimore: Lippincott Williams & Wilkins; 2004:315–356.

Clement L, Boylan M, Miller VG, et al. Serum levels of folate and cobalamin are lower in depressed than in nondepressed hemodialysis subjects. J Ren Nutr 2007;17:343–349.

Hsieh YY, Shen WS, Lee LY, et al. Long-term changes in trace elements in patients undergoing chronic hemodialysis. Biol Trace Elem Res 2006;109:115–121.

Jamison RL, Hartigan P, Kaufman JS, et al. Veterans Affairs Site Investigators. Effect of homocysteine lowering on mortality and vascular disease in advanced chronic kidney disease and end-stage renal disease: a randomized controlled trial. JAMA 2007;298: 1163–1170. Erratum. JAMA 2008;300:170. Comment: Am J Kidney Dis. 2008;51:549–553. JAMA 2007;298:1212–1214. JAMA 2008; 299:287–288; author reply 288.

Kalantar-Zadeh K, Kopple JD. Trace elements and vitamins in maintenance dialysis patients. Adv Renal Replace Ther 2003;10:170.

Kanakiriya S, De Chazal I, Nath KA, et al. Iodine toxicity treated with hemodialysis and continuous venovenous hemodiafiltration. Am Jour Kidney Dis 2003;41:702.

Kopple JD, Mercurio K, Blumenkrantz MJ, et al. Daily requirement for pyridoxine supplements in chronic renal failure. Kidney Int 1981;19:694–704.

Krachler M, Scharfetter H, Wirnsberger GH. Exchange of alkali trace elements in hemodialysis patients: a comparison with Na(+) and K(+). Nephron 1999;83:226.

Nanayakkara PW, van Guldener C, ter Wee PM, et al. Effect of a treatment strategy consisting of pravastatin, vitamin E, and homocysteine lowering on carotid intima-media thickness, endothelial function, and renal function in patients with mild to moderate chronic kidney disease: results from the Anti-Oxidant Therapy in Chronic Renal Insufficiency (ATIC) Study. Arch Int Med 2007;167: 1262–1270.

Navarro JA, Granadillo VA, Rodriguez-Iturbe B, et al. Removal of trace metals by continuous ambulatory peritoneal dialysis after desferrioxamine B chelation therapy. Clin Nephrol 1991;35:213.

Navarro-Alarcon M, Reyes-Pérez A, Lopez-Garcia H, et al. Longitudinal study of serum zinc and copper levels in hemodialysis patients and their relation to biochemical markers. Biol Trace Elem Res 2006;113:209–222.

Nomura S, Osawa G, Karai M. Treatment of a patient with end-stage renal disease, severe iron overload and ascites by weekly phlebotomy combined with recombinant human erythropoietin. Nephron 1990;55:210.

Padovese P, Gallieni M, Brancaccio D, et al. Trace elements in dialysis fluids and assessment of the exposure of patients on regular hemodialysis, hemofiltration and continuous ambulatory peritoneal dialysis. Nephron 1992;61:442.

Podda GM, Lussana F, Moroni G, et al. Abnormalities of homocysteine and B vitamins in the nephrotic syndrome. Thromb Res 2007; 120:647–652.

Porrini M, Simonetti P, Ciappellano S, et al. Thiamin, riboflavin and pyridoxine status in chronic renal insufficiency. Int J Vitam Nutr Res 1989;59:304.

Rodger RS, Sheldon WL, Watson MJ, et al. Zinc deficiency and hyperprolactinemia are not reversible causes of sexual dysfunction in uremia. Nephrol Dial Transplant 1989;4:888.

Siddiqui J, Freeburger R, Freeman RM. Folic acid, hypersegmented polymorphonuclear leukocytes and the urermic syndrome. Am J Clin Nutr 1970;23:11.

Van Renterghem D, Cornelis R, Vanholder R. Behaviour of 12 trace elements in serum of uremic patients on hemodiafiltration. J Trace Elem Electrolytes Health Dis 1992;6:169.

11

Nutritional Requirements in Hemodialysis Patients

T. Alp Ikizler

Among the risk factors that affect patients with end-stage renal disease (ESRD) and especially those receiving maintenance hemodialysis (MHD), metabolic and nutritional derangements designated as protein-energy wasting (PEW) of chronic kidney disease (CKD) plays an important role. PEW is associated with major adverse clinical outcomes such as increased rates of hospitalization and death in patients undergoing MHD. For these reasons, the prevention and treatment options of PEW are both critical and complex in MHD patients. Because of the large number of factors affecting nutritional and metabolic status of patients undergoing MHD (Fig. 11-1), prevention and treatment of PEW requires a comprehensive combination of strategies to prevent protein and energy depletion and to institute therapies that will avoid further losses.

DIAGNOSIS OF PROTEIN-ENERGY WASTING IN PATIENTS UNDERGOING MAINTENANCE HEMODIALYSIS

A summary of nutritional parameters for detecting PEW in patients undergoing conventional hemodialysis (CHD) and their applicability for guiding nutritional therapies is provided in Table 11-1. Recently, the International Society of Renal Nutrition and Metabolism organized an expert panel to re-examine the terms and criteria used for the diagnosis of PEW; the recommendations for the four main, established categories for the diagnosis of PEW are in Chapter 14 (Table 14-1).

Assessment of Visceral Protein Stores

Serum albumin has been used most widely as a nutritional marker in patients receiving MHD. This is primarily because of its easy availability and strong association with hospitalization and death risk. Unfortunately, there are many nonnutritional factors that influence serum albumin concentrations such as decreased synthesis from liver diseases, increased transcapillary losses, and increased losses from the gastrointestinal tract and kidneys and from tissue injuries such as wounds, burns, and peritonitis. Serum albumin has also been shown to decrease with volume overload, a highly prevalent condition in patients undergoing MHD. Serum albumin (a "negative acute-phase reactant") is also affected by conditions such as inflammation, infection, and trauma, which decrease albumin synthesis, leading to prompt decreases in serum albumin concentration. Consequently, the decrease in serum albumin can reflect the degree of illness and inflammation, rather than nutritional status. Because a low serum albumin is highly predictive of poor clinical outcomes at all stages of CKD, it is still considered a reliable index that there can be abnormalities in a patient's nutritional status.

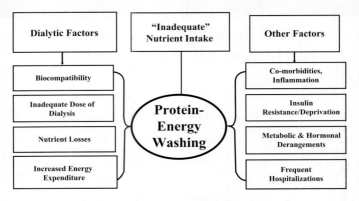

Figure 11-1. Causes of protein–energy wasting in advanced kidney disease.

Serum transferrin is another potential nutritional biomarker, but its level is influenced by changes in iron stores, the presence of inflammation, and changes in extracellular volume. Consequently, it is not a good indicator of nutritional status. Although very responsive to dietary nutrient intake, serum prealbumin levels may also rise because of decreased kidney function. In addition, prealbumin is a negative acute-phase reactant, so its utility in monitoring nutritional status in MHD patients is questionable. Since serum albumin is also a negative acute phase reactant like prealbumin, it is reasonable to measure the C-reactive protein (CRP), an acute-phase reactant and an index of inflammation when serum levels of albumin or prealbumin are low.

Assessment of Body Composition

The assessment of body composition and somatic protein stores is based on the measurement of different body compartments (water, fat, bone, muscle, and visceral organs). The fat-free mass (mainly composed of muscle) is the major somatic protein mass. Generally, somatic protein stores are preserved, but when there are catabolic illnesses, depletion of fat-free mass will occur. We use body composition techniques to diagnose protein depletion and to monitor efficacy of nutritional therapies. Simple anthropometric measures can provide a guide over long-term treatment, and bioelectrical impedance analysis (BIA) and dual-energy x-ray absorptiometry (DEXA) can be used for research purposes as long as it is recognized that both of these techniques are greatly influenced by changes in body water, a complication that is common in MHD patients.

Composite Indices of Nutritional Status

The diagnostic measures based on changes in body composition and dietary intake assessment have been accompanied by a subjective assessment of overall nutritional status, especially when large numbers of patients are being evaluated. The most com-

Table 11-1. Suggested table to monitor nutritional status and guide therapy in kidney failure

Simple (monthly) Assessment	Findings	Possible Interventions
BW	Continuous decline or <85% IBW	Suspect of PEW and perform more detailed nutritional assessment
Serum albumin	<4.0 g/dL	Consider preventive measures
Serum creatinine	Relatively low predialysis values	No specific intervention needed at this point
Detailed assessment	Findings	Possible interventions (simple)
Serum prealbumin	<30 mg/dL, and/or	Dietary counseling: DPI ≥1.2 g/kg/day, energy intake 30–35 kcal/day
Serum transferrin	<200 mg/dL, and/or	Increase dialysis dose to Kt/V >1.4
IGF-I	<200 ng/mL, and/or	Use biocompatible membranes
LBM and/or fat mass	Unexpected decrease	Upper GI motility enhancer
SGA	Worsening	Consider timely initiation of CDT
Repeat detailed assessment (2 to 3 months from previous)	Findings	Possible interventions (moderate to complex)
Serum prealbumin	<30 mg/dL, and/or	Nutritional supplements: Oral, enteric tube feeding, IDPN (requires Medicare approval)
Serum transferrin	<200 mg/dL, and/or	Anabolic Factors: Anabolic steroids
IGF-I	<200 ng/mL, and/or	rhGH (experimental)
Serum creatinine	Relatively low predialysis values, and/or unexpected decrease	Appetite stimulants
LBM and/or fat mass	unexpected decrease	Megase; ghrelin (experimental)
C-reactive protein	>10 mg/L	Anti-inflammatory (experimental)

BW, body weight; CDT, chronic dialysis therapy; DPI, dietary protein intake; GI, gastrointestinal; IBW, ideal body weight; IDPN, intradialytic parenteral nutrition; IGF-I, insulin-like growth factor 1; LBM, lean body mass; PEW, protein-energy wasting; rhGH, recombinant human growth hormone; SGA, subjective global assessment.
Adapted from Pupim LB, Cuppari L, Ikizler TA. Nutrition and metabolism in kidney disease. Semin Nephrol 2006;26:134–157, with permission.

monly used composite indices include subjective global assessment (SGA) or its modified or expanded versions such as the composite nutritional index (CNI) and the malnutrition-inflammation score (MIS). These measures can only provide a general assessment because they evaluate nutritional status from a broader perspective, including medical history, symptoms, and physical parameters.

SGA was originally used to evaluate outcomes in surgical patients with gastrointestinal disease. The evaluation included a history of weight changes, nutritional intake and gastrointestinal symptoms, nutrition-related functional impairment plus a physical examination to assess subcutaneous fat, muscle stores, and the presence or absence of edema. The surgical patients were divided into three categories: (i) well-nourished; (ii) mild to moderately malnourished; or (iii) severely malnourished. In the surgical patients, the SGA was found to correlate with other measures of nutritional status and clinical outcome. The use of the SGA was expanded to include patients undergoing MHD, but the SGA does not reliably detect sarcopenia (based on total body nitrogen), and even though it has some utility in discriminating between best- versus worst-nourished patients, the SGA does not separate patients undergoing MHD with mild or moderate PEW. Despite these shortcomings, the National Kidney Foundation Disease Outcomes Quality Initiative (NKF K/DOQI) guidelines included a recommendation that the modified SGA should be performed every 6 months in patients receiving MHD. However, its subjective nature, the absence of measures of visceral protein stores, and its relative insensitivity to small changes in nutritional status greatly limit the usefulness of the SGA. We believe that if used, the SGA should be accompanied by parameters that include body weight and weight-for-height, skinfold measures, and serum albumin concentration plus other estimates of protein stores.

The Malnutrition Inflammation Score (MIS) incorporates components of the SGA and includes components related to nutritional status (body mass index) and inflammation (serum albumin concentration and total iron binding capacity) plus indices that are not directly related to nutritional status, such as comorbidities and functional status. We recommend that the MIS should be used in conjunction with other methods as proposed for SGA.

The critical point is that the nutritional status of patients undergoing MHD should be monitored regularly to detect nutritional disturbances early. In addition, regular monitoring is needed to evaluate the response of nutritional interventions and to motivate and improve patient's compliance to the dietary therapy. Overall, we recommend routine follow-up measurements that include body weight and nPNA plus values of serum albumin, prealbumin, and cholesterol every 3 months in clinically stable patients. Some investigators include anthropometric measurements, dietary interviews, and SGA every 6 months for those patients who are at risk of developing PEW or with established PEW, but the utility of this strategy has not been evaluated carefully. Figure 11-2 depicts a proposed algorithm for the assessment and management of nutritional status in patients receiving MHD.

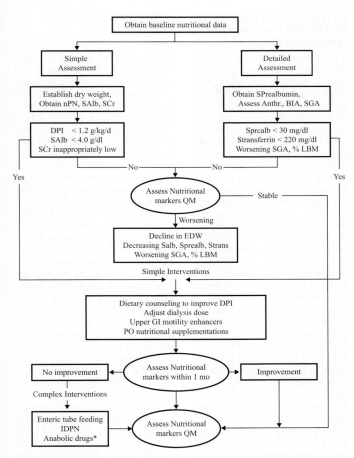

Figure 11-2. **A proposed algorithm for the assessment and manage-ment of nutritional status in patients receiving MHD.** Anthr, anthro-pometric measurements; BIA, bioelectrical impedance analysis; DPI, dietary protein intake; EDW, estimated dry weight; GI, gastro-intes-tinal; IDPN, intradialytic parenteral nutrition; LBM, lean body mass; nPNA, normalized protein nitrogen appearance rate; QM, every month; SAlb, serum albumin; SCr, serum creatinine; SGA, subjective global assessment; SPrealb, serum prealbumin. * Mostly experi-mental.

EPIDEMIOLOGY OF PROTEIN-ENERGY WASTING IN PATIENTS UNDERGOING MAINTENANCE HEMODIALYSIS

Virtually every study evaluating the nutritional status of MHD patients reports some degree of abnormalities in the nutritional status. Unfortunately, many different diagnostic tools were used in the separate studies, so the actual prevalence of PEW in MHD patients varies widely, ranging from 20% to 60%. Although there is evidence that nutritional parameters improve within 3 to 6 months following initiation of hemodialysis, there also is evidence that PEW is present in up to 40% or more of the MHD population; the prevalence seems to increase with time of MHD treatment.

As noted above, there are serious shortcomings in the use of serum albumin as a principal measure of nutritional status. Unfortunately, serum albumin has been the major basis for epidemiologic reports on nutrition in patients undergoing MHD. For example, in the baseline phase of the Hemodialysis (HEMO) Study, 29% of the patients had albumin levels below 3.5 g/dL. Results from the Dialysis Outcomes and Practice Patterns Study (DOPPS) suggest there is a lower prevalence of hypoalbuminemia in countries other than United States, with the lowest mean value of serum albumin occurring in the United Kingdom for Europe and the U.S. value being significantly lower compared with European countries (3.60 versus 3.72 g/dL [36 versus 37 g/L]). Japan also had significantly higher albumin values compared with U.S. values even when adjusted for patient age, sex, and the timing of the measurement (i.e., during the week or over the weekend). In DOPPS II, 20.5% of U.S. patients had a serum albumin level less than 3.5 g/dL (35 g/L). Based on the serum albumin and the SGA, it was concluded that the prevalence of moderate malnutrition ranged from 7.6% (United States) to 18% (France) and for severe malnutrition, from 2.3% (Italy) to 11% (United States). Because these conclusions are made based on inaccurate assessments of nutritional status, their usefulness in understanding what occurs in patients undergoing MHD is very limited. On the other hand, the relevance of these measurements is that practically every marker has been associated with hospitalization and death risk. Recent epidemiologic data also indicate there is an improvement in survival when these markers are corrected.

Etiology of Protein-Energy Wasting in Patients Receiving Maintenance Hemodialysis

The mechanisms leading to PEW in advanced kidney disease are still being elucidated; they can not be attributed to any single factor in patients receiving MHD (Fig. 11-1). Still, it appears that the common pathway for all the metabolic derangements is related to exaggerated protein degradation relative to decreased protein synthesis. There are no agreed upon mechanisms relating dietary protein and energy intake and the development of nutritional and metabolic abnormalities in CHD, but there is an epidemiological association between inadequate nutrient intake and the abnormalities associated with PEW.

Dietary Nutrient Intake, Hemodialysis, and Development of Protein–Energy Wasting in Patients Receiving Maintenance Hemodialysis

The observation that patients with CKD decrease their protein and energy intake as they progressively lose kidney function has led some to conclude that uremia per se causes protein catabolism stimulated by decreased nutrient intake. This conclusion has been challenged because even in patients with advanced CKD, balance studies show that there is a concomitant decrease in both protein synthesis and degradation that is at least uncomplicated by acidosis. The dual change in protein synthesis and degradation results in a net nitrogen balance that is not different from matched healthy controls. Conversely, accelerated protein degradation stimulated by acute illnesses or stress conditions is not suppressed, and there is no adequate compensatory increase in protein synthesis partly caused by insufficient dietary nutrient intake. For example, hospitalized patients undergoing MHD can be provided limited protein and energy and may not be able to adjust rates of protein turnover leading to loss of cellular protein stores.

An additional stimulus for protein losses is the dialytic treatment per se. Recent measurements of protein synthesis and degradation unequivocally demonstrate the catabolic effects of hemodialysis. Both whole-body and skeletal muscle protein homeostasis are disrupted, and there is a consistent finding of decreased protein synthesis at the whole-body level and an additional increase in whole-body protein breakdown. There also is evidence for a significant increase in net skeletal muscle protein breakdown. Notably, these undesirable effects persist for at least 2 hours following the completion of hemodialysis.

Chronic Inflammation as a Catabolic Stimulus in Advanced Chronic Kidney Disease

Recent epidemiologic studies have pointed out that there is a high prevalence of increased levels of inflammatory markers in patients with advanced CKD. The metabolic and nutritional responses to chronic inflammation are many (vide infra) and closely mimic the PEW that appears to be common in patients with advanced CKD, including exaggerated protein catabolism. This raises the potential that there is a "cause and effect" relationship between inflammation and loss of protein stores. Inflammation, more correctly termed the systemic inflammatory response syndrome, is a complex combination of physiologic, immunologic, and metabolic effects occurring in response to a variety of stimulators such as tissue injury or disease processes. Certain cytokines, such as interleukin (IL)-1, IL-6, and tumor necrosis factor-alpha (TNF-α) are the potential mediators of these effects. Therefore, it is important to limit their biological activities, but in conditions where the inflammatory response is ongoing and cannot be controlled effectively, adverse effects are highly likely.

Etiology of Chronic Inflammation in Patients with End-Stage Renal Disease

The etiology of inflammation is multifactorial in patients with advanced CKD (Fig. 11-3). For example, in patients with CKD

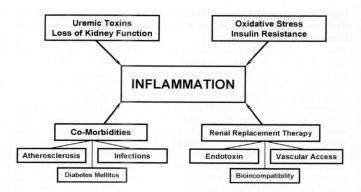

Figure 11-3. Several modifiable and nonmodifiable factors lead to the chronic inflammatory state of advanced kidney disease.

who are not yet receiving MHD, the progression of kidney disease is associated with inflammatory response. It is not clear how loss of kidney function leads to whole body inflammation and impairment of protein metabolism. Secondly, moderate to advanced CKD can be associated with increased oxidative stress burden leading to formation of advanced glycosylation end products (AGEs). The interaction of AGE with its receptor for advanced glycation end products (RAGE) stimulates the production of IL-6 by monocytes and indirectly leads to excess production of C-reactive protein in the liver. These interactions are discussed in more detail in Chapter 2.

Besides the accumulation of proinflammatory compounds in advanced CKD, the type of dialysis can result in inflammatory responses. For example, the hemodialysis procedure is associated with activation of an inflammatory cascade with increases in the synthesis of C-reactive protein, IL-6, and fibrinogen. The activation of the inflammatory cascade has been attributed to exposure of blood to dialysis membranes and/or back-leakage of lipopolysaccharide through the dialysis membranes from the use of less-than-sterile dialysate. Indeed, it has been shown that use of ultrapure, endotoxin-free dialysate is associated with reduced blood concentrations of proinflammatory cytokines. Infection is another common occurrence in patients undergoing MHD, which can cause significant inflammation; this is especially common in patients with a hemodialysis catheter.

Effects of Inflammatory Response on Metabolism and Nutrition

Although not proven, proinflammatory cytokines are thought to play an integral role in the muscle catabolism of MHD patients. For example, elevated levels of IL-6 are associated with increased muscle proteolysis, and the administration of IL-6 receptor antibody can block this catabolism. In surgical patients with sepsis with abundant levels of proinflammatory cytokines, there is increased whole body protein catabolism. Further, injection of animals with TNF-α stimulates skeletal muscle protein breakdown, but exposure of the muscle to TNF-α does not cause protein catabolism. This indicates the complexity of these interactions. One mechanism that could tie these observations together is that impaired insulin/IGF-1 signaling can stimulate muscle protein breakdown. In fact, there is evidence that involvement of proinflammatory cytokines with muscle protein catabolism is because of suppression of insulin receptor -1 (IRS-1)-associated phosphatidylinositol 3-kinase (PI3K) activity. This suppression stimulates the activity of the ubiquitin-proteasome proteolytic system (UPS) and activates caspase-3, the two proteolytic pathways that cause degradation of muscle protein.

Anorexia or suppressed nutrient intake is a well-established metabolic response to inflammation; IL-1 and TNF-α can cause anorexia through their effects on the satiety center in the central nervous system. Again, this is complicated because prostaglandins may be involved; prophylactic use of anti-inflammatory agents blunts the anorectic effects of cytokines. It should be noted that the combined presence of decreased nutrient intake plus increased protein breakdown in the setting of exaggerated inflammatory response worsens overall nitrogen balance, predisposing the patients to accelerated loss of skeletal muscle mass and overall poor nutritional state.

Several indirect responses to chronic inflammation can also predispose patients receiving CHD to hypercatabolism. It is known that a prolonged decrease in muscular activity is associated with muscle weakness, muscular atrophy, and negative nitrogen balance, all leading to loss of lean body mass. Finally, there are hormonal derangements associated with chronic inflammation. These include disruption of the growth hormone and IGF-1 axis leading to decreased anabolism and increased leptin concentrations (a potential contributor to anorexia).

Insulin Resistance and Deprivation as Catabolic Stimuli in Advanced Chronic Kidney Disease

Patients with CKD secondary to diabetes mellitus (DM), the leading cause of ESRD in the United States, have a higher incidence of PEW when compared with nondiabetic patients. The degree of insulin resistance and/or insulin deprivation seems to play the most critical role in this process (see Chapter 16 for additional discussion of Sarcopenia of Obesity).

As with inflammation, decreased insulin or decreased sensitivity to insulin can cause muscle protein losses. Multiple in vitro and in vivo studies have demonstrated that the metabolic effects of insulin extend beyond carbohydrate metabolism; specifically, insulin deprivation stimulates protein breakdown and administration of insulin suppresses protein degradation. With adequate amino acid availability, insulin also regulates protein synthesis. These actions are mediated through IRS-1-associated PI3K activity. A deficiency of insulin stimulates the UPS and caspase-3 activity to break down muscle protein. It is believed that regulatory abnormalities in these pathways are responsible for the muscle catabolism observed in patients with diabetes or insulin resistance undergoing MHD. Several reports demonstrate that among patients undergoing MHD, muscle protein breakdown is enhanced in patients with type II DM when compared with patients without DM undergoing CHD. This abnormality translates into a greater loss of lean body mass within the first year of MHD in diabetic patients receiving MHD compared with nondiabetic patients receiving MHD. In the absence of severe obesity, insulin resistance is still detectable in patients undergoing CHD and is strongly associated with increased muscle protein breakdown, even after controlling for inflammation.

In addition to the protein catabolism that occurs with insulin resistance, diabetic patients undergoing MHD are likely to be more prone to protein depletion because of associated gastrointestinal symptoms (e.g., gastroparesis, nausea and vomiting, bacterial overgrowth in the gut, and pancreatic insufficiency).

The Dose of Dialysis and Protein–Energy Wasting Development in Patients Receiving Maintenance Hemodialysis

Underdialysis can lead to anorexia and decreased taste acuity, and there does appear to be a relationship between underdialysis and decreased dietary protein intake. Not surprisingly, patients with stage 5 CKD experience a significant improvement in their protein intake within 3 to 6 months of initiation of MHD. Because uremic anorexia usually develops when the dose of dialysis is below acceptable levels (single pool Kt/V <1.2), it follows that adequate dialysis will raise appetite, and this was found in the National Institutes of Health (NIH)-sponsored study, HEMO. In addition, it was found that patients undergoing MHD who were dialyzed more frequently (6 times a week) had an improved nutrient intake. The conclusion is that a significant increase in dialysis dose might be beneficial in improving the nutritional status of patients undergoing MHD.

METABOLIC AND HORMONAL DERANGEMENTS LEADING TO PROTEIN-ENERGY WASTING IN PATIENTS RECEIVING MAINTENANCE HEMODIALYSIS

Metabolic acidosis, a common abnormality in patients with progressive CKD, promotes PEW by increasing protein catabolism, especially in muscle. In addition, acidosis stimulates the oxidation of essential amino acids (as shown for leucine oxidation) to raise protein requirements in patients receiving MHD. Even a small correction of a low serum bicarbonate concentration will improve nutritional status by correcting essential amino acid catabolism and down-regulating muscle proteolysis via the ubiquitin-proteasome system. As with the other abnormalities that stimulate muscle protein catabolism, metabolic acidosis acts in large part by suppressing insulin/IGF-1 signaling in muscle. Currently, we recommend that the predialysis serum bicarbonate level should be greater than 24 mmol/L in patients undergoing MHD although very high levels should be avoided, especially if the dialysate bicarbonate levels are high as well.

Increased concentrations of parathyroid hormone have been implicated as a protein catabolic factor in ESRD, although evidence for this response in humans is sparse. In addition, there are abnormalities in thyroid hormone-stimulated metabolism in

MHD patients, specifically, low circulating thyroxine and triiodothyronine concentrations. Because similar changes resemble those found in patients with prolonged malnutrition, it has been suggested that the thyroid hormone response to malnutrition (and possibly to advanced CKD), is a maladaptive response to a decrease in energy intake. There are no trials of correcting thyroid hormone levels with documentation of improved nutritional improvements in patients undergoing MHD. Finally, abnormalities in the growth hormone and Insulin-like growth factor 1 (IGF-I) axis could be important factors in the development of PEW in patients undergoing MHD. For example, growth hormone administration does improve the growth of children with CKD. Growth hormone stimulates beneficial responses such as enhancing protein synthesis, reducing protein degradation, increasing fat mobilization, and increasing gluconeogenesis. Although there generally is an increase in the plasma concentrations of growth hormone during progressive kidney disease, it appears that this is because of the development of resistance to growth hormone at cellular levels. Interestingly, administration of recombinant human growth hormone can induce a net anabolic effect in patients undergoing MHD (see below).

NUTRITIONAL SUPPORT IN PATIENTS RECEIVING MAINTENANCE HEMODIALYSIS

Given the significance of the problem, as well as the complexity of the pathophysiologic basis of PEW in advanced CKD, it is evident that the prevention and treatment options of PEW in patients receiving MHD are complex. Table 11-2 provides daily dietary recommendations for patients undergoing MHD. In MHD with PEW or at risk for PEW, there is no single treatment approach that will alleviate the multiple adverse consequences of PEW. An overview of prevention and treatment options for patients who have CKD with PEW plus specific therapeutic options for patients undergoing MHD are provided in Table 11-3.

General Aspects of Nutritional Management

Management of nutritional aspects of patients undergoing MHD includes a comprehensive combination of preventive maneuvers to prevent protein and energy depletion. Unfortunately, for some therapies, there are only empiric data suggesting benefits. Standard therapies for patients with PEW who are undergoing MHD include provision of adequate dialysis, treatment of metabolic acidosis, adjustments of dietary factors, and treatment of infections. Factors that are not so closely linked to the nutritional status include correction of fluid overload and treatment of comorbid conditions such as diabetes and cardiovascular diseases. Likewise, a search for signs of chronic inflammation is required, and all attempts must be made to eliminate inflammatory responses, especially the use of central venous catheters.

Nutritional Supplementation

The susceptibility toward PEW from decreased protein and energy intake could be ameliorated by increasing nutrient intake through dietary supplements, especially during hemodialysis. Nutritional supplementation of patients undergoing MHD should

Table 11-2. Daily dietary recommendations for patients undergoing maintenance hemodialysis*

Nutrient or Substance	Recommended Intake
Protein (g/kg)	1.2–1.4
Calories (sedentary, kcal/kg)	30–35†
Protein (%)	15–25
Carbohydrate (%)	50–60‡
Fat (%)	25–35
Cholesterol	<200 mg (0.52 mmol)
Saturated fat (%)	<7
Crude fiber (g)	20–30
Sodium	<2.0 g (<80 mmol)§
Calcium	2.0 g (50 mmol)¶
Phosphorus	0.8–1.0 g (26–32 mmol)**

*All intakes calculated on the basis of normalized body weight (i.e., the average body weight of normal persons of the same age, height, and sex as the patient).
†35 kcal/kg body weight per day if <60 years of age; 30–35 kcal/body weight per day if greater than 60 years of age.
‡Carbohydrate intake should be decreased in patients with hypertriglyceridemia.
§Lower sodium intakes in the range of 1.0–1.5 g (40–60 mmol) may result in better control of blood pressure.
¶The total dose of elemental calcium provided by the calcium-based phosphate binders should not exceed 1500 mg (37 mmol) per day, and the total intake of elemental calcium (including dietary calcium) should not exceed 2000 mg (50 mmol) per day.
**For patients with serum phosphorus level >5.5 mg/dL (1.8 mmol/L).

be delivered by the oral route if at all possible, but if not, parenteral nutritional supplements can be provided.

Oral Nutritional Supplementation
Both the short- and long-term benefits of oral nutritional supplements for patients undergoing MHD can be accomplished especially when the supplements are provided around the time of hemodialysis, including intradialytic administration. For example, oral feeding can be associated with a robust improvement in whole-body and skeletal muscle protein balance. Whether the beneficial protein metabolic responses persist during long-term administration has not been examined systematically. Studies assessing beneficial responses to prolonged oral nutritional supplementation in patients undergoing MHD can be found in a recent publication (Stratton 2005). In brief, the outcome measures examined included clinical (quality of life, complications, and mortality), biochemical (serum albumin and electrolyte levels), and nutritional (dietary intake and anthropometry). The analysis included 18 studies (5 randomized controlled trials [RCTs], 13 non-RCTs), and the conclusion was that enteral nutritional support can increase total (energy and protein) intake and raise serum albumin concentrations by an average of 0.23 g/dL, with no adverse effects on electrolyte status (serum phosphate and potassium). The practical implication is that oral nutritional

Table 11-3. Proposed nutritional and anti-inflammatory interventions in chronic disease states

Nutritional interventions:

Chronic Kidney Disease (Stage 3–5 not on dialysis)
- Close supervision and nutritional counseling (especially for patients on protein-restricted diets)
- Initiation of dialysis or renal transplant in patients with advanced chronic renal failure with apparent protein-energy wasting despite vigorous attempts

Chronic Dialysis Patients
- Continuous dietary counseling
- Appropriate amount of dietary protein and calorie intake (dietary protein and energy intake >1.2 g/kg/day and >30 kcal/kg/day, respectively)
- Optimal dose of dialysis
- Use of biocompatible hemodialysis membranes
- Nutritional support in chronic dialysis patients who are unable to meet their dietary needs
  - Oral supplements
  - Tube feeds (if medically appropriate)
  - Intradialytic parenteral nutritional supplements for patients receiving hemodialysis
  - Amino acid dialysate for peritoneal dialysis patients
  - Resistance exercise combined with nutritional supplementation
- Anabolic steroids
- Appetite stimulants (not proven or experimental)
  - Megestrol acetate, dronabinol, melatonin, thalidomide, and ghrelin)
- Growth Factors (Experimental):
  - Recombinant human growth hormone
  - Recombinant human insulin-like growth factor - 1

Anti-inflammatory Interventions:

- Pentoxifylline
- Resistance exercise
- Targeted anticytokine therapy
  - IL-1 receptor antagonist
  - TNF-α blocker
- Statins
- Thiazolidinediones
- ACE inhibitors
- Resistance exercise
- Thalidomide
- Fish oil and vitamin E

supplementation is effective, especially when administered during hemodialysis, and is practical, convenient, and well-tolerated.

Intradialytic Parenteral Nutrition

While the gastrointestinal route is always preferred for nutritional supplementation, parenteral provision of nutrients, especially during the dialysis procedure (intradialytic parenteral nutrition [IDPN]), is safe, effective, and convenient for individuals who can not tolerate oral or enteral administration of nutrients. Several but not all reports provide evidence that nutritional status can improve with IDPN. Unfortunately, the sample sizes in most reports have been small and did not allow appropriate stratification of patients undergoing MHD and were carried out over a short period of time. These shortcomings contribute to the observed inconsistency of results. Notably, there is a high cost of IDPN, and these considerations plus regulatory concerns have limited the utilization of this potentially beneficial treatment.

Recent metabolic studies show that the net effect of IDPN is a remarkable change from negative (muscle loss) to positive (muscle accretion) balance at least during IDPN administration. This is important because it can be estimated that during the 3.5 hours of IDPN, approximately 51.5 g of whole-body protein can be obtained. If the fat-free mass is 73% water, there could be an additional 191 g of fat-free mass gain because of the IDPN treatment. IDPN has also been shown to increase the hepatic synthesis of albumin, contributing to an improvement in the whole-body protein homeostasis. But it must be recognized that dialysis stimulates protein catabolism, and even when IDPN was provided, the increase in protein catabolism recurred when the IDPN was terminated. This would diminish the benefits of IDPN at least until a method is found to block protein catabolism.

Results from a recent study (FINEs) have provided insights into effects from long-term use of nutritional supplementations in patients with PEW undergoing MHD. In this study, 186 patients with PEW undergoing MHD were randomly assigned to receive intradialytic parenteral nutrition (for 1 year) plus standard oral supplements providing 500 kcal/day and 25 g/day protein and were compared with those receiving oral supplements only. The nutritional goal was to bring the intakes up to the recommended amounts of 30 to 35 kcal/kg/day and 1.2 g/kg/day, respectively. The primary outcome, 2-year mortality, was similar in the 2 groups (39% in the control group and 43% in the IDPN group), suggesting that oral nutritional supplementation is equally effective as IDPN when oral intake is possible. When there was an increase in serum prealbumin, it was associated with a decrease in the 2-year mortality and hospitalization rate. This large study provides the first prospective evidence of a link between a positive response to nutritional therapy and improved outcomes.

The other conclusion is that oral or combined oral–parenteral methods of delivering supplements are the same in terms of mortality of patients with PEW undergoing MHD, if equal and adequate amounts of protein and calories are provided. Despite the lack of an appropriate control group, these results imply that nutritional supplementation can improve nutritional markers in patients with PEW undergoing CHD, and this conclusion is consistent with the recommendations of the NKF K/DOQI (>1.2 g/kg/day and >30 kcal/kg/day, respectively) (Fig. 11-4). Although these results imply that nutritional interventions can improve the survival of patients undergoing MHD, caution is needed in this interpretation because the study lacked a no-intervention arm, and the nutritional improvements may just reflect a regression-to-the-mean phenomenon. Compared with the overall 2-year mortality rate in the FINE study (42%) with the published mortality rate from the European registry data after adjustment for a serum albumin <35 g/L, there could be as much as a 15% improvement in overall mortality. Such a survival benefit would be unmatched by any other proposed therapy for high-risk patients undergoing MHD to date.

PHARMACOLOGIC INTERVENTIONS FOR TREATMENT OF PROTEIN-ENERGY WASTING IN PATIENTS RECEIVING MAINTENANCE HEMODIALYSIS

Growth Hormone and IGF-1

Growth hormone and its major mediator, IGF-1, could have several anabolic properties. Besides the well-documented benefits of growth hormone in children with CKD, short-term administration of the hormone to patients undergoing MHD can have anabolic responses. Most if not all long-term studies indicate there is a significant increase in lean body mass in the growth hormone-treated patients undergoing MHD. For example, growth hormone was associated with statistically significant gains in lean body mass in a trial consisting of 139 patients. There also were statistically significant beneficial changes in other biomarkers of mortality (homocysteine, transferrin, high-density lipoprotein [HDL]) as well as quality of life (QOL). Finally, there was a trend toward increased levels of serum albumin as compared with placebo administration.

Regarding IGF-1, a preliminary report of nitrogen balance studies in patients receiving CAPD suggested that anabolism occurred. However, the side effects of this agent may impede its widespread use at this time. The long-term responses to rhIGF-1in patients with PEW undergoing MHD have not been tested.

Appetite Stimulants

Examples of pharmacologic agents that may stimulate appetite include megestrol acetate, dronabinol, cyproheptadine, melatonin, thalidomide, and ghrelin. Most of these drugs have not been studied systematically in patients with PEW undergoing MHD but have been used in other catabolic illnesses. For example, megestrol acetate, a steroid-like progestagen, led to increased appetite and weight gain in breast cancer patients. In elderly men, the orexigenic and weight gaining effects of megestrol acetate have been recently attributed to its anticytokine effects via reduced levels of IL-6 and TNF-α. The increase in appetite was associated with an increase in weight, mainly because of increased fat and not lean body mass. Moreover, megestrol acetate has been associated with side effects including hypogonadism, impotence, and increased risk of thromboembolism. In patients

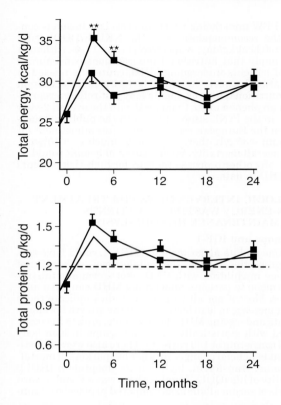

Figure 11-4.   Changes in total energy and protein intakes during the 2-year follow-up in control (*bottom line*) and IDPN (*top line*) groups (means ± SEM) in the FINE study participants. While there were between-group differences in energy intake at months 3 and 6 (p <0.01), both groups achieved the minimum K/DOQI recommended thresholds for protein and energy intake in maintenance patients undergoing hemodialysis (*dotted lines*). In both groups, nutritional support induced comparable increases in serum albumin at months 3, 6, 12, and 18 (p <0.01) and in serum prealbumin at months 3 to 24 (p <0.02). (Adapted from Cano NJ, Fouque D, Roth H, et al. Intradialytic parenteral nutrition does not improve survival in malnourished hemo-dialysis patients: a 2-year multicenter, prospective, randomized study. J Am Soc Nephrol 2007;18:2583–2591, with permission.)

undergoing MHD, megestrol acetate can stimulate appetite and induce small increases in serum albumin, but large-scale prospective studies are needed to assess whether these drugs provide adjunctive nutritional therapy for patients undergoing MHD or patients with CKD patients. We know of no long-term systematic evaluation of other appetite-stimulating and weight gain responses to dronabinol, cyproheptadine, melatonin, ghrelin, and thalidomide in patients undergoing MHD.

Anabolic Steroids

There are reports of significant improvements in body composition and physical function of patients undergoing MHD who are given nandrolone decanoate. In addition, there was an increase in quadriceps muscle cross-sectional area (magnetic resonance imaging [MRI] measurements) and an increase in lean body mass by DEXA. Curiously, the combination of resistance exercise with nandrolone deaconate did not improve the beneficial effects of the drug.

Exercise as an Anabolic Intervention in Patients Receiving Maintenance Hemodialysis

Exercise training can maintain and/or improve exercise capacity and endurance in the general population. In addition, resistance exercise can increase muscle mass, strength, and appetite as well as lessen muscle weakness and frailty in elderly patients (see Chapter 17). Resistance exercise can increase oxygen consumption, but whether this response only occurs when there is a positive muscle protein balance is unknown. The rates of both muscle synthesis and breakdown increase during a resistance exercise session in normal adults, and if resistance exercise is combined with nutrient supplementation, anabolism is maximized while muscle breakdown declines somewhat. Short-term (i.e., a single hemodialysis session) metabolic studies indicate that exercise when combined with intradialytic oral or parenteral nutrition will increase net protein balance in patients undergoing MHD, but longer-term evaluations of resistance exercise performed during hemodialysis in patients receiving MHD have not shown significant nutritional benefits. Nonetheless, the beneficial effects of exercise on quality of life and physical functioning must be taken into account when considering an exercise regimen for a patient undergoing MHD. We recommend an adequate nutritional supplement during exercise unless the patient is considered for supervised weight loss.

Anti-inflammatory Interventions

Anti-inflammatory interventions aimed at ameliorating the changes in nutritional status in patients with ESRD (see Table 11-3) include pentoxifylline and resistance exercise. Pentoxifylline, a drug that blocks TNF-α release, was administered intravenously to patients with stage 4–5 CKD. There was not only an improvement in protein breakdown but also improvement in the anabolic effects of a balanced amino acid mixture given concurrently. While pentoxifylline did not significantly affect TNF-α levels, it did decrease TNF-α -soluble receptors and hence could block the influence of TNF-α. In a study of resistance exercise training over 12 weeks, there was simultaneous improvement in whole-body protein balance and inflammatory markers in patients with stage 3–4 CKD.

Besides pentoxifylline and resistance exercise, thalidomide, IL-1 receptor antagonists, TNF-α receptor blockers, fish oil, statins, angiotensin-converting enzyme (ACE) inhibitors, peroxisome proliferator-activated receptor (PPAR)-gamma agonists plus certain antioxidants have been proposed as anti-inflammatory strategies in patients undergoing MHD. Combined administration of γ-tocopherol and docosahexaenoic acid over 3 months was associated with a significant decrease in IL-6 and the white blood cell count in patients undergoing MHD. These results indicate the need for further, larger-scale studies.

Obesity in Patients Receiving Maintenance Hemodialysis

Another important nutritional issue in terms of patients receiving MHD is obesity. The most recent United States Renal Data System (USRDS) results of 2006 showed that the average body mass index (BMI) of patients receiving MHD is 28.5 kg/m2. A detailed discussion of the impact of obesity in kidney disease is in Chapter 16. This issue is important because there is a plethora of epidemiologic studies indicating that higher BMI, regardless of its etiology (i.e., increased adiposity and/or lean body mass) is associated with an improved survival of patients with ESRD. While the exact mechanism(s) underlying this association has not been elucidated, there is a potentially beneficial effect of increasing protein and energy intakes because weight gain might be a potentially beneficial outcome.

Selected Readings

Cano NJ, Fouque D, Roth H, et al. Intradialytic parenteral nutrition does not improve survival in malnourished hemodialysis patients: a 2-year multicenter, prospective, randomized study. J Am Soc Nephrol 2007;18:2583–2591.

Feldt-Rasmussen B, Lange M, Sulowicz W, et al. Growth hormone treatment during hemodialysis in a randomized trial improves nutrition, quality of life, and cardiovascular risk. J Am Soc Nephrol 2007;18:2161–2171.

Fouque D, Kalantar-Zadeh K, Kopple J, et al. A proposed nomenclature and diagnostic criteria for protein-energy wasting in acute and chronic kidney disease. Kidney Int 2008;73:391–398.

Ikizler TA. Nutrition, inflammation and chronic kidney disease. Curr Opin Nephrol Hypertens 2008;17:162–167.

Kalantar-Zadeh K, Block G, McAllister CJ, et al. Appetite and inflammation, nutrition, anemia, and clinical outcome in hemodialysis patients. Am J Clin Nutr 2004;80:299–307.

Kaysen GA. The microinflammatory state in uremia: causes and potential consequences. J Am Soc Nephrol 2001;12:1549–1557.

Lecker SH, Goldberg AL, Mitch WE. Protein degradation by the ubiquitin-proteasome pathway in normal and disease states. J Am Soc Nephrol 2006;17:1807–1819.

Lim VS, Ikizler TA, Raj DS, et al. Does hemodialysis increase protein breakdown? Dissociation between whole-body amino acid turnover and regional muscle kinetics. J Am Soc Nephrol 2005;16:862–868.

Majchrzak KM, Pupim LB, Flakoll PJ, et al. Resistance exercise augments the acute anabolic effects of intradialytic oral nutritional supplementation. Nephrol Dial Transplant 2008;23:1362–1369.

Pupim LB, Cuppari L, Ikizler TA. Nutrition and metabolism in kidney disease. Semin Nephrol 2006;26:134–157.

Pupim LB, Majchrzak KM, Flakoll PJ, et al. Intradialytic oral nutrition improves protein homeostasis in chronic hemodialysis patients with deranged nutritional status. J Am Soc Nephrol 2006;17: 3149–3157.

Siew ED, Ikizler TA. Determinants of insulin resistance and its effects on protein metabolism in patients with advanced chronic kidney disease. Contrib Nephrol 2008;161:138–144.

Stenvinkel P, Heimburger O, Paultre F, et al. Strong association between malnutrition, inflammation, and atherosclerosis in chronic renal failure. Kidney Int 1999;55:1899–1911.

Stratton RJ, Bircher G, Fouque D, et al. Multinutrient oral supplements and tube feeding in maintenance dialysis: a systematic review and meta-analysis. Am J Kidney Dis 2005;46:387–405.

12

Nutritional Considerations in Patients on Peritoneal Dialysis

Sharon J. Nessim and Joanne M. Bargman

INTRODUCTION

Nutritional status in patients with kidney disease has garnered increasing attention over the last several years. A major reason for this is the recognition that the prevalence of signs of protein energy wasting (PEW) increases as glomerular filtration rate (GFR) declines; these signs persist even after maintenance dialysis is initiated. Not only are signs of PEW highly prevalent among patients receiving peritoneal dialysis (PD), but evidence of a poor nutritional status is associated with adverse outcomes. In the CANUSA study, which prospectively followed a cohort of 680 patients undergoing PD, evidence of a poor nutritional status was associated with reduced patient and technique survival and increased hospitalization. Other results support a link between nutritional status and mortality. Given that PEW (or malnutrition as it was previously called) is not the direct cause of death in the majority of patients undergoing PD, the presence of nutritional abnormalities is likely a marker of comorbid illnesses that are more likely to lead to adverse outcomes. Nevertheless, recognizing the relationship between PEW and a higher morbidity and mortality reminds clinicians of the importance of nutrition in PD.

We will review some commonly used markers of the nutritional status of patients undergoing PD, the factors that may contribute to an abnormal nutritional state, as well as potential management options. We will also briefly discuss the problem of obesity in PD.

COMMON METHODS USED TO ASSESS NUTRITIONAL STATUS

An ideal marker of nutritional status would be one that is easily measured, reliable, inexpensive, and unaffected by the patient's underlying diseases or inflammatory status. There is no ideal marker, so we are forced to rely on surrogate measures and each has important limitations. A more detailed discussion of this subject can be found in Chapter 18.

Physical Examination

The best starting point in an assessment of nutritional status is the careful physical examination. Features that may be suggestive of PEW include wasting of the temporalis, interosseous, quadriceps, or deltoid muscle groups and loss of subcutaneous fat. While the presence of edema may be suggestive of protein malnutrition in the general population, it cannot be relied upon in patients with end-stage renal disease (ESRD) who frequently have extracellular fluid volume expansion that is unrelated to their nutritional status.

Subjective Global Assessment

The subjective global assessment (SGA) is a clinical tool that incorporates information elicited from the patient's history (weight change, dietary intake, gastrointestinal symptoms, and functional impairment) as well as a physical examination. This information is then scored and patients are divided into one of 3 categories: well nourished, mild/moderate malnutrition, or severe malnutrition. While SGA can be used to distinguish severe malnutrition from normal nutrition, it is neither a sensitive nor reliable predictor of the degree of malnutrition.

Anthropometry

Anthropometric measures are among the simplest methods of assessing nutritional status. These include weight, the calculated body mass index (BMI), mid-arm circumference, and skinfold thickness. While easy to measure, these indices are relatively insensitive to changes in body composition; they may be helpful when used in conjunction with other tests.

Albumin/Prealbumin

Serum albumin is the most frequently used measure of nutrition in patients with chronic kidney disease (CKD) or ESRD. Advantages of using serum albumin include its ease of measurement and low cost. The primary limitation is that albumin is a negative acute phase reactant, so albumin decreases in response to inflammation. Consequently, a low albumin cannot reliably distinguish signs of PEW from inflammation. Even a normal albumin level cannot be taken as a sign of adequate nutrition, because a normal albumin has been reported in patients with marked malnutrition in association with eating disorders.

Prealbumin is the precursor of the more abundant plasma protein, albumin. It has a shorter half-life and hence, is a more sensitive measure of changes in visceral protein stores compared with albumin. Despite this potential benefit, prealbumin levels are subject to the same changes in response to inflammation as is albumin, and the cost of a prealbumin assay is higher.

Bioelectrical Impedance Analysis

Bioelectrical impedance analysis (BIA) is a technique used to determine body composition by providing an estimate of total body water and can then be used to estimate lean body mass and fat mass. While the device is easy to use, it is not readily available in all PD units, and its use requires a trained operator. For the BIA to be accurate, a patient must be edema-free, a state that is not always present in patients undergoing dialysis. In addition, the estimates of lean body mass are based on comparisons of the BIA of the patient undergoing PD with estimates made in healthy individuals. The estimates should be compared with those made in well-nourished patients undergoing PD.

Normalized Protein Equivalent of Total Nitrogen Appearance

Ingested proteins are metabolized to several nitrogenous products, the principal one being urea. As a result, the normalized protein equivalent of total nitrogen appearance (nPNA) can be calculated from the urea appearance rate. The utility of the nPNA is that in a metabolically stable patient, it is an accurate reflection of the dietary protein. There are several important concerns with the use of nPNA in the assessment of nutritional status. While the information provided by the nPNA is helpful, dietary protein intake is only one component of nutritional status. Furthermore, factors other than dietary protein intake may influence the generation of urea. For example, a catabolic patient will have increased urea generation resulting in an overestimation of dietary protein. The process of normalizing the PNA to body weight is of concern because the nPNA is lowest in well nourished or obese patients.

Despite the limitations associated with each of these markers, their use (either in isolation or in combination) can give the clinician a general sense of the nutritional status in the patient undergoing PD. Unfortunately, the lack of a criterion standard has limited our ability to identify malnutrition with certainty and to quantitate its severity in patients with ESRD.

FACTORS THAT CONTRIBUTE TO PROTEIN–ENERGY WASTING IN PATIENTS RECEIVING PERITONEAL DIALYSIS

Several factors can influence the nutritional status of patients undergoing PD, only some of which are common to all patients with ESRD. These factors will be discussed in detail below. Other conventional factors affecting nutrition that are unrelated to renal disease should also be considered, but are not discussed further.

Factors Present in All Patients with End-Stage Renal Disease

One of the most important contributors to inadequate nutrition is the constellation of abnormalities present in uremia. As GFR declines, uremic toxins accumulate, leading to symptoms of nausea and diminished appetite. This is particularly evident in terms of dietary protein because it can decline in patients with advancing CKD. While there are likely several mediators of the anorexia seen in advanced CKD and ESRD, increased levels of the anorexigenic hormone, leptin, may play an important role. Uremic symptoms and decreased protein intake can lead to PEW. The corollary is that providing "adequate" solute clearance will ameliorate these symptoms. While there may be incremental benefit associated with increasing dialysis dose, there is likely a threshold above which increased clearance does not provide added nutritional benefit (as shown in ADEMEX study of patients undergoing PD). The effect of uremia on appetite is, therefore, most relevant among predialysis patients and dialysis patients who are being under dialyzed.

Concomitant with increasing levels of uremic toxins, patients with advancing CKD frequently develop metabolic acidosis. This acidosis is because of a combination of impaired ammoniagenesis and the accumulation of dietary sulfates and phosphates. Based on several animal and human studies, it has become clear that acidosis leads to protein catabolism and results in negative nitrogen balance. A major mediator of this protein catabolic effect is the ubiquitin-proteasome proteolytic pathway. If not corrected, metabolic acidosis will contribute to malnutrition in predialysis patients. Once dialysis is initiated, however, the high concentration of lactate or bicarbonate in the dialysate usually resolves the acidosis, and it should not be a major factor in most patients with apparent PEW once PD has been initiated. One group of patients receiving dialysis who may be at risk of persistent metabolic acidosis is the group taking sevelamer HCl as a phosphate binder; in this case, the use of the carbonate form of sevelamer may avoid this problem.

Independent of the protein catabolism caused by metabolic acidosis, patients receiving dialysis appear to have chronic catabolism. While the basis for the increased protein breakdown present in patients with uremia is not fully understood, a major mechanism is resistance to anabolic hormones such as insulin and insulin-like growth factor 1 (IGF-1). This may explain why protein catabolism is further accelerated among diabetic patients receiving dialysis, who are known to have a high degree of insulin resistance.

Another important mechanism for protein catabolism in ESRD is chronic inflammation. The basis for inflammation is often multifactorial and may involve uremia per se, infection, periodontal disease, bioincompatibility of dialysis solutions, as well as genetic factors. The result of chronic inflammation is the release of proinflammatory cytokines. One such proinflammatory cytokine that has been implicated is tumor necrosis factor-alpha (TNF-α), which can induce NF-kappa B activation, promoting skeletal muscle wasting via the ubiquitin-proteasome proteolytic system. Proinflammatory cytokines such as TNF-α have also been shown to suppress appetite, possibly by increasing leptin production. While malnutrition and inflammation frequently coexist in certain disease states, the above data suggest that inflammation may also be causally linked to the PEW found in some patients with kidney disease.

Advanced CKD and ESRD also impose a major psychological burden on patients. Some patients experience depressive symptoms or a sense of apathy. These feelings can contribute to decreased appetite and a decline in nutritional status.

In addition to the above issues, dietary management of patients with advanced CKD and ESRD can be challenging because of hyperphosphatemia. Unfortunately, foods that are high in phosphorus are often excellent sources of protein, and caution is required when advising these patients about dietary restrictions that improve phosphate control because it may come at the expense of excessive protein restriction.

Factors Specific to Peritoneal Dialysis

As a renal replacement modality, PD takes advantage of the fact that the peritoneum provides an excellent membrane for diffusive and convective clearance. The instillation of fluid into the peritoneal cavity may, however, contribute to PEW in some patients through several mechanisms.

Firstly, while the movement of uremic toxins and potassium down a concentration gradient from the peritoneal capillaries into the dialysate is advantageous, the movement of protein and amino acids in the same direction is not. It is known that protein losses into the peritoneal dialysate can be quite variable. In one study, protein losses ranged from 3.5 to 13.2 g/day and unless protein intake at least matches protein losses, patients undergoing PD will be prone to a chronic state of negative protein balance in a manner that is similar to the nephrotic syndrome. Some of the variability in the degree of protein loss relates to peritoneal transport status, with rapid transporters losing more protein compared with slow transporters. Certain factors increase protein losses above a patient's usual baseline rate; peritonitis causes peritoneal capillaries to become "leaky" and with prolonged peritoneal inflammation, the protein lost and the cytokines released can have an important adverse impact on nutritional status. Another cause of protein losses in the effluent is ascites. Protein loss in patients with ascites may exceed 30 g/day in the weeks after PD initiation; there are data suggesting that the amount of losses diminishes over time. When initiating PD in a patient with ascites, careful attention must be paid to the risk of protein malnutrition.

The instillation of fluid into the peritoneal cavity may have other adverse effects. It is known that intraperitoneal pressure rises when a patient has dialysate in their peritoneum, and that the increase in pressure is related to the size of the patient, the volume of fluid instilled, and the position of the patient. This increased intra-abdominal pressure may lead to symptoms of early satiety and consequent reduced dietary intake. This hypothesis is supported by results of two small studies in which gastric emptying was significantly slower in patients with dialysate in the abdomen compared to those with an empty abdomen. The most extreme delays in gastric emptying occurred in those with small body surface area. Delayed emptying may be most noticeable in diabetic patients undergoing PD who frequently have pre-existing gastroparesis.

An additional risk factor for PEW relates to the primary constituent of the PD fluid being instilled. Most patients undergoing PD are dialyzed with dextrose-based solutions that contain concentrations of dextrose ranging from 76 mmol/L for a 1.5% dextrose solution to 215 mmol/L for a 4.25% dextrose solution. A high dextrose concentration in the peritoneum leads to net absorption of dextrose, and the amount of dextrose absorbed will vary widely, depending on the dextrose concentration, the time that the fluid is left to dwell, and the peritoneal transport status (rapid transporters absorbing the most). This is relevant because the caloric load from a single dextrose exchange ranges from approximately 50 to 300 kcal. This high carbohydrate load can reduce the appetite and hence the consumption of foods rich in protein and other nutrients.

MANAGEMENT OF PATIENTS RECEIVING PERITONEAL DIALYSIS WITH PROTEIN–ENERGY WASTING

In managing PEW in patients undergoing PD, it is of paramount importance to identify the primary contributors to PEW in an individual patient. This leads to the design of a multifactorial management plan that is most likely to be successful.

General Measures

While dialysis adequacy is intuitively important, there is little evidence that increasing dialysis dose improves nutritional status. In the ADEMEX study, a higher dialysis dose did not improve nutritional parameters. Still, it is uncertain whether these results can be generalized to patients undergoing PD who have PEW. One study showed modest nutritional benefit to increasing dialysis dose in malnourished patients without comorbidity, while two other studies showed increased nPNA when the number of exchanges was increased from 3 to 4 per day. The use of nPNA must be interpreted with caution because Kt/V and nPNA are mathematically coupled so nPNA can rise artificially with an increase in Kt/V.

The Kidney Disease Outcomes Quality Initiative (K/DOQI) of the National Kidney Foundation in the U.S. has suggested a minimum weekly Kt/V of 1.7 for PD adequacy. Despite conflicting evidence about the benefits of increasing dialysis dose and nutrition, if a patient has symptoms of anorexia or evidence of PEW despite a Kt/V greater than 1.7, a trial of aiming for a higher dialysis dose is warranted.

The importance of correcting metabolic acidosis was highlighted in a randomized controlled trial in which prevalent patients with serum bicarbonate less than 25 mmol/L receiving continuous ambulatory peritoneal dialysis (CAPD) were randomized to receive oral sodium bicarbonate or placebo. At 12 months, the bicarbonate group had a higher SGA score and an increase in nPNA as compared with placebo. Therefore, persistent metabolic acidosis should be corrected with oral sodium bicarbonate if hypervolemia is not a limiting factor.

Early involvement of a renal dietician to provide counseling and longitudinal follow-up is invaluable. In a stable chronic patient receiving PD, the recommended total daily caloric intake is 30 to 35 kcal per kg of body weight per day. Because of protein losses in the PD effluent, the recommended dietary protein intake is 1.2 to 1.3 g per kg of body weight per day, which is higher than the 0.75 g/kg/day recommended for the general population. At least 50% of ingested dietary protein should be of high biological value, meaning that it contains an appropriate balance of essential amino acids necessary for protein anabolism. High biological value proteins are generally provided by animal sources of protein, such as meat, poultry, fish, eggs, and milk products.

If daily protein and caloric requirements are not being met despite dietary counseling and a seemingly adequate dose of dialysis, other sources of nutritional supplementation should be considered. These include oral supplements, enteral nutrition via nasogastric feeding tubes, and intraperitoneal supplementation with amino acid-based dialysate.

Oral Supplementation and Enteral Feeding

When patients undergoing PD cannot achieve their daily calorie and/or protein requirement through a combination of dietary ingestion and absorption of calories from the dialysate, a trial of oral supplements is recommended. There are several preparations available, allowing the choice of a supplement to be tailored to the patient's needs; there are high calorie supplements for those with inadequate caloric intake and high protein supplements for those with inadequate dietary protein. Despite the common availability of these agents, there are few systematic examinations of their efficacy in patients undergoing PD. The use of an egg albumin-based protein supplement was assessed in an open-label randomized trial involving 28 patients receiving CAPD followed for 6 months. The supplement resulted in an increase in serum albumin, calorie and protein intake, and nPNA when baseline and follow-up measurements were compared. The frequency of moderate or severe PEW as assessed by SGA was significantly reduced in the supplement group compared with results from the control group. Based on the potential benefits and the noninvasiveness of this approach, a trial of oral supplementation in an ESRD patient with ESRD who has PEW regardless of the dialytic modality is warranted.

Unfortunately, there is a subgroup of patients with PEW who may be unable to comply with oral supplementation, particularly if there is a poor appetite. In these patients, enteral feeding via a nasogastric tube may be tried, although the efficacy is unproven. Insertion of a percutaneous gastrostomy tube in patients who have already initiated PD is not advisable because the incidence of peritonitis is extremely high. If insertion is absolutely necessary, the patient should have dialysis fluid drained during the insertion procedure and be kept dry for at least 24 hours afterward. Prophylactic antibiotics should be considered, and, if possible, the stomach should be fixed to the anterior abdominal wall to minimize the risks of contamination.

Amino Acid-based Dialysate

The above strategies rely on the classic paradigm of delivering protein via the gastrointestinal tract. The alternative is to use an amino acid-based dialysis solution to supplement protein intake. One 2 L exchange of a 1.1% amino acid solution will contain 22 g of amino acids, or for a 70 kg patient, approximately 0.3 g/kg/day if provided in one exchange daily.

Several studies have addressed the role of amino acid solutions, with conflicting results (Table 12-1). Inconsistent findings in these studies likely relate to the small patient numbers as well as heterogeneity in the patient populations, the duration of follow-up time, and differences in measures used to assess nutritional status. In one study, 105 patients were randomized to receive their usual dextrose-based dialysate or substitution of one to two amino acid exchanges daily. At the end of the 3-month follow up, the amino acid group had higher levels of IGF-1, prealbumin, and serum transferrin. A second trial randomized 60 malnourished patients undergoing CAPD to receive either dextrose-based dialysate alone or dextrose-based dialysate with substitution of 1 amino acid exchange daily. After 3 years, there was no benefit in terms of patient survival or a composite nutritional index. However, the amino acid group demonstrated stabilization of serum albumin levels and a sustained increase in nPNA. Short-term, crossover studies of both fasting and fed patients receiving PD have suggested that using a mixture of amino acid-based solutions and dextrose-based solutions during cycler therapy is an alternative approach to improving protein synthesis.

While these results suggest potential benefit, there are concerns regarding intraperitoneal amino acid supplementation.

Table 12-1. Studies of intraperitoneal amino acid supplementation*

Author, Year	Study Design	Patients (n)	Patient Population	Duration of Follow-up (months)	No. of Amino Acid Exchanges/Day	Result
Schilling, 1985	PC	12	Postperitonitis	1	2	*No effect
Faller, 1995	PC	15	Unselected	3	1	*Increased albumin, transferrin levels
Chertow, 1995	RCT, crossover	183	Unselected	2–19	1	*Increased albumin
Misra, 1996	RCT, crossover	18	Unselected	6	1	*Improved composite nutrition score *No change in albumin or transferrin overall *Increase in albumin in those who started with albumin <30
Jones, 1998	RCT	105	Malnourished	3	1–2	*Increased IGF-1, prealbumin, transferrin
Gonzalez, 1999	PC	14	2 groups: malnourished, well nourished	12	1	*Increased albumin in malnourished patients
Taylor, 2002	RC	22	Malnourished	6–26	1	*Increased albumin, nPCR
Li, 2003	RCT	60	Malnourished	36	1	*No change in composite nutritional index *Increased nPNA and DPI

*Includes only studies with at least 10 adult patients and a minimum of 1 month of follow-up.
DPI, dietary protein intake; IGF-1, insulin-like growth factor 1; nPCR, normalized protein catabolic rate; nPNA, normalized protein equivalent of total nitrogen appearance; PC, prospective cohort study; RC, retrospective cohort study; RCT, randomized controlled trial.

Firstly, patients receiving amino acid solutions can develop metabolic acidosis. If uncorrected, this acidosis may itself promote protein catabolism (see above). Secondly, the provision of supplemental amino acids may not reverse PEW if there is an insufficient concomitant caloric intake. In fact, sufficient carbohydrate intake may be a prerequisite for protein anabolism, even with amino acid supplementation. This was illustrated in a study of prevalent patients undergoing PD in which positive nitrogen balance was more tightly correlated with total energy intake than with protein intake. Among patients with similar protein intakes, the most positive nitrogen balance occurred in patients who had the highest total caloric intake. In summary, larger studies with longer term follow up are required to confirm the safety and efficacy of amino acid solutions in malnourished patients undergoing PD.

Other Novel Treatment Options

Given that protein catabolism in uremic patients is in part related to resistance to the effects of anabolic hormones, the possible role of exogenous administration of hormones to reverse this catabolism has been examined. Both recombinant human growth hormone (rhGH) and recombinant human IGF-1 (rh-IGF-1) have been shown in small, short-term studies to have a protein anabolic effect. The androgen, nandrolone decanoate, given by intramuscular injections was associated with improvement in both anthropometric and biochemical nutritional markers in a study lasting 6 months. As with the amino acid-based dialysates, longer-term studies of these agents to evaluate safety and efficacy are required to support these preliminary findings.

The best-studied appetite stimulant is megestrol acetate; it has been used successfully in patients with cachexia related to cancer or acquired immunodeficiency syndrome. One of the limitations of its use, however, has been its side effects, including suppression of the hypothalamic-pituitary-adrenal axis, hypogonadism, and an increased risk of thromboembolism. In one study of 32 patients undergoing PD, two thirds of patients receiving megestrol reported improved appetite along with weight gain and a trend toward a higher albumin. Another study of 10 dialysis patients showed significant increases in weight, albumin, and tricep skinfold thickness. While the positive results and lack of side effects are encouraging, larger-scale placebo-controlled trials are required to verify the safety and efficacy of megestrol acetate before recommending its widespread use.

Another potential therapeutic agent is ghrelin, a hormone secreted by the stomach that that seems to function as an appetite enhancer. In a randomized, placebo-controlled crossover study of 9 patients undergoing PD, subcutaneous administration of single dose ghrelin before a meal led to a doubling of energy intake. As with other appetite-stimulating agents, further study is required before recommending widespread use.

Given the important role of inflammation in anorexia and protein catabolism, a method of blocking inflammation would be welcome. To date, there are no effective anti-inflammatory strategies beyond trying to reverse the underlying condition causing the inflammatory state.

OBESITY IN PERITONEAL DIALYSIS

Among patients undergoing PD, the increasing prevalence of obesity is an emerging problem; 34% of prevalent patients undergoing PD from a U.S. Medicare cohort had a BMI >28. The rising prevalence of PD patients may be due, in part, to the fact that the average BMI at dialysis initiation is rising. Other factors could also be involved in patients who gain weight after PD is initiated. One major contributor to obesity is the dextrose that is absorbed from the peritoneal cavity. In a randomized controlled study in which 175 patients undergoing PD were given 2.5% dextrose or 7.5% icodextrin for the long, nighttime dwell period, the dextrose group gained on average 2 kg over a 1-year period in contrast to no average gain of weight in the icodextrin-treated group. Weight gain may be particularly problematic among rapid transport patients because they absorb dextrose more rapidly and require higher dextrose concentrations to maintain ultrafiltration. In a single center study of 114 patients on PD for at least 2 years, the unifying characteristics of the 8 patients who gained at least 10 kg were the presence of minimal residual renal function and high average transport status. Both characteristics could have mandated the use of higher concentrations of dextrose.

Weight gain in patients undergoing PD is not a universal phenomenon even though all patients are exposed to dextrose-based dialysate. Possibly, genetic differences in metabolic rates may contribute to fat accumulation in some patients. In fact, a polymorphism within the uncoupling protein 2 (UCP2) gene is associated with significantly greater weight gains and increases in body fat mass in patients treated with PD. Interestingly, when both patients undergoing PD and patients undergoing hemodialysis (HD) bearing the polymorphism were studied, an increase in total and truncal fat mass during the first year of therapy was only observed among patients treated by PD, suggesting a possible role for defective UCP2 in dissipating the excess energy of the high glucose environment that is unique to PD.

Whether obesity in patients undergoing PD has an adverse effect on outcome is a matter of debate. A higher BMI has been shown to be associated with lower mortality in patients receiving hemodialysis, but the results in patients undergoing PD are more heterogeneous. This may relate to the inability of BMI to distinguish muscle mass from fat mass. In one study among patients with a high BMI, a high muscle mass conferred a protective effect, whereas a high body fat was associated with higher all-cause and cardiovascular mortality (91).

There are several important considerations in managing obese patients undergoing PD. As a result of their high fat mass, it becomes difficult to predict reliably the urea distribution volume (V) in obese patients, rendering Kt/V a less accurate marker of dialysis adequacy in this setting. In addition, given that obese patients have increased intraperitoneal pressure at baseline, they may be at higher risk for pericatheter or abdominal leaks and subsequently for hernias. With this in mind, nocturnal intermittent PD can be used when there is significant residual renal function. Alternatively, smaller volume exchanges could be added during the day if additional clearance is required. Efforts should be made to limit the dextrose load. The first strategy for limiting dextrose accumulation and metabolism is to minimize the amount of peritoneal ultrafiltration required to maintain euvolemia. This includes salt restriction and the promotion of salt and water loss in the urine with diuretics in patients with residual renal function. If these strategies are inadequate and high dextrose concentrations are required to control fluid accumulation, icodextrin, which is not associated with weight gain, can be used in the long dwell. If glucose is still excessive, amino acid solutions for PD can be considered to replace one dextrose exchange daily. However, both icodextrin and amino acid dialysis fluids represent caloric loads for patients. An experienced renal dietician can help obese patients undergoing PD make informed decisions about proper food choices and the optimal daily caloric intake considering the dextrose delivered during the dialysis.

CONCLUSION

Nutritional derangements are common in patients on peritoneal dialysis and are often multifactorial. An awareness of the prevalence of PEW is particularly important, because patients with poor nutritional status have been shown to have increased morbidity and mortality relative to those who are well nourished. While several markers of nutrition may be helpful in the assessment of nutritional status, all are subject to important limitations. In the absence of a criterion standard, however, we rely on these markers to decide which patients would benefit from more intensive strategies to treat PEW. While some general preventive and management strategies are currently utilized, further research is required to delineate the role of amino-acid based dialysate, as well as novel agents such as appetite stimulants and anabolic agents.

Selected Readings

Bargman JM. The rationale and ultimate limitations of urea kinetic modelling in the estimation of nutritional status. Perit Dial Int 1996;16:347–351.

Canada-USA (CANUSA) Peritoneal Dialysis Study Group. Adequacy of dialysis and nutrition in continuous peritoneal dialysis: association with clinical outcomes. J Am Soc Nephrol 1996;7:198–207.

Cano F, Azocar M, Cavada G, et al. Kt/V and nPNA in pediatric peritoneal dialysis: a clinical or a mathematical association? Pediatr Nephrol 2006;21:114–118.

Chung SH, Heimbürger O, Stenvinkel P, et al. Influence of peritoneal transport rate, inflammation, and fluid removal on nutritional status and clinical outcome in prevalent peritoneal dialysis patients. Perit Dial Int 2003;23:174–183.

Costero O, Bajo MA, del Peso G, et al. Treatment of anorexia and malnutrition in peritoneal dialysis patients with megestrol acetate. Adv Perit Dial 2004;20:209–212.

Fein PA, Madane SJ, Jorden A, et al. Outcome of percutaneous endoscopic gastrostomy feeding in patients on peritoneal dialysis. Adv Perit Dial 2001;17:148–152.

González-Espinoza L, Gutiérrez-Chávez J, del Campo FM, et al. Randomized, open label, controlled clinical trial of oral administration of an egg albumin-based protein supplement to patients on continuous ambulatory peritoneal dialysis. Perit Dial Int 2005;25:173–180.

Ikizler TA, Wingard RL, Breyer JA, et al. Short-term effects of recombinant human growth hormone in CAPD patients. Kidney Int 1994; 46:1178–1183

Jones M, Hagen T, Boyle CA, et al. Treatment of malnutrition with 1.1% amino acid peritoneal dialysis solution: results of a multicenter outpatient study. Am J Kidney Dis 1998;32:761–769.

Kopple JD, Greene T, Chumlea WC, et al. Relationship between nutritional status and the glomerular filtration rate: results from the MDRD study. Kidney Int 2000;57:1688–1703.

Kramer HJ, Saranathan A, Luke A, et al. Increasing body mass index and obesity in the incident ESRD population. J Am Soc Nephrol 2006;17:1453–1459.

Li FK, Chan LY, Woo JC, et al. A 3-year, prospective, randomized, controlled study on amino acid dialysate in patients on CAPD. Am J Kidney Dis 2003;42:173–183.

McDonald SP, Collins JF, Johnson DW. Obesity is associated with worse peritoneal dialysis outcomes in the Australia and New Zealand patient populations. J Am Soc Nephrol 2003;14:2894–2901.

Mitch WE, Du J, Bailey JL, et al. Mechanisms causing muscle proteolysis in uremia: the influence of insulin and cytokines. Miner Electrolyte Metab 1999;25:216–219.

NKF-K/DOQI Clinical Practice Guidelines for Peritoneal Dialysis Adequacy: update 2006. Available at: http://www.kidney.org/ professionals/KDOQI/guideline_upHD_PD_VA/. Accessed May 1, 2008.

Paniagua R, Amato D, Vonesh E, et al. Mexican Nephrology Collaborative Study Group. Effects of increased peritoneal clearances on mortality rates in peritoneal dialysis: ADEMEX, a prospective, randomized, controlled trial. J Am Soc Nephrol 2002;13:1307–1320.

Prasad N, Gupta A, Sinha A, et al. Changes in nutritional status on follow-up of an incident cohort of continuous ambulatory peritoneal dialysis patients. J Ren Nutr 2008;18:195–201.

Ramkumar N, Pappas LM, Beddhu S. Effect of body size and body composition on survival in peritoneal dialysis patients. Perit Dial Int 2005;25:461–469.

Szeto CC, Wong TY, Chow KM, et al. Oral sodium bicarbonate for the treatment of metabolic acidosis in peritoneal dialysis patients: a randomized placebo-control trial. J Am Soc Nephrol 2003;14: 2119–2126.

Wang X, Axelsson J, Nordfors L, et al. Changes in fat mass after initiation of maintenance dialysis is influenced by the uncoupling protein 2 exon 8 insertion/deletion polymorphism. Nephrol Dial Transplant 2007;22:196–202.

Wolfson M, Piraino B, Hamburger RJ, et al. Icodextrin Study Group. A randomized controlled trial to evaluate the efficacy and safety of icodextrin in peritoneal dialysis. Am J Kidney Dis 2002;40: 1055–1065.

Nutritional Requirements of Kidney Transplant Patients

Simin Goral and Melissa B. Bleicher

Successful kidney transplantation can be a liberating experience for the recipient. In addition to being freed from the rigors of maintenance dialysis, a recipient is freed from the strict limitation of the "renal" diet. This, along with an improved overall sense of well-being and improved appetite, results in an increase in body weight. The kidney transplant recipient now faces a new set of dietary challenges related to pre-existing comorbidities, potential new metabolic abnormalities, and nutritional requirements, which vary in the immediate and long-term posttransplant period. Along with these challenges, some patients never achieve optimal kidney function posttransplant, and most will eventually suffer from a decline in allograft function over time. In light of all of these dynamic factors, it behooves those caring for kidney transplant recipients to become knowledgeable in proper nutritional therapy for this population.

OBESITY

Obesity at the Time of Transplantation

The National Health and Examination Survey in 2003–2004 indicated that approximately 66% of U.S. adults were either overweight (BMI 25–29.9 kg/m2) or obese (BMI 30–34.9 kg/m2). Obesity is considered a risk factor for the development and progression of certain etiologies of chronic kidney disease (CKD). Impressively, weight loss in the predialysis population either by means of lifestyle modification or surgically mediated weight loss can sometimes halt progression or even improve kidney function. As expected, the prevalence of obesity among patients listed for a kidney transplant has increased significantly. Importantly, there is a general reluctance among transplant surgeons and nephrologists in transplanting obese patients. In the United States, the likelihood of receiving a kidney transplant progressively decreased between 1995 and 2006 with increasing degrees of obesity. To justify this trend and refute any possibility of obesity discrimination, the transplant community must demonstrate any difference in survival between transplantation and maintenance dialysis across degrees of obesity as well as any difference in patient and allograft survival across all levels of BMI. Despite the limitations of retrospective design, large epidemiologic studies analyzing United States Renal Data System (USRDS) and Scientific Registry of Transplant Recipients (SRTR) databases support a survival benefit of transplantation over dialysis in the obese population.

In the setting of a shortage of transplantable kidneys, it is incumbent upon the medical community to allocate this resource so as to maximize the benefit for society at large, and not just

Table 13-1.   Contributors to posttransplant weight gain

- Loss of anorectic factors
- Loss of the dietary restriction of advanced kidney disease
- Improvement in taste of food
- Effect of immunosuppressive agents

each individual or small cohort of individuals. There is conflicting data in the literature in regard to any adverse effect of BMI at the time of transplantation on patient and allograft outcome. An analysis of 51,927 primary adult kidney transplants in the USRDS database demonstrated a strong association between BMI and both patient and allograft survival at both ends of the BMI spectrum, yet elevated BMI was associated with a worse graft survival independent of patient survival as well as delayed graft function (DGF). In contrast, a more recent analysis of the Australian and New Zealand Dialysis and Transplant Registry assessed the relationship between BMI at transplant and allograft outcomes in 5684 patients transplanted between 1991 and 2004 and did not demonstrate a significant relationship of elevated BMI and inferior patient or allograft survival on multivariate analysis. Furthermore, underweight patients had greater late ($\geq$5 year) death-censored graft loss, which was attributed to greater chronic allograft nephropathy. Nevertheless, it remains unclear whether obesity itself or factors related to obesity are associated with poorer allograft outcomes. In addition, the effect of intentional weight loss in this population in preparation for transplantation remains unknown.

Posttransplant Obesity

Weight gain is quite common in the posttransplant period. Mean weight gains seem to fall within the range of 8% $+/-$ 10% at 1 year and slightly greater thereafter. The impact of weight changes on patient and allograft survival remains unclear. A retrospective analysis revealed a correlation of poor weight gain and low BMI posttransplant with worse kidney function and a greater incidence of chronic allograft nephropathy. In contrast, two retrospective studies found that patients with better kidney function, measured by the Cockcroft-Gault equation, gained more weight posttransplant. Whether poor weight gain is a marker of other confounding factors associated with either an acute or a chronic inflammatory state and not a direct function of weight itself is unknown. Similarly, it is well-established that weight gain is strongly associated with increased risk of an unfavorable metabolic milieu including hyperglycemia, hypertension, and hyperlipidemia, which are all highly prevalent posttransplantation. Prospective studies are necessary to clarify the correlation between allograft function and posttransplant weight gain as well as what degree of change in weight correlates with worse clinical outcomes.

The stimulus for posttransplant weight gain is thought to be multifactorial (Table 13-1). The impact of immunosuppressive therapy on posttransplant weight gain is of particular interest because this is one area in which a physician may intervene in an attempt to impact a change in weight. Over the past two decades, patients have classically remained on triple therapy including low-dose prednisone, a calcineurin inhibitor (CNI), and an antiproliferative agent. Many in the transplant community believed that, based on the physiologic effects of excessive exogenous corticosteroid administration, chronic steroid therapy had an adverse effect on new-onset diabetes, hyperlipidemia, and weight gain posttransplant. Beliefs regarding the effect of either CNI or antiproliferative agents, both as a class or individually, remained unclear. A recent retrospective analysis evaluated the difference in posttransplant weight gain over the first 3 years posttransplant in 95 patients treated with standard triple immunosuppression and those with either complete steroid avoidance or early steroid withdrawal. Using a chi-square analysis there was no significant difference among percentage of patients who gained weight after transplantation between groups ($p = 0.27$). However, the largest retrospective analysis of the association between chronic steroid exposure and posttransplant weight gain, which included 328 patients, found that while all patients gained weight during the first posttransplant year, there was a significant difference between the steroid withdrawal and maintenance steroid group. In light of these studies as well as a few other small retrospective analyses, it appears that posttransplant weight gain is multifactorial and the relative contribution of steroids, if present, is small.

The most common cause of allograft loss in the U.S. is currently death with a functioning graft secondary to cardiovascular diseases (CVD). It is established within the general population that obesity and comorbidities related to increased adiposity increase the risk for CVD and death. While this has not been prospectively confirmed in the kidney transplant population, it is reasonable to speculate that minimizing all modifiable cardiovascular risk factors including obesity in transplant recipients could improve both patient and allograft survival. Strategies to either maintain or lose weight posttransplant include lifestyle modification with caloric restriction and increased physical activity, pharmacotherapy, and surgery. A prospective study to assess the efficacy of a weight reduction program in motivated overweight, obese, and severely obese transplant recipients through lifestyle medication demonstrated less weight gain in the motivated group who met with a healthcare professional for 40 minutes and reviewed a detailed three-day food diary and had anthropometric measurements taken yet received no dietary recommendations. While the group was too small to draw any conclusions, these encouraging findings suggest that simply making patients conscious of their dietary habits and making them aware of weight gain posttransplant without any further active intervention may have a significant impact.

There are few medications currently available in the U.S. approved for weight loss. One such medication, Orlistat, is a reversible inhibitor of pancreatic lipase. Inhibition of this enzyme results in some degree of fat malabsorption and reduced net caloric consumption. Patients must follow a low-fat diet as well, or they will suffer from steatorrhea. While no studies currently exist evaluating the safety or efficacy of orlistat in the kidney transplant population, a small prospective study was performed in liver transplant patients. As there is evidence in the literature of cyclosporine malabsorption with orlistat, this study exclusively included patients taking tacrolimus. There were no documented cases of rejection with orlistat treatment. While weight did not change with orlistat use, there was a significant decrease in waist circumference following 6 months of therapy. As with all gastrointestinal conditions associated with fat malabsorption, the risk for enteric hyperoxaluria with secondary nephrolithiasis and even nephrocalcinosis remains a concern as well. Formal evaluation of both safety, especially at high doses of orlistat, and efficacy are necessary in the kidney transplant population.

Sibutramine is a serotonin and epinephrine reuptake inhibitor that acts centrally to affect satiety. Efficacy of this agent for weight loss in the general population has been established. The efficacy of sibutramine in the kidney transplant population remains unknown, but one should monitor CNI levels closely with introduction of this medication for weight loss management because both are metabolized by the cytochrome P450 3A4 pathway.

Surgery, either in the form of gastric banding or gastric bypass, remains the most invasive option for weight loss. Case reports and small case series are present in the literature; however, formal documentation of the effect of Roux-en-y gastric bypass on the bioavailability of immunosuppressive agents is lacking. Should it be felt that the morbidity and mortality risk from severe obesity be sufficient to justify the risk of allograft rejection secondary to immunosuppressive malabsorption, the patient must be informed of these risks and serum immunosuppressive drug levels must be followed closely.

HYPERGLYCEMIA

Abnormalities in glucose metabolism following kidney transplantation have been recognized as common complications that may adversely affect long term both allograft and patient outcomes. Transplant-associated hyperglycemia (TAH) has been proposed as terminology that encompasses new onset diabetes mellitus (NODM), impaired fasting glucose, and impaired glucose tolerance. The incidence of NODM posttransplantation falls within the range of 2% to 53%. While prospective, randomized, controlled interventional trials are absent in the posttransplant population, abundant evidence exists within the general population supporting the benefit of aggressive glycemic control on limiting microvascular and possibly cardiovascular events.

The pathogenesis of TAH is complex and multifactorial. In brief, TAH is the end result of an imbalance between insufficient insulin secretion, increased insulin metabolism, and insulin resistance by target organs. Often, some degree of impaired glucose tolerance may be present but unrecognized in the pretransplant setting, because the kidney contributes to insulin degradation and loss of kidney function results in decreased insulin metabolism. In such situations, placement of a functioning allograft will then restore normal insulin metabolism and unmask this imbalance. Nonmodifiable risk factors for TAH include advanced age, male gender, nonwhite ethnicity, family history, and polycystic

Table 13-2.   Contributors to transplant-associated hyperglycemia

Etiology:
   Imbalance between:
      Insufficient insulin secretion
      Increased insulin metabolism
      Insulin resistance by target organs
   Pretransplant impairment unmasked by increased renal insulin
      metabolism

Nonmodifiable risk factors	Modifiable Risk Factors
Advanced age	Hepatitis C infection
Male gender	Obesity
Nonwhite ethnicity	Physical inactivity
Family history	Weight gain
Polycystic kidney disease	Immunosuppressive medications

kidney disease. Modifiable risk factors include hepatitis C (HCV) infection, obesity, physical inactivity, weight gain, and immuno-suppressive regimens (Table 13-2).

Screening strategies for impaired glucose metabolism varies across transplant centers. Screening should begin during the initial transplant evaluation through taking a thorough medical and family history along with assessment of fasting plasma glucose. Those with normal fasting plasma glucose (glucose <100 mg/dL) or impaired fasting glucose (100<glucose<126 mg/dL) should have follow-up screening by an oral glucose tolerance test (OGTT) either annually or biannually while waiting for a transplant. Screening by OGTT will identify those with isolated postprandial hyperglycemia and those with diabetes mellitus (DM), which is masked by decreased insulin metabolism secondary to advanced CKD. Such screening strategy will identify those in need of treatment as well as those with prediabetic states, including impaired glucose tolerance or impaired fasting glucose, which may benefit from initiation of lifestyle changes to impede progression to overt DM. Pretransplant evaluation will also identify HCV-positive patients and provide an opportunity for a trial of viral clearance with interferon therapy. Attainment of a sustained viremic response pretransplant may then reduce the risk of TAH.

Hyperglycemia is very common in the immediate posttransplant setting. Most patients receive some form of induction therapy, which includes high-dose corticosteroids, and this along with the stress of surgery is implicated as the main contributors to impaired glycemic control during the first posttransplant week. Monoclonal antibodies against CD25, the IL2 receptor, used for induction immunosuppression have been associated with a greater incidence of TAH. Within 1 week of surgery the dose of steroids is tapered or completely withdrawn, making it less of a contributor to hyperglycemia.

Maintenance immunosuppression, which often includes low-dose prednisone, a CNI, an antiproliferative agent, or mammalian target of rapamycin inhibitor, is yet another contributor to TAH. Inferences from the transplantation literature seem to suggest that low-dose maintenance glucocorticoid therapy has minimal if any effect on long-term glucose metabolism. Cyclosporine was immediately recognized to negatively impact numerous metabolic parameters. With the approval of tacrolimus, a newer CNI, the transplant community had the feeling that this agent had a more favorable metabolic profile, with uncertainty in the area of glycemic control. A large international prospective randomized controlled trial that compared the glycemic influence of cyclosporine and tacrolimus showed that tacrolimus was associated with a significant increased risk of TAH and impaired fasting glucose at 6 months posttransplant without any difference in efficacy between the 2 agents. While less diabetogenic than tacrolimus, cyclosporin has also been recognized as a risk factor for TAH. Sirolimus has been reported to be more diabetogenic than cyclosporine, making conversion to sirolimus a less attractive option to the transplant physician seeking to minimize modifiable risk factors for TAH.

Hyperglycemia that persists once the steroid dosing is under 20 mg/day is predictive of long-term glycemic impairment. Diabetic education should begin prior to discharge from the hospital, and each patient with hyperglycemia should monitor both fasting and 2 hours' postprandial glucose concentrations. As always, treatment should include intensive education for lifestyle modifications including daily moderate exercise such as walking for at least 30 minutes daily, weight loss mediated by caloric restriction and increased energy expenditure, and dietary modification. The currently recommended diet should limit the daily carbohydrate intake to 130 to 180 grams as part of an 1800 to 2000 Kcal diet, with complete avoidance of concentrated sweets. Along with lifestyle modification, pharmacologic therapy is necessary as well. In the immediate posttransplant period exogenous insulin remains the treatment of choice; when both dosing of glucocorticoids as well as daily caloric intake varies from day to day, glycemic management is most safely and quickly attained with "sliding scale" dosing of rapid-acting insulin every 6 hours. Once postoperative stress subsides and the patient's diet and steroid dosing begins to stabilize, the cumulative insulin requirement is calculated and administered as a combination of basal and bolus insulin. Usually, one third to one half of the daily insulin requirement is administered as basal long-acting insulin, whereas the remaining insulin is administered as rapid-acting insulin immediately before each meal. When the 24-hour insulin requirement falls below 20 units/day, one can then consider transitioning the patient to oral insulin secretagogues like sulfonylurea or meglitinide. Because glycemic management is complex and dynamic in the early posttransplant period, a time when transplant recipients find themselves taking many new medications, collaboration with an endocrinologist would be helpful to achieve safe and effective glycemic control.

Kidney transplant recipients are felt to remain at increased risk for TAH throughout the lifespan of their allograft and therefore, continued diabetic screening is recommended in this population. For those patients who are not hyperglycemic on discharge from the hospital, international consensus guidelines recommend weekly assessment of fasting plasma glucose for the first post-transplant month and then every 3 months thereafter. Our institution, however, favors a more vigorous surveillance program with assessment of fasting plasma glucose monthly from month 1 through 6 and bimonthly through the remainder of the first posttransplant year. In addition, we screen all patients with an oral glucose tolerance test at 3 months posttransplant and then yearly thereafter, because OGTT was recently shown to be a more sensitive means of diagnosing NODM and impaired fasting glucose. Long-term management of TAH is similar to management in the general population. Minimizing exposure to diabetogenic maintenance immunosuppressive agents like glucocorticoids, CNI, and sirolimus may improve glycemic control. The adjunctive use of mycophenolic acid to spare tacrolimus exposure may reduce the incidence of TAH. Pharmacologic options in the long-term kidney transplant recipient are similar to that of the CKD population, with occasional dose adjustment necessary with deteriorating kidney function. Sulfonylureas directly stimulate insulin secretion from beta cells of the pancreas, thereby improving both fasting and postprandial glycemic control. Glipizide, a second-generation sulfonylurea, is predominantly metabolized by the liver and as such can be used with advanced kidney disease. However, such patients remain at increased risk for hypoglycemic events in the setting of a failing allograft and consequently will often require a dose adjustment. Meglitinides, including repaglinide and nateglinide, are insulin secretagogues with a rapid onset and short duration of action. These agents are most effective in treatment of postprandial hyperglycemia. As both agents are metabolized by the liver, the drugs may be used across all degrees of kidney function. The thiazolidinediones (TZD) improve glycemic control by increasing peripheral insulin sensitivity. Both rosiglitazone and pioglitazone do not have any apparent interaction with CNI metabolism and are considered both safe and effective for treatment in the kidney transplant recipient. Metformin is cleared by renal tubular secretion, and there are case reports of lactic acidosis in the setting of advanced renal impairment, limiting use of this agent in the setting of severe allograft dysfunction. A new class of agents available for diabetic management exerts their effect by promoting glucagon-like peptide 1 (GLP1) receptor activation. GLP1 stimulates insulin secretion in a glucose-dependent manner with minimal hypoglycemic potential. Additionally, it slows gastric emptying thereby suppressing appetite. Exenatide, the only GLP1 receptor agonist currently available, improves postprandial hyperglycemia and thus favorably improves HbA1c in diabetics along with a mean 4 to 5 kg weight loss over 18 months of treatment in the general population. Because this medication causes weight loss by delaying gastric emptying, immunosuppressive dosing may require adjustment and drug levels should be monitored closely with initiation of therapy. Exenatide is metabolized by the kidney and should not be used with a creatinine clearance <30 mL/minute. Sitagliptin, another drug with similar actions, inhibits the activity of dipeptidyl peptidase-IV (DPP-IV), the enzyme responsible for metabolism of GLP1. This agent, a pill administered once daily as compared with exenatide, which is a twice-daily injection, raises endogenous levels of GLP1 thereby resulting in improved fasting and postprandial glycemic control. Sitagliptin, however, does not have the added benefit of promoting weight loss. Dose adjustment is required in the setting of impaired kidney function, and information regarding the impact of this agent on immunosuppression drug dosing is currently unknown. As such, drug levels should be carefully monitored with initiation of therapy.

HYPERLIPIDEMIA

Hyperlipidemia after transplantation is a multifactorial phenomenon resulting from genetic and environmental factors, some of which are iatrogenic. Dyslipidemia and long-standing vascular disease from pre-existing hyperlipidemia, prolonged dialytic support, or diabetes mellitus are nonmodifiable factors in contrast to immunosuppressive therapy, diet, and weight gain posttransplantation. The prevalence of dyslipidemia is reported within the range of 16% to 60% after kidney transplantation. Whereas hypertriglyceridemia is the more common abnormality in lipid metabolism among patients undergoing dialysis, transplantation is associated with an elevation in total and low-density lipoprotein (LDL) cholesterol. A strong family history of dyslipidemia among first-degree relatives as well as apolipoprotein E polymorphisms are predictive of dyslipidemia posttransplantation and perhaps may be useful to preemptively identify patients at increased risk.

Exposure to different immunosuppressive agents appears to influence the incidence and severity of dyslipidemia postkidney transplant. The dyslipidemic effect of glucocorticoids is well recognized. This effect is mediated through increased insulin resistance in peripheral tissues, impaired synthesis and activity of lipoprotein lipase, increased activity of HMG CoA reductase, decreased LDL receptor activity, and enhanced hepatic lipoprotein synthesis. Over the past decade, there has been a global trend toward minimization of chronic glucocorticoid use with strategies ranging from lower dose daily administration, alternate day administration, early steroid withdrawal, and complete steroid avoidance. Several retrospective studies have demonstrated a beneficial association between this decrement in glucocorticoid exposure and dyslipidemia.

The mechanism by which cyclosporine adversely affects lipid metabolism is not entirely clear, although evidence supports a dose- and duration-dependent effect. Cyclosporine has been implicated in inhibiting bile acid synthesis, increasing hepatic lipase activity while decreasing lipoprotein lipase activity resulting in impaired very-low–density lipoprotein (VLDL) and LDL clearance. In addition, cyclosporine, which is complexed with LDL particles in the plasma, binds with the LDL receptor, thereby preventing the host particle from being metabolized. In contrast to tacrolimus, cyclosporin is associated with a greater incidence of dyslipidemia. The mechanisms responsible for these within-class drug differences are unknown. A prospective randomized trial comparing the effect of tacrolimus and cyclosporin in kidney transplant recipients demonstrated lower total cholesterol, LDL cholesterol, and triglyceride level in those treated with tacrolimus without any significant difference in high-density lipoprotein

Table 13-3.   Adult treatment panel III guidelines

Diet
    Saturated fats <7% of total calories
    Dietary cholesterol <200 mg/day
LDL lowering options
    10–25 g/day soluble fiber
    2 g/day plant stanol/sterol
Weight loss
Increased physical activity

LDL, low-density lipoprotein.

(HDL) cholesterol levels. In addition, a prospective multicenter study demonstrated that conversion from cyclosporine to tacrolimus in patients with hyperlipidemia resulted in a significant improvement in both lipid profile and blood pressure control, thereby improving their 10-year estimated risk of coronary heart disease. These studies support the potential benefit to deliberate use of tacrolimus in patients at greater risk of posttransplant dyslipidemia. This is yet another area where prospective studies are necessary to demonstrate any true benefit.

Hyperlipidemia is a well-known consequence of sirolimus, a newer immunosuppressive agent that inhibits the mammalian target of rapamycin, which occurs in a dose-dependent manner. The incidence is cited within the range of 40% in kidney transplant recipients, with hypertriglyceridemia being the predominant feature. Studies show that this effect is fully reversible within 2 months of cessation of this medication. While the exact mechanism is not entirely clear, in vitro studies show reduced expression of the LDL receptor on human hepatocytes cultured with sirolimus. While this dramatic change in lipid metabolism remains a big concern for the transplant community, the composite physiologic effect of this agent remains unclear at this time. An observational study failed to detect a difference in the incidence of cardiovascular events over 4 years among kidney transplant recipients treated with either sirolimus or a calcineurin inhibitor. In addition, sirolimus may have additional antiatherogenic properties, including inhibition of vascular smooth muscle proliferation, which may offset the hyperlipidemic effect. Additional studies with longer follow-up are necessary before any conclusion may be drawn.

The Kidney Disease Outcomes Quality Initiative (K/DOQI) published an extensive guideline addressing dyslipidemias in the kidney transplant recipient. They classified transplant recipients in the highest cardiovascular risk category per the Adult Treatment Panel III classification; a combination of lifestyle modification and pharmacotherapy should be utilized to achieve a target LDL <100 mg/dL (Table 13-3).

While hyperlipidemia may largely be a result of unavoidable factors including genetics and unavoidable use of certain medications, both pharmacologic and lifestyle modifying therapies are available to us for possible treatment. Kidney transplant recipients with hyperlipidemia are more commonly above their ideal body weight and more likely to have gained more weight in the 6 months following transplantation. This observation suggests that intensive pre- and posttransplant education and encouragement to increase energy expenditure through regular exercise may exert beneficial effects. Prospective studies are necessary to characterize this effect. Conversely, many small prospective observational studies have assessed the effect of dietary modification on hyperlipidemia in the kidney recipient. One prospective study of kidney recipients with BMI >27 kg/m2 and hyperlipidemia assessed the effect of a 6-month dietary intervention with a moderate calorie-restricted American Heart Association "step 1" diet and found an improvement in serum cholesterol along with weight loss. These changes, along with those found in similar studies, while statistically significant, are not clinically significant enough to be confidently used as monotherapy. A similar significant but clinically small benefit was found with adherence to a Mediterranean diet rich in olive oil and polyunsaturated fatty acids.

In addition to the traditional focus on caloric and fat intake, use of vegetable as opposed to animal-derived proteins has different physiologic effects on the kidney and on metabolism. Soy protein, which is rich in mono and polyunsaturated fatty acids and phytoestrogens, which exert weak estrogenic activity with antioxidant and antiproliferative effects, have been shown to significantly decrease total cholesterol and LDL cholesterol without any effect on HDL cholesterol in a small group of kidney transplant patients.

Fish oils, which contain omega-3 polyunsaturated fatty acids including alpha-linolenic acid, eicosapentaenoic acid, and docosahexaenoic acid, have been found to be beneficial in preventing cardiovascular disease in the general population. A recent meta-analysis of randomized controlled trials of fish oil treatment on kidney transplant recipients on chronic CNI therapy found a beneficial effect on diastolic blood pressure and HDL cholesterol. The effect on lipids was not significantly different than low-dose statins. Fish oil use was not associated with any difference in patient or allograft survival, acute rejection, or CNI toxicity. At the current time, the available data is insufficient to globally recommend routine use in kidney transplant recipients.

The results of Assessment of Lescol in Renal Transplantation (ALERT) trial demonstrated that statin use was both safe and effective in this patient population. The study was underpowered to detect a significant reduction in cardiac events, but they demonstrated a 35% reduction in the secondary endpoints of cardiac death and nonfatal myocardial infarction with statin therapy. Further post hoc analysis demonstrated the greatest benefit with early initiation of therapy. The cumulative benefits of statin therapy may extend beyond that of lipid lowering and may include decreases in interstitial fibrosis, proteinuria, and inflammatory response, which require further studies.

PROTEIN METABOLISM

The immediate posttransplant period is associated with a negative nitrogen balance secondary, in part, to the increased stress of surgery, increased requirement for wound healing, and increased hepatic gluconeogenesis stimulated by pulse dose steroids used for induction immunosuppression. Investigators have shown that one can prevent the generation of a negative nitrogen balance by increasing a patient's dietary protein intake. The current recommended postoperative protein intake falls within the range of 1.3 to 1.5 g/kg ideal body weight. In the case of a patient with apparent pretransplant protein energy wasting, it would be prudent to adjust his or her dietary intake to the upper range. Daily caloric intake must be sufficient for the protein to be utilized for anabolic needs as opposed to gluconeogenesis. The caloric requirement of the average patient is within the range of 35 kcal/kg ideal body weight for the first several weeks following transplantation. Obese patients may benefit from caloric restriction to the range of 25 to 30 kcal/kg ideal body weight in an attempt to avoid excessive posttransplant weight gain. Adequate protein intake during administration of high-dose glucocorticoids has been shown to minimize some steroid-induced side effects including a cushingoid appearance and steroid-induced myopathy.

While increased protein intake is beneficial in the immediate posttransplant period, optimal long-term dietary protein intake is less well established. The relatively low doses of steroid use are not felt to strongly impact protein catabolism. The knowledge that a high protein diet causes glomerular hyperfiltration along with one theory of chronic allograft nephropathy centering around nephron-underdosing and chronic hyperfiltration injury has led some to believe that protein restriction be beneficial in prolonging allograft function. One study, which compared stable kidney transplant recipients who were adherent with a protein (0.8 g/kg/day), sodium (3 g/day), and fat (<30% caloric intake) with those who were nonadherent, found a decline in allograft function in the nonadherent group as measured by creatinine clearance and renal scintigraphy. In the setting of a lack for evidence to support any specific recommendation, dietary protein intake is recommended in the range of 1 g/kg/day, similar to patients with stage 2–3 CKD.

BONE AND MINERAL METABOLISM

CKD is associated with a spectrum of bone disease, ranging from high-bone turnover osteitis fibrosa, low-bone turnover including osteomalacia and adynamic bone disease, and mixed uremic osteodystrophy. It is not surprising that the spectrum of posttransplant bone disease is variable as well, likely secondary to preexisting pretransplant bone disease along with posttransplant factors. Diagnosis of particular pathologic processes is challenging. Bone biopsy remains the criterion standard of diagnosis, and such analyses are becoming more common. In a recent review characterizing the pathology of bone biopsies from 57 kidney transplant recipients with a mean dialysis vintage of 43 months and mean interval between transplantation and bone biopsy of 53 months, high turnover bone disease was most prevalent, with 47% of patients having mild or moderate osteitis fibrosa; approximately 12% having mixed bone disease; 9% having low turnover bone disease, either adynamic bone disease or osteomalacia; 23% had reduced bone mass in the absence of pathology associated with renal osteodystrophy; and only 9% having normal bone morphology. Bone disease is often assessed using the noninvasive dual energy x-ray absortiometry (DEXA) scan. However, interpretation of this test is very difficult in the CKD and kidney transplant population because it does not provide any information on microarchitecture or the volume of either cortical or trabecular bone. Furthermore, interpretation of a standard DEXA of lumbar vertebrae is confounded by calcification of the overlying abdominal aorta, which will seemingly increase the mineralization score. Newer techniques, including micro magnetic resonance imaging (MRI), are emerging as better noninvasive modalities of differentiating between high- and low-bone turnover diseases.

Alterations in bone metabolism posttransplant are attributed to a complex interplay of allograft function, the parathyroid gland, posttransplant immunosuppression, vitamin D synthesis as well as polymorphism of the vitamin D receptor, along with calcium and phosphate metabolism. While serum calcium levels tend to fall within the lower end of the normal range, it most often rises posttransplant, occasionally resulting in mild hypercalcemia. This change is attributed to elevated parathyroid hormone (PTH) levels. Similarly, hypophosphatemia is common following kidney transplant, affecting up to 93% of patients in the early posttransplant period. While it usually resolves within the first few months posttransplant, hypophosphatemia may persist for many years in some patients. Initially, hypophosphatemia was attributed to elevated PTH levels as a consequence of secondary hyperparathyroidism and persistent hypophosphatemia attributed to tertiary hyperparathyroidism. Recent investigation has uncoupled this relationship, because renal phosphate wasting may be found in the absence of an elevated PTH. Other factors that support the uncoupling of this association is the concomitant finding of inappropriately low serum calcitriol levels in the presence of normal allograft function and hypophosphatemia, a potent stimulus of calcitriol synthesis. FGF 23 is known to induce renal phosphate wasting and inhibit 1-alpha hydroxylation of 25-OH vitamin D. FGF 23 levels typically increase with advancing stages of CKD, thereby increasing the capacity of the diseased kidney to excrete phosphate at the expense of inhibiting calcitriol synthesis. A longitudinal study of 27 living donor kidney recipients confirmed the association between excess FGF 23 at the time of transplantation and both renal phosphate excretion and serum phosphate level posttransplant. Serum phosphate levels should be followed in the posttransplant period, and repletion should be considered for those with persistent hypophosphatemia. However, vigorous repletion may exacerbate existing secondary hyperparathyroidism, and therefore the minimal necessary supplemental dose should be administered.

The main concern regarding posttransplant bone disease centers around an increased risk of fracture compared with both the general population as well as the dialysis population. Therapeutic options for treating posttransplant osteodystrophy include the use of bisphosphonates, vitamin D analogues, calcitonin, and hormone replacement therapy. A Cochrane systematic review found that no individual intervention was associated with a reduction in fracture risk compared with placebo. Bisphosphonates had greater efficacy at minimizing loss of bone mineral density when compared with vitamin D supplementation. However, because these studies did not include bone biopsy and low-turnover bone disease is not uncommon in this population, many experts are hesitant about the use of bisphosphonates because the inhibitory effect of bisphosphonates on osteoclast-mediated bone resorption persists far beyond the duration of drug administration, and lack of loss of bone mineral density does not necessarily indicate the presence of structurally stable healthy bone.

ACID-BASE AND ELECTROLYTES

Metabolic acidosis is a common finding in the kidney transplant recipient. A cross-sectional analysis of 823 transplant recipients revealed a mean venous serum bicarbonate of 22.5 ± 4 mmol/L, with 58.1% of patients having a bicarbonate less than 24 mmol/L. The pathogenesis is attributed in part to reduced nephron mass, impaired acid excretion in the distal nephron, and impaired ammoniagenesis secondary to insulin resistance. Acidosis may adversely impact bone metabolism and muscle function. However, the effect of correcting the acidosis with bicarbonate supplementation remains unknown at this time.

Electrolyte abnormalities, including potassium and magnesium, are common following kidney transplant. Hypomagnesemia (serum magnesium <1.5 mg/dL) has been reported to occur in up to 25% of cyclosporine-treated patients and up to 43% of tacrolimus-treated patients. Tacrolimus level is the best predictor of urinary magnesium excretion, and serum magnesium levels inversely correlate with tacrolimus concentration and creatinine clearance. In addition to CNIs, sirolimus is also associated with renal magnesium loss in animals; any effect on human renal magnesium handling remains unknown at this time. Consequences of hypomagnesemia include hypokalemia, hypocalcemia, muscle weakness, and elevated LDL. Levels should be monitored routinely after kidney transplantation and with complaints of muscle fatigue and weakness, and oral supplementation prescribed if hypomagnesemia develops or persists.

Both hyper- and hypokalemia may be found in a kidney transplant recipient. Hyperkalemia is the more dominant disorder of potassium regulation, being found across the spectrum of excellent and impaired GFR. Calcineurin inhibitors cause hyperkalemia, with the incidence highest in the setting of higher serum levels common to the early posttransplant period. The primary mechanism of hyperkalemia is a defect in distal tubular potassium secretion, often along with insensitivity to mineralocorticoids. Treatment usually begins with dietary potassium restriction; however, because most protein-rich foods are rich in potassium and liberal protein intake in the range of 1.3 to 1.5 g/kg is necessary in the early posttransplant period, other means of potassium reduction may be necessary. These include the use of diuretics, sodium bicarbonate, and ion-exchange resins.

CONCLUSION

Recommended diets for the immediate posttransplantation period and for long-term therapy are summarized in Table 13-4. A recurrent theme in the preceding discussion of nutritional and metabolic abnormalities in recipients of kidney transplants is the

Table 13-4.   Recommended nutritional intake for kidney transplant recipients

First Month After Transplantation and During Therapy for
Acute Rejection

Protein	1.3–1.5 g/kg b.w./day
Calories	30–35 kcal/kg b.w./day

After First Month

Protein	1.0 g/kg b.w./day
Calories	Sufficient to achieve and maintain optimal weight for height

At All Times

Carbohydrates	50% of calories
Fats	Not >30% of calories
Cholesterol	Not >300 mg/day
Calcium	1200 mg/day
Phosphorus	1200 mg/day
Exercise	>30 minutes most days of the week

lack of prospective randomized interventional studies with long-term follow-up to assess the benefit of most treatments. We believe that all kidney transplant recipients should be educated and continuously encouraged and motivated to maintain a healthy lifestyle through adherence to a heart-healthy diet along with regular exercise.

Selected Readings

Alexander JW, Goodman H. Gastric bypass in chronic renal failure and renal transplant. Nutr Clin Pract 2007;22:16–21.

Barbagallo CM, Cefalù AB Gallo, S, et al. Effects of Mediterranean diet on lipid levels and cardiovascular risk in renal transplant recipients. Nephron 1999;82:199–204.

Bayes B, Pastor MC, Lauzurica R, et al. Do anti-CD25 monoclonal antibodies potentiate posttransplant diabetes mellitus? Transplant Proc 2007;39:9–20.

Bernardi A, Biasia F, Pati T, et al. Long-term protein intake control in kidney transplant recipients: Effect in kidney graft function and in nutritional status. Am J Kidney Dis 2003;41:S146–S152.

Bhan I, Shah A, Holmes J, et al. Post-transplant hypophosphatemia: Tertiary 'Hyper-Phosphatoninism'? Kidney Int 2006;70:1486–1494.

Bloom RD, Crutchlow MF. New-onset diabetes mellitus in the kidney recipient: diagnosis and management strategies. Clin J Am Soc Nephrol 2008;Suppl 2:S38–S48.

Cassiman D, Roelant, M, Vandenplas G, et al. Orlistat treatment is safe in overweight and obese liver transplant recipients: a prospective, open label trial. Transpl Int 2006;19:1000–1005.

Chang SH, Coates PT, McDonald SP. Effects of body mass index at transplantation on outcomes of kidney transplantation. Transplantation 2007;84:981–987.

Colman E, Fossler M. Reduction in blood cyclosporine concentrations by orlistat. N Engl J Med 2000;342:1141.

Cupisti A, D'Alessandro C, Ghiadoni L, et al. Effect of a soy protein diet on serum lipids of renal transplant patients. J Ren Nutr 2004; 14:31–35.

Elster EA, Leeser DB, Morrissette C, et al. Obesity following kidney transplantation and steroid avoidance immunosuppression. Clin Transplant 2008;22:354–359.

Fellström B, Holdaas H, Jardine AG, et al. Effect of fluvastatin on renal end points in the Assessment of Lescol in Renal Transplant (ALERT) trial. Kidney Int 2004;66:1549–1555.

Jezior D, Krajewska M, Madziarska K, et al. Weight reduction in Renal Transplant Recipients Program: the first successes. Transplant Proc 2007;39:2769–2771.

Joss N, Staatz CE, Thomson AH, et al. Predictors of new onset diabetes after renal transplantation. Clin Nephrol 2007;21:136–143.

Lehmann G, Ott U, Stein G, et al. Renal osteodystrophy after successful renal transplantation: a histomorphometric analysis in 57 patients. Transplant Proc 2007;39:3153–3158.

Lim AKH, Manley KJ, Roberts MA, et al. Fish oil treatment for kidney transplant recipients: a meta-analysis of randomized controlled trials. Transplantation 2007;83:831–838.

Lopes IM, Martinm M, Errasti P, et al. Benefits of a dietary intervention on weight loss, body composition, and lipid profile after renal transplantation. Nutrition 1999;15:7–10.

Marcén R, Chahin J, Alarcón A, et al. Conversion from cyclosporine microemulsion to tacrolimus in stable kidney transplant patients with hypercholesterolemia is related to an improvement in cardiovascular risk profile: a prospective study. Transplant Proc 2006; 38:2427–2430.

Pelletier RP, Akin B, Henry ML, et al. The impact of mycophenolate mofetil dosing patterns on clinical outcome after renal transplantation. Clin Transplant 2003;17:200–205.

Rogers CC, Alloway RR, Buell JF, et al. Body weight alterations under early corticosteroid withdrawal and chronic corticosteroid therapy with modern immunosuppression. Transplantation 2005;80:26–33.

Segev DL, Simpkins CE, Thompson RE, et al. Obesity impacts access to kidney transplantation. J Am Soc Nephrol 2008;19:349–355.

Subramanian S, Trence DL. Immunosuppressive agents: effects on glucose and lipid metabolism. Endocrinol Metab Clin North Am 2007;36:891–905.

Vincenti F, Friman S, Scheuermann E, et al. DIRECT (Diabetes Incidence after Renal Transplantation: Neoral C Monitoring Versus Tacrolimus) Investigators. Results of an international, randomized trial comparing glucose metabolism disorders and outcome with cyclosporine versus tacrolimus. Am J Transplant 2007;7:1506–1514.

Yakupoglu HY, Corsenca A, Wahl P, et al. Posttransplant acidosis and associated disorders of mineral metabolism in patients with a renal graft. Transplantation 2007;84:1151–1157.

Nutritional Aspects
of Kidney Stones

Gary C. Curhan

INTRODUCTION

Nephrolithiasis (kidney stone disease) is common. The lifetime risk of stone formation in the United States is 12% in men and 6% in women. The prevalence is rising in the United States and other countries; lifestyle factors, including diet and obesity, are likely responsible for this increase.

Stone disease is morbid and costly, and recurrence rates may be as high as 30% to 50% after 5 years. Consequently, efforts to prevent stone formation are essential. Tailored dietary recommendations to prevent stone recurrence should be offered to every patient and be based on a metabolic evaluation. In many patients, medication will be necessary to reduce stone risk optimally, but use of medications does not obviate the need for an effective dietary and fluid prescription.

Most data on the relation between diet and stone disease come from observational and physiologic studies rather than randomized trials. There is not yet a consensus on the specifics of dietary modification, but several important concepts should be kept in mind when designing a therapeutic regimen. First, short-term intervention studies examining changes in urine composition are of interest, but clinical recommendations should be based on studies using actual stone formation as the desired outcome. This is recommended because stone formation cannot be perfectly predicted by urinary composition, and it is likely that many factors influence urinary supersaturation but are not identified by the formulas used to calculate supersaturation (e.g., phytate). Second, it is important to individualize recommendations based on stone type and urinary composition (two 24-hour urine collections obtained at least 6 weeks after a stone episode are required for the initial evaluation). For example, we do not recommend dietary oxalate restriction to individuals with pure uric acid stones. Third, the impact of dietary risk factors varies by age, sex, and body mass index. Fourth, patients must provide follow-up 24-hour urine collections to evaluate the impact of dietary recommendations. If the urine composition does not change in response to a dietary change, then alternative approaches should be tried. Finally, it is important to distinguish stone passage from new stone formation. If a patient implements dietary changes and then passes a pre-existing stone, this does not indicate treatment failure.

DIETARY RISK FACTORS FOR CALCIUM STONE DISEASE

More than 80% of kidney stones contain calcium, and the majority of calcium stones consist primarily of calcium oxalate. Less common types of calcium stones include calcium phosphate, uric acid, struvite, and cystine. Consequently, the majority of studies have

Table 14-1. Putative dietary factors associated that may increase or decrease calcium oxalate kidney stones*

Dietary Factor	Proposed Mechanism(s)
Increased risk	
Oxalate	Increased urinary oxalate excretion
Sodium	Increased urinary calcium excretion
Animal protein	Increased urinary calcium and uric acid excretion; reduced urinary citrate excretion
Vitamin C	Increased oxalate generation and excretion
Carbohydrates	Increased urinary calcium excretion
Decreased risk	
Dietary calcium	Binding of dietary oxalate in gut
Potassium	Increased urinary citrate excretion; reduced urinary calcium excretion
Phytate	Inhibition of calcium oxalate crystal formation
Magnesium	Reduced dietary oxalate absorption; inhibition of calcium oxalate crystal formation
Vitamin B6	Vitamin B6 deficiency may increase oxalate production and oxaluria

*Phosphorus and n-3 fatty acids are discussed in the text.

focused on the prevention of calcium oxalate stones. Dietary factors purported to be associated with increased or decreased risk of calcium oxalate stone are listed in Table 14-1.

Calcium

In the past, a high calcium intake was incorrectly believed to increase the risk of stone formation. This was primarily based on the observation that approximately 20% of ingested calcium is absorbed; this proportion increases in individuals with idiopathic hypercalciuria. However, substantial evidence demonstrates that a higher calcium diet is associated with a *reduced* risk of stone formation. One potential mechanism to explain this apparent paradox is that the higher calcium intake will bind dietary oxalate in the gut, thereby reducing oxalate absorption and urinary excretion. It is also possible that dairy products (the major source of dietary calcium) may contain factors that inhibit stone formation.

Several large prospective observational studies in men and women consistently support a reduced risk of stone formation with increasing dietary calcium intake: compared with individuals in the lowest quintile of dietary calcium intake, those in the highest quintile had more than a 30% lower risk of forming a stone. These results were adjusted for multiple factors, including age, body mass index, total fluid intake, the use of thiazide diuretics, and the intake of nutrients such as animal protein, magnesium, phosphorous, sodium, and potassium. The risk of stone formation associated with calcium intake is an example of how the impact of a risk factor can vary by age: there was no association between dietary calcium and stone formation in men aged 60 years or older.

The observational findings were subsequently confirmed by a 5-year randomized, controlled clinical trial which compared stone recurrence in individuals with a history of calcium oxalate nephrolithiasis and idiopathic hypercalciuria assigned to a diet low in calcium (400 mg/day) or to a diet with "normal" calcium content (1200 mg/day) plus lower amounts of animal protein and sodium. The risk of developing a recurrent stone on the higher calcium diet was 51% lower than for the low-calcium diet. Because both dietary sodium and animal protein can contribute to the formation of calcium stones, these results, although suggestive, did not directly address the independent role of dietary calcium in the pathogenesis of kidney stones. Nonetheless, there is overwhelming evidence that dietary calcium should not be restricted; such a diet increases the risk of stone formation and may be harmful to bone health by inducing negative calcium balance.

The impact of supplemental calcium on stone risk differs from the influence of dietary calcium. In an observational study of older women, calcium supplement users were 20% more likely to form a stone than women who did not take supplements. The Women's Health Initiative randomized trial also found an increased risk with calcium supplementation, although in this case, the supplements also contained vitamin D. In younger women and men, there was no association between calcium supplement use and the risk of stone formation. This discrepancy between the risks from dietary calcium versus calcium supplements may be because of the timing of calcium intake; calcium supplements are not typically taken with meals, which would diminish the binding of dietary oxalate.

It should be mentioned that for the calcium supplement user, the absolute risk of forming the first kidney stone is only slightly increased (1.2 cases/1000 women per year compared with 1.0/1000 per year) indicating that supplement use is not a major contributor to stone risk. However, for an individual who has had a stone, the impact of calcium supplementation on urine composition should be evaluated before recommending calcium supplement use. Specifically, a patient with calcium nephrolithiasis who wishes to continue calcium supplementation should collect 24-hour urine samples on and off the supplement, and recommendations about supplements should be based on the changes, if any, in urine composition and relevant clinical issues (e.g., osteoporosis, lactose intolerance, vitamin D deficiency).

Oxalate

Urine oxalate concentration is clearly an important risk factor for calcium oxalate stone formation, but the role of dietary oxalate in the pathogenesis of calcium oxalate nephrolithiasis is less clear. First, the proportion of urinary oxalate derived from dietary oxalate is controversial: estimates range from 10% to 50%. Thus, a substantial proportion of urinary oxalate is derived from the endogenous production from the metabolism of glycine, glycolate, and hydroxyproline. Second, other dietary factors influence oxalate in urine. For example, vitamin C supplementation appears to be an important contributor because it can be metabolized to oxalate. Third, much of the oxalate in food may not be readily absorbed because of low bioavailability. Finally, there is significant variation in the gastrointestinal (GI) tract absorption of oxalate. For instance, up to one third of patients who have calcium oxalate nephrolithiasis may experience increased absorption of dietary oxalate, while those colonized with Oxalobacter formigenes, an intestinal bacterium that degrades oxalate, can decrease oxalate availability for absorption.

Older reports of the oxalate content in food may be unreliable because of measurement issues related to the quality of the assay procedure as well as the variability in oxalate content of different foods. More reliable assays for the direct determination of the oxalate content of food, including ion chromatography and capillary electrophoresis, have been developed, and large-scale prospective studies of the relationship between dietary oxalate and kidney stone formation have revealed that the impact of dietary oxalate was minimal in men and older women and not associated with stone formation in younger women.

We recommend that calcium oxalate stone formers should limit their intake of certain nuts (including almonds, peanuts, cashews, walnuts, and pecans), certain vegetables (including beets and spinach), wheat bran, and rice bran. Most types of chocolate are not high in oxalate. A list of the oxalate content of several hundred food items can be found at https://regepi.bwh.harvard.edu/health/Oxalate/files.

Sodium

Higher sodium intakes result in decreased proximal sodium reabsorption with subsequent reduction in calcium reabsorption in the distal nephron. There is a powerful effect of concomitant dietary sodium and animal protein restriction on reducing urinary calcium excretion. Observational studies reveal a positive, independent association between sodium consumption and new kidney stone formation in women but not men. In 24-hour urine collections, urine sodium excretion appeared to be associated with an increased risk in men but not consistently in women. Thus, there appears to be differences in the impact by age and gender. While the importance of sodium restriction to <2.5 g/day is clear for lowering of blood pressure (justifying the recommendation to limit sodium intake for the general population), its role in calcium stone formation requires further study.

Potassium

Dietary potassium restriction can increase urinary calcium excretion. In addition, hypokalemia stimulates citrate reabsorption, decreasing the urinary excretion of citrate, an important inhibitor of calcium oxalate stone formation. Potassium in food also accompanies organic anions such as citrate that are metabolized to bicarbonate. Thus, the consumption of potassium-containing foods such as fruits and vegetables represents an alkali load that increases the urinary excretion of citrate. A high potassium intake is inversely associated with kidney stones in men and older women but not younger women.

Animal Protein

From a metabolic standpoint, animal protein should be divided into dairy (e.g., milk, yogurt) and nondairy (meat, chicken, seafood) sources. The metabolism of sulfur-containing amino acids in animal flesh generates sulfuric acid, so nondairy animal protein provides an acid load that may increase urinary calcium excretion and reduce urinary citrate excretion. Nondairy animal protein can also increase calcitriol production. A positive association between total animal protein consumption and new kidney stone formation occurs in men but not women, but these studies did not explicitly look at the two separate sources of animal protein. Because the amount of dietary calcium is inversely associated with stone formation and dairy foods are a major source of dietary calcium, it is likely that dairy protein would be inversely associated with risk. But restriction of nondairy animal protein may be beneficial.

Phytate

Dietary phytate (inositol hexaphosphate) may play a role in preventing the formation of calcium-containing stones. Phytate is found in many foods high in fiber, such as cereals, legumes, and vegetables, and it binds strongly to calcium in the intestine. Phytate is also absorbed from the GI tract and is excreted in the urine where it inhibits urinary crystallization of calcium salts. This is relevant because urinary levels of phytate in some calcium oxalate stone formers appear to be low.

Observational data from younger women showed that dietary phytate was inversely associated with incident kidney stone formation, but there was no similar relationship in men.

Magnesium

Magnesium may reduce oxalate absorption in the gastrointestinal tract and can form soluble complexes with oxalate in the urine, potentially decreasing calcium oxalate supersaturation. The few randomized trials of magnesium supplementation on stone recurrence yielded inconclusive results because magnesium was given in combination with other compounds (e.g., thiazide diuretic or potassium citrate), and patient dropout rates were high. In observational studies, higher dietary magnesium was associated with a 30% lower risk of stone formation in men but not in women.

Carbohydrates

Carbohydrate ingestion can increase urinary calcium excretion, an effect that may be at least partially mediated by insulin. A positive association between sucrose intake and new kidney stone formation has been shown to occur in women but not men. Recently, higher fructose intake was found to increase the risk of stone formation in men and women.

Vitamin C

Vitamin C (ascorbic acid) can be metabolized to form oxalate. A supplement of 1000 mg of vitamin C consumed twice daily increased urinary oxalate excretion by 22%. Thus, a high vitamin

C intake could increase the risk of calcium oxalate stone formation, and in support of this possibility, there was a 40% higher risk of stone formation in men who consumed 1000 mg or more per day of vitamin C compared with men who consumed less than 90 mg/day (the recommended dietary allowance). This relationship was observed only after adjusting for dietary potassium. We do not recommend restricting *dietary* vitamin C (because foods high in vitamin C are also high in inhibitory factors such as potassium), but a calcium stone former should be instructed to discontinue vitamin C supplements.

Vitamin D

The role of vitamin D in stone formation is also unclear. While very high intakes of vitamin D and calcium can increase urine calcium excretion, the impact of usual levels of intake is uncertain. In the Women's Health Initiative Study, the increase in stone risk was ~20% higher in women who were given calcium supplements (1000 mg/day) and vitamin D_3 (400 IU/day), so it unclear if the increase in risk was because of the calcium supplement (most likely), the vitamin D (less likely), or the combination. Given the high prevalence of vitamin D deficiency in the United States even among healthy individuals and the adverse impact on bone health, it is reasonable to measure plasma 25(OH) vitamin D and replete in deficient individuals, even if they have high urine calcium.

Vitamin B_6

Vitamin B_6 is a cofactor in oxalate metabolism, and vitamin B_6 deficiency increases oxalate production and oxaluria. Although a very high dose of vitamin B_6 can reduce urine oxalate in selected patients with type 1 primary hyperoxaluria, the use of vitamin B_6 in other settings remains unclear. While substantial vitamin B_6 supplements may reduce the risk of kidney stone formation in women, this relationship was not found in men.

Phosphorus

Higher levels of dietary phosphate will decrease intestinal absorption of dietary calcium. One of the challenges of studying independent associations of dietary phosphate with kidney stone formation is its high correlation with calcium in the diet. For patients who have calcium phosphate stones, there is a theoretical benefit to reducing phosphate intake to reduce phosphate excretion, but there are no data documenting benefits in stone formation.

N-3 Fatty Acids

It has been proposed that dietary fatty acids can modulate the urinary excretion of calcium and oxalate and that fish oil supplementation will lower urinary calcium and oxalate. However, a prospective study showed there was no association between the intake of n-3 fatty acids and the risk of kidney stone formation in men or women.

Calories

There are no data on the direct relation between total caloric intake and stone risk. However, higher body weight, a larger waist circumference, and a higher body mass index plus weight gain are associated with an increased risk of kidney stone formation, independent of diet. Although there are no available data to support weight loss as preventive treatment for stone disease, stone formers should be encouraged to exercise and modulate their intake of calories to maintain a healthy weight.

BEVERAGES AND CALCIUM STONES

Total Fluid

Nephrolithiasis is a disease arising from increased concentration of the urine and its constituents. Even if the total amounts of lithogenic substances excreted in the urine are reasonable, a low urine volume can raise the concentrations leading to stone formation. Thus, modifying the concentration of the lithogenic factors is the focus of stone prevention, and fluid intake, the main determinant of urine volume, is a critical component of stone prevention. Observational studies and a randomized controlled trial have demonstrated that a higher fluid intake reduces the risk of stone formation. Patients must be given specific advice on how much to drink to form at least 2 liters of urine per day. In addition to fluid intake, other factors such as insensible losses and the water contained in foods influence urine volume. Rather than arbitrarily specifying a certain amount of fluid intake (e.g., 8 glasses of water per day), the recommendation should be tailored based on the total volume of 24-hour urine collections of each individual patient. For example, if an individual produces 1.5 liters of urine per day, consuming an additional two 8-ounce (240 mL) glasses of water would raise their output to the target of 2 liters. Patients should be reminded that consistency of fluid intake is important: producing 3 liters of urine on 1 day will not cancel out the crystal forming potential from 1 liter of output on the previous day. While some clinicians suggest that a patient should have urine that is very light in color and should wake up at least once per night, there are no data to support such guidelines, and the desire to have constantly dilute urine needs to be balanced against the harm of sleep disruption.

Individual Beverages

When advised to increase to their fluid intake, patients often want to know what they should and should not drink. The associations of specific beverages, beyond fluid intake, with kidney stone formation are presented in Table 14-2. Despite previous beliefs to the contrary, alcoholic beverages, coffee, and tea do not increase the risk of stone formation. In fact, observational studies have found that coffee, tea, beer, and wine *reduce* the risk of stone formation. The mechanism for this protective association is likely related to the impact on antidiuretic hormone (ADH) in the kidney by caffeine and the inhibition of ADH secretion by alcohol. The role of tea deserves special mention. There is a widespread belief that tea is high in oxalate and should be avoided. A cup of tea contains 14 mg of oxalate. While this is not insignificant, the bioavailability does not appear to be high and when tested, there was a negligible impact on urinary oxalate. Citrus juices, such as orange and grapefruit juice, theoretically could reduce the risk

Table 14-2. Select beverages, risk, and mechanism for calcium oxalate stone formation*

Beverage Type	Risk	Proposed Mechanism(s)
Coffee and tea	Decreased	Caffeine interferes with antidiuretic hormone action, leading to decreased urinary concentration
Alcohol	Decreased	Alcohol inhibits secretion of antidiuretic hormone, leading to decreased urinary concentration
Milk	Decreased	Binding of dietary oxalate in gut
Grapefruit juice	Increased	Possible increased oxalate production

*Orange juice and soda are discussed in the text.

of stone formation by increasing urine citrate, but prospective studies found no association with orange juice; and in fact, grapefruit juice intake was associated with a 40% higher risk of stone formation. Grapefruit juice can affect several intestinal enzymes, but the mechanism for the observed increased risk is unknown. One feeding study found that grapefruit consumption did increase urine citrate but also substantially increased urine oxalate.

The relation between soda ("soft drink") consumption and stone risk is complicated. Dietary patterns associated with sweetened soda consumption were found to increase the risk of stone formation. Because sweetened sodas contain fructose, which increases the risk of stone formation, these beverages should be avoided.

Dietary Patterns

Beyond specific nutrient information, some patients prefer to receive advice about an overall dietary approach. One such dietary pattern is the DASH diet. The Dietary Approaches to Stop Hypertension Study, or DASH, found that a diet rich in fruits, vegetables, nuts, legumes plus low-fat dairy and low-sodium food substantially reduces blood pressure. While this pattern theoretically should reduce the risk of stone formation (in addition to lowering blood pressure), there are no published studies that have specifically examined this question. In contrast, high animal protein diets promoted to cause weight loss may increase the risk of stone formation, but this has not been formally tested.

PREVENTION OF STONE RECURRENCE—OTHER STONE TYPES

For the less common types of stones, there are few data supporting specific dietary manipulations. The following recommendations, therefore, are based on pathophysiology, but these suggestions may prove to be incorrect as shown for older recommendations about calcium oxalate stone prevention.

Uric Acid Stones

The two driving forces for uric acid crystal formation are the uric acid concentration and urine pH (the solubility of uric acid in-

Table 14-3. Dietary recommendations for calcium oxalate stone prevention according to urinary risk factor

Urinary Abnormality	Dietary Changes
High calcium	Adequate dietary calcium intake Reduce nondairy animal protein intake (5–7 servings of meat, fish, or poultry/week) Reduce sodium intake to <2.5 g/day Reduce sucrose intake
High oxalate	Avoid high-oxalate foods Avoid vitamin C supplements Adequate dietary calcium intake
Low citrate	Increase fruit and vegetable intake Reduce nondairy animal protein intake
Low volume	Increase total fluid intake to maintain urine volume ≥ 2 L/day

creases substantially as the urine pH increases from 5.0 to 6.5). Decreasing the consumption of meat, chicken, and seafood will decrease purine intake and, therefore, uric acid production; it may also increase urinary pH. Higher intake of fruits and vegetables should raise the urine pH and reduce the risk of uric acid crystal formation.

Cystine Stones
Patients with cystine stone disease nearly always require medications, but dietary modification may also help. Restricting sodium intake can reduce the urinary excretion of cystine, and the solubility of cystine increases as urinary pH rises. Thus, a higher fruit and vegetable consumption may be beneficial. There is little evidence to support the dietary restriction of proteins high in cystine, although reducing animal protein intake may be beneficial by increasing urine pH.

Calcium Phosphate Stones
Information on dietary factors related to calcium phosphate stone formation is limited. Because patients with type 1 renal tubular acidosis and stone disease may benefit from alkali supplementation, generally as potassium citrate, they may also benefit from a diet high in fruits and vegetables. It should be noted, however, that an increase in urinary pH can increase the risk of calcium phosphate crystal formation. Dietary maneuvers directed at decreasing urinary calcium excretion (Table 14-3) and urinary phosphate excretion would be expected to decrease calcium phosphate stone recurrence.

CONCLUSION
Dietary factors play an important role in kidney stone formation, and dietary modification can reduce the risk of stone recurrence. Because stone recurrence rates may be as high as 30% to 50% after 5 to 10 years, individualized dietary intervention to prevent stone recurrence should be offered to every patient willing to par-

ticipate in a diagnostic workup and to adhere to treatment recommendations. The necessity of prescribing medications should not obviate the need for an effective dietary and/or fluid prescription. Dietary interventions and subsequent evaluations of therapeutic efficacy should be based on results from multiple 24-hour urine collections. Adequate fluid intake and appropriate dietary modifications based on the increasingly available scientific evidence may substantially reduce the morbidity and costs that are associated with recurrent nephrolithiasis.

Selected Readings

Baggio B, Priante G, Brunati AM, et al. Specific modulatory effect of arachidonic acid on human red blood cell oxalate transport: clinical implications in calcium oxalate nephrolithiasis. J Am Soc Nephrol 1999;10(Suppl 14):S381–S384.

Borghi L, Meschi T, Amato F, et al. Urinary volume, water and recurrences in idiopathic calcium nephrolithiasis: a 5-year randomized prospective study. J Urol 1996;155:839–843.

Borghi L, Schianchi T, Meschi T, et al. Comparison of two diets for the prevention of recurrent stones in idiopathic hypercalciuria. N Engl J Med 2002;346:77–84.

Curhan GC, Willett WC, Knight EL, et al. Dietary factors and the risk of incident kidney stones in younger women: Nurses' Health Study II. Arch Intern Med 2004;164:885–891.

Curhan GC, Willett WC, Rimm EB, et al. A prospective study of dietary calcium and other nutrients and the risk of symptomatic kidney stones. N Engl J Med 1993;328:833–838.

Curhan GC, Willett WC, Rimm EB, et al. A prospective study of the intake of vitamins C and B6, and the risk of kidney stones in men. J Urol 1996;155:1847–1851.

Frick KK, Bushinsky DA. Molecular mechanisms of primary hypercalciuria. J Am Soc Nephrol 2003;14:1082–1095.

Goldfarb DS, Asplin JR. Effect of grapefruit juice on urinary lithogenicity. J Urol 2001;166:263–267.

Hess B, Ackermann D, Essig M, et al. Renal mass and serum calcitriol in male idiopathic calcium renal stone formers: role of protein intake. J Clin Endocrinol Metab 1995;80:1916–1921.

Holmes RP, Assimos DG. The impact of dietary oxalate on kidney stone formation. Urol Res 2004;32:311–316.

Jackson RD, LaCroix AZ, Gass M, et al. Calcium plus vitamin D supplementation and the risk of fractures. N Engl J Med 2006;354:669–683.

Sacks FM, Svetkey LP, Vollmer WM, et al. Effects on blood pressure of reduced dietary sodium and the Dietary Approaches to Stop Hypertension (DASH) diet. DASH-Sodium Collaborative Research Group. N Engl J Med 2001;344:3–10.

Stamatelou KK, Francis ME, Jones CA, et al. Time trends in reported prevalence of kidney stones in the United States: 1976–1994. Kidney Int 2003;63:1817–1823.

Taylor EN, Curhan GC. Fructose consumption and the risk of kidney stones. Kidney Int 2008;73:207–212.

Taylor EN, Stampfer MJ, Curhan GC. Dietary factors and the risk of incident kidney stones in men: new insights after 14 years of follow-up. J Am Soc Nephrol 2004;15:3225–3232.

Taylor EN, Stampfer MJ, Curhan GC. Obesity, weight gain, and the risk of kidney stones. JAMA 2005;293:455–462.

15

Dietary Salt Intake for Patients with Hypertension or Kidney Disease

Christopher S. Wilcox

INTRODUCTION

Our genes were selected to adapt us to life in the African continent where the climate is hot and dry, perspiration substantial, and dietary salt intake was low. Presently, individuals living in rural African communities have very low levels of blood pressure until they migrate to an urban environment, where salt intake rises steeply and, with it, the incidence of hypertension. These observations suggest that we are adapted to retain, rather than eliminate, salt through a salt appetite and renal mechanisms for avid salt retention. Despite these evolutionary adaptations, most normal subjects maintain an extracellular fluid volume that changes by less than 1 liter (1 kilogram of body weight) and a blood pressure that changes by less than 10%, despite wide variations in daily salt intake. These subjects are termed "salt resistant" and encompass the majority of healthy adolescents and young adults. However, a minority are unable to maintain a normal, low level of blood pressure in face of a steep rise in salt intake and are termed "salt-sensitive." Salt sensitivity precedes hypertension. It is a cardiovascular risk factor, complicates antihypertensive therapy, contributes to progressive loss of kidney function in patients with chronic kidney disease (CKD), exacerbates proteinuria, and diminishes the antiproteinuric response to drugs in those with renal disease. Thus, the evaluation and management of dietary salt intake is an essential component of care for patients with high blood pressure, kidney disease, or cardiovascular risk. Regrettably, many physicians erroneously believe that dietary salt intake does not require attention in the era of modern diuretics. This chapter will outline arguments for a more comprehensive assessment of dietary salt intake than is presently customary and provide goals and steps to appropriate management.

Most sodium is ingested as salt. Moreover, the increase in blood pressure in salt-sensitive subjects fed salt is not apparent if an equivalent quantity of sodium is given with another anion. However, intake is usually quantitated as sodium. A daily intake of 100 mmol of sodium is equivalent to 5.8 g of salt.

EPIDEMIOLOGY OF DIETARY SALT INTAKE

Daily sodium intake varies widely in modern Western societies but is generally between 80 and 250 mmol. A multinational IN-TERSALT study concluded that the mean level of blood pressure of individuals in a country increases with ambient salt intake. Because hypertension is the leading cause of cardiovascular death and cardiovascular disease is the leading cause of death, any increase in population blood pressure is a cause for concern.

A reduction of salt intake in patients with pre- or established hypertension is recommended by the World Health Organization and the Joint National Commission on Prevention, Detection, Evaluation, and Treatment of High Blood Pressure (JNC). Clandestine promotion of high salt intake by food and beverage companies in the United States, for example by the Salt Institute, has unfortunately been highly successful. Whereas prior to 1980, the total sales of food salt and the prevalence of hypertension in the United States were decreasing, since then the use of salt has increased by as much as 90%. This has been accompanied by an increase in age-adjusted prevalence of high blood pressure in the U.S. population. The relationship between salt intake and blood pressure varies between individuals. This obscures the overall effect of dietary salt on blood pressure and cardiovascular disease and has complicated the public health case for salt restriction in food.

ASSESSMENT OF SALT SENSITIVITY

Salt sensitivity is defined arbitrarily as a greater than 10% increase in blood pressure on passing from a low to a high salt intake. Salt-sensitive individuals constitute approximately 30% of the young adult population. A shortened protocol to assess salt sensitivity has been developed whereby individuals are given dietary advice to achieve a 150 mmol per day sodium intake for 3 days. They then receive 2 L of 0.9% saline intravenously over 4 hours to provide high salt intake. The following day, they receive a salt-restricted diet of 10 mmol daily and 3 oral doses of 40 mg furosemide. The blood pressure is compared at the end of the high and low salt periods. This shortened protocol is reproducible in defining salt-sensitive and salt-resistant individuals. However, there is a normal distribution of salt-induced blood pressure. Therefore, division into salt resistant and salt sensitive is arbitrary.

Unfortunately, this protocol is too cumbersome for routine clinical use. The proportion of subjects who are salt sensitive is rather greater in African Americans than Caucasians, is associated with a low plasma renin activity, increases with age, and increases markedly with declining renal function. Salt sensitivity is more frequent in hypertensive than normotensive subjects. Therefore, elderly or African American hypertensives, and especially those with chronic kidney disease can reasonably be assumed to be salt sensitive. In practice, salt sensitivity often becomes apparent as a large fall in blood pressure with dietary salt restriction and thiazide diuretic therapy.

SALT INTAKE, BLOOD PRESSURE, AND CHRONIC KIDNEY DISEASE

The degree of salt sensitivity increases exponentially with declining kidney function. As patients approach end-stage renal disease, the great majority are salt sensitive. The exceptions are those with primary tubulointerstitial disease who typically do not retain sodium chloride (NaCl) and have normal blood pressure.

Because the level of blood pressure determines the progression of kidney disease in those with more than 1–3 g/24 hours of protein excretion, attention to dietary salt and proper use of diuretics are essential in hypertensive patients with chronic proteinuric kidney disease. Moreover, a high level of dietary salt increases protein excretion in patients with proteinuric kidney disease and appears to enhance the progression of underlying CKD. Therefore, dietary salt restriction and proper use of diuretics are an important component of the management of the great majority of patients with CKD. Indeed, because proper management of blood pressure (often with a lower than normal blood pressure goal) is required for optimum control of progressive proteinuric kidney disease, control of salt intake and proper use of diuretics should be a part of the initial clinical management of these patients. This follows from the observations that salt intake determines blood pressure, whereas blood pressure determines not only the progression of chronic kidney disease but the rapidity and severity with which cardiovascular events develop in this high-risk population.

SALT INTAKE AND CARDIOVASCULAR DISEASE

Current estimates suggest that the high level of dietary salt in the United States presently accounts for up to 15% of strokes and 8% of coronary artery disease. In countries such as Finland where national programs to reduce salt intake have been effective, there is a reduction in blood pressure and a greater than 70% decrease in stroke and coronary heart mortality in the population younger than 65 years.

PATHOPHYSIOLOGY

Normal Responses to Changes in Dietary Salt

A healthy individual whose daily dietary salt intake is changed abruptly from a low level (for example, 20 mmol) to a high level (for example, 200 mmol) achieves dietary salt balance within 2 to 3 days. During this nonequilibrium time, renal sodium excretion, although increasing, remains below the level of sodium intake, accounting for a net positive balance of approximately 150 mmol of sodium and chloride matched by an increase in body weight of approximately 1 kg. Thereafter, the high level of salt intake is matched by an equivalent level of sodium and chloride excretion (200 mmol/day in this example). Homeostasis is achieved by integrated changes in renal hemodynamics and tubular function, key hormones, the sympathetic nervous system, and cardiovascular function.

An increase in dietary salt intake in healthy subjects is accompanied by an initial increase in renal blood flow without a change in glomerular filtration rate (GFR). The accompanying reduction in filtration fraction reduces proximal tubular sodium chloride and fluid reabsorption. Because there is little or no increase in plasma sodium concentration or GFR, the increase in renal sodium excretion is because of a reduction in tubular sodium chloride reabsorption. The nephron segments responsible have been studied indirectly in human subjects from changes in the clearance of lithium, which is reabsorbed almost exclusively in the proximal tubule in parallel with sodium. Such techniques demonstrate a modest reduction in proximal sodium reabsorption accompanied by a larger fractional reduction in distal sodium reabsorption.

Within the first 1 to 2 days of increased dietary salt intake, there is a sharp decline in plasma renin activity, serum aldosterone concentration, and plasma catecholamine levels. Plasma levels of atrial natriuretic peptide (ANP) increase in response to an increase in central blood volume and stretch of cardiac atria. Because angiotensin II and alpha adrenergic activation enhance reabsorption throughout most of the nephron and reabsorption in the collecting ducts is enhanced by aldosterone but reduced by ANP, these neurohumoral changes dictate appropriate changes in tubular sodium chloride reabsorption with dietary salt intake.

Because the changes in renal sodium and fluid excretion lag behind the changes in intake, an increase in dietary salt is associated with some increase in the extracellular and plasma fluid volumes. The ensuring increase in venous return enhances cardiac output. In salt-resistant subjects, this is offset by a reduction in peripheral resistance such that blood pressure changes little.

Similar studies in patients who are salt sensitive document two linked abnormalities. First, most studies indicate that patients who are salt sensitive retain a slightly greater fraction of dietary NaCl during adaption to a high salt intake. Because infusion of saline into salt-resistant normotensive subjects leads to little or no increase in blood pressure, this by itself is insufficient to explain the rise in blood pressure in salt-sensitive individuals. The second difference is that salt-resistant subjects, although showing an early rise in cardiac output during salt loading, have a blunted or absent reduction in peripheral resistance thereby leading to a rise in blood pressure. Presently, the causes for the defective renal sodium and chloride elimination and the defective reduction in peripheral resistance with salt intake in salt-sensitive subjects are poorly understood.

Salt Intake and Elimination in Patients with Renal Disease

Patients with CKD have several differences in their response to a high dietary salt intake. First, the majority of such patients are salt sensitive and therefore have a rise in blood pressure with dietary salt. As the GFR declines, salt balance can only be achieved by a parallel reduction in the fraction of the filtered sodium reabsorbed. This restricts the capacity of the tubule for rapid and effective achievement of salt balance during large changes in salt intake. Accordingly, patients with moderate or advanced CKD are unable to change renal salt excretion as rapidly or effectively during changes in salt intake as normal subjects. This results in greater gains of salt and body fluids during high salt intake and, especially in those with tubulointerstitial disease, greater losses of salt and body fluids during reductions in salt intake. Therefore, salt intake should be adjusted carefully and incrementally in patients with advanced CKD, and the patients must be carefully followed. Second, unlike normal individuals, patients with CKD typically experience reductions in GFR with low dietary salt and increases in GFR with high salt intake.

Patients with heavy proteinuria and the nephrotic syndrome respond poorly to an increase in salt intake. The underlying avid renal salt retention, together with the low plasma oncotic pressure, increases the body weight and the peripheral edema. Moreover, increases in dietary salt increase proteinuria. Therefore, dietary salt restriction is especially important in patients with CKD with heavy proteinuria and the nephrotic syndrome. The exception may be some younger subjects with minimal change nephropathy in whom the plasma volume is already contracted and the edema due almost entirely to the low plasma oncotic pressure. These subjects respond poorly to salt restriction.

DIURETICS

Effects of Salt Intake on the Fluid Depleting and Antihypertensive Responses to Diuretics

Studies in normal human subjects given a daily dose of a loop diuretic such as 40 mg of furosemide show the anticipated sharp increase in sodium excretion after the diuretic that leads initially to a negative balance for sodium and fluid. However, because of the short duration of loop diuretics of 4 to 6 hours, this is followed by 18 to 20 hours during which renal function is no longer dictated by the direct effects of the diuretic on the kidney. During this postdiuretic period, dietary salt and fluid may be retained sufficiently to counteract the immediate effects of the diuretic on the kidney. Studies at a high daily level of dietary salt intake (for example, 300 mmol) demonstrate that this postdiuretic renal sodium retention is sufficient to prevent any negative loss of sodium or fluid over 24 hours. In contrast, studies at a low daily level of dietary salt intake (for example, 20 mmol) show that negative salt balance is ensured because the diuretic-induced loss of salt is greater than the total daily intake. During dietary salt restriction, sodium balance is achieved by a declining natriuretic response to the drug (tolerance).

Salt restriction in normal subjects to a level of 100–120 mmol daily is required to induce any sustained loss of body salt and fluid. Thiazide and distal potassium-sparing diuretics generally have longer durations of action than loop diuretic. This restricts the capacity of the kidney to restore salt loss with once daily diuretic dosing. This likely accounts for the greater effectiveness of thiazide and distal diuretics, compared with loop diuretics, as antihypertensives. Clearly, dietary salt restriction is required to ensure negative salt balance, especially with the short-acting loop diuretics despite their extreme acute natriuretic potency.

All antihypertensive agents, with the possible exception of calcium channel blockers, are less effective in reducing the blood pressure during high dietary salt intake. Dietary salt restriction is especially important for patients receiving diuretics and drugs that inhibit the renin-angiotensin-aldosterone system (RAAS).

Drug-resistant hypertension is defined as sustained hypertension despite the use of three or more antihypertensive agents. Almost invariably, drug-resistant hypertension can be ascribed to inappropriate, ongoing high levels of salt intake and insufficient use of diuretics.

Angiotensin-converting enzyme inhibitors (ACEIs) and angiotensin receptor blockers (ARBs) are widely used to reduce protein excretion in patients with proteinuric kidney disease. This antiproteinuric action is lost during high levels of dietary salt intake, whereas a reduction in dietary salt itself produces a fall in protein excretion.

These observations lead to the proposal that dietary salt intake requires assessment and attention in all patients with more than the most modest levels of hypertension or CKD and any with heavy proteinuria.

GOALS OF DIETARY SALT RESTRICTION

The aim of salt restriction is to combat salt-sensitive hypertension, enhance antihypertensive drug responsiveness, achieve an appropriate level of blood pressure, prevent progressive loss of kidney function, limit proteinuria, and reduce cardiovascular risk. The level of salt intake required to achieve these goals varies with the clinical circumstance and the severity of the underlying condition.

An ideal daily level of dietary sodium intake for healthy, normotensive individuals is not clearly established but is likely 80–120 mmol. The first step in antihypertensive therapy, and the only step presently recognized for patients with prehypertension, is nonpharmacologic therapy of which dietary salt restriction is a key component. The goal daily salt intake for these individuals should be 100 mmol or less. Patients with drug-resistant hypertension and those with edema, nephrotic syndrome, or heavy proteinuria require a greater degree of dietary salt restriction. In practice, a goal of 80 mmol of sodium daily is often chosen. However, patients who are able to achieve lower levels of salt intake have a further reduction in blood pressure or protein excretion. Therefore, more severe levels of salt restriction should be encouraged in those willing and able to comply. This requires careful monitoring because patients with CKD not infrequently experience an initial reduction in GFR as salt intake is reduced. This reduction in GFR should reverse within weeks. Indeed salt restriction should slow the progressive loss of GFR over time.

ASSESSMENT OF DIETARY SALT INTAKE

A dietary history, even with the help of a skilled nutritionist, provides only an approximate insight into salt intake. Because greater than 95% of sodium ingested normally is excreted by the kidneys, a properly collected 24-hour urine for sodium excretion is the best indication of sodium intake. Patients should be instructed in how to undertake a 24-hour collection and cautioned against changes in dietary intake or diuretic therapy in the week preceding the collection. The completeness of collection should be assessed from measurements of creatinine excretion, which should be 14–22 mg/kg for women and 20–25 mg/kg for men (with allowance for body size and muscle mass). Subjects with fever, a strenuous aerobic exercise program, diarrhea, and especially those with an ileostomy have significant extrarenal sodium losses. Renal sodium excretion in these subjects is not an accurate measure of sodium intake. Because sodium excretion fluctuates widely during the day in response to meals, spot urine collection for sodium/creatinine ratio is a poor indication of dietary salt intake. A 24-hour urine collection also provides an opportunity to assess creatinine clearance, microalbumin or protein excretion, and the excretion of other food constituents such as potassium and calcium, which also can contribute to the level of blood pressure.

During accommodation to diuretic therapy in a subject without edema, there is initially a loss of body fluids resulting in approximately a 1 kg weight loss that is complete within 1 to 3 days. Negative sodium and fluid balance in patients with edema may persist for days or weeks during diuretic therapy. Dietary salt intake reflects renal sodium excretion in patients on diuretics only during the steady state. Therefore, patients should be provided adequate time to accommodate to diuretic therapy. Their body weight should have stabilized for some days before the 24-hour collection is undertaken. Because restriction of dietary salt is recommended even for patients with prehypertension and for most patients with CKD, especially those with proteinuria, a 24-hour urine collection for sodium excretion is an important initial assessment in all such subjects. If the level of sodium excretion is above goal, the 24-hour collection should be repeated about 1 month after providing dietary advice to assess compliance. A 24-hour urine collection for sodium excretion is essential in patients with drug-resistant hypertension and those accumulating edema, because inappropriate salt intake is a frequent contribution to these problems.

SALT CONTENT OF FOODS

Unfortunately, more than 80% of the salt ingested presently in the United States is already added to food prior to serving. Therefore, abolition of table salt cannot make more than a modest contribution to reducing salt intake. Reductions in dietary salt require changes in food intake and in eating habits. Dietary salt restriction is most effective in those individuals who can consume their meals in their own home from foods prepared in the household from fresh ingredients. These subjects should be able to reduce salt intake to recommended goals. The use of low salt-containing flour and other ingredients can reduce daily salt intake in subject eating home-prepared foods to less than 50 mmol. Unfortunately, most individuals eat food that is already prepared for them in restaurants or fast food outlets or prepared from processed or tinned foods in the home. These sources usually contain much higher levels of dietary salt, which may not be acknowledged explicitly by the food provider. Individuals eating in this manner have a much harder task to restrict dietary salt. They may require advice from a nutritionist or insight from reading nutritional pamphlets or books.

A critical component of success in dietary salt restriction is the motivation of the physician to assess salt intake regularly from 24-hour sodium excretion and to encourage patients as their salt intake improves or identify problem areas of salt intake in those in whom sodium excretion is not falling to goal levels. Obese subjects who have an excessive intake of food almost invariably have an excessive intake of salt. Such subjects are unlikely to be successful with salt restriction unless this is matched by restriction of calorie intake as part of a weight reduction program.

The body salt burden can also be reduced modestly by regular aerobic exercise with perspiration. A regime of 30 minutes of daily aerobic exercise is an important component of nonpharmacologic

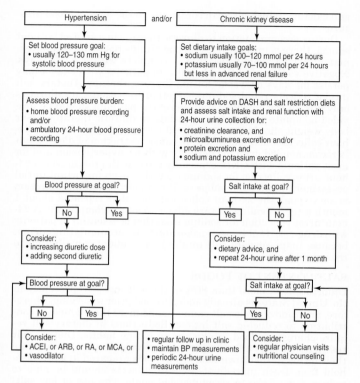

Figure 15-1. A proposed algorithm for the management of dietary salt intake in patients with hypertension or chronic kidney disease.

therapy for patients with hypertension and may also reduce progression of CKD, although this has been less well studied. Therefore, diet and exercise should be considered together and exercise adjusted appropriately within a subject's capacity.

Subjects accustomed to a high level of dietary salt intake may experience salt craving as they adapt to a lower salt intake. This salt-seeking behavior normally adjusts to meet the new level of salt intake after 1 to 2 weeks. Therefore, advice about a low-salt diet should contain a warning that the subject may experience a salt-seeking drive in the first few weeks but that this will abate with time. Salt can be substituted in the food by potassium chloride, providing there is no hyperkalemia or advanced CKD, or by a highly spiced diet. Nevertheless, most patients require advice about what foods contain an intrinsically high level of salt and must be avoided or their consumption restricted.

A National Institutes of Health (NIH)-funded controlled study of dietary advice to stop hypertension (DASH) demonstrated that over a relatively short period of months, a healthy diet with a

Table 15-1. Salt content of common foods

Food that contain *much* salt:
- Constituents of fast food, especially hamburgers,* pizza,* Thai,* and Mexican food*
- Olives in brine,* salted nuts,* potato chips*
- Canned beans,* corn,* and peas*
- Sauerkraut,* tomato ketchup,* or tomato puree*
- Peanut butter
- Corn flakes
- Bread,* crackers,* donuts, muffins, pies, pretzels,* scones*
- Cheese (especially Roquefort,* processed cheese,* camembert*)
- Bacon,* ham, pate,* sausages,* salami*
- Pickled, smoked, or canned fish
- Sardines

Foods that contain *little* salt:
- Fruits and fruit juices
- Vegetables and salads
- Unsalted nuts
- Grains and pasta
- Eggs, milk, yogurt, ice cream
- Chocolate
- Most fresh meats, fish, and shellfish
- Cottage cheese
- Carbonated drinks and alcoholic beverages

*Food especially rich in salt.

high intake of fruits, vegetables, nuts, and skimmed mild products with fish and white meat but little processed foods and red meat led to a remarkable reduction in blood pressure in normotensive and mildly hypertensive subjects. This DASH diet is an excellent basis for a healthy dietary intake but is not very low in salt. Therefore, it may need to be combined with advice on salt restriction for those with severe hypertension. Studies have shown that the blood pressure lowering effect of the DASH diet and of salt restriction are additive.

RECOMMENDATIONS
The management of dietary salt intake starts with setting appropriate goals for blood pressure, sodium, and sometimes potassium intakes (Fig. 15-1). Blood pressure should be assessed prior to changing the diet. The blood pressure burden is best assessed by home blood pressure recordings or ambulatory 24-hour blood pressure recording. Dietary advice then should be given. This can include advice about the DASH diet, together with referral to appropriate literature sources on the DASH diet or foods to avoid because of high salt content (Table 15-1). The effectiveness of this advice should be assessed by a 24-hour urine collection for sodium excretion, which can be combined with creatinine clearance and excretion of microalbumin and other minerals. If salt intake and blood pressure are at goal, regular follow-up in the clinic can be scheduled with measurements of blood pressure and periodic measurements of 24-hour sodium excretion to assess long-term

compliance. Where sodium excretion is not at goal, especially if blood pressure remains elevated, patients require further dietary advice and repeated 24-hour urine collection after approximately 1 month. Persistent failure to achieve goal sodium excretion requires regular physician visits and a nutritional consult.

Sources of Dietary Advice for Patients

Ellis P. The Cleveland Clinic Foundation creative cooking for renal diets. Chesterland, OH: Senay Publishing Inc; 1985.

Lentner C. Geigy scientific tables: units of measurement, body fluids, composition of the body, nutrition, Vol. 1. Basel, Switzerland: Ciba Geigy; 1981:243–260.

Mattes RD, Donnelly D. Relative contributions of dietary sodium sources. J Am Coll Nutr 1991;10:383–393.

Moore T, Svetkey L, Lin P-H, et al. The DASH diet for hypertension: Lower your blood pressure in 14 days without drugs. New York: The Free Press; 2001.

U.S. Department of Health and Human Services, NIH, NHLBI, NIH Publication No. 06-4082, 2006. *Your guide to lowering your blood pressure with DASH eating plan.*

Willett WC. Eat, drink and be healthy: The Harvard Medical School guide to healthy eating. New York: The Free Press; 2001.

Suggested Readings

Adrogue HJ, Madias NE. Sodium and potassium in the pathogenesis of hypertension. N Engl J Med 2007;356:1966–1978.

Cappuccio FP. Dietary salt reduction. In: Wilcox CS, ed. Therapy in Nephrology and Hypertension, 3rd ed. Philadelphia: Elsevier; 2008;583–590.

Cappuccio FP. Salt and cardiovascular disease. Br Med J 2007;334: 859–860.

Esnault VL, Ekhlas A, Delcroix C, et al. Diuretic and enhanced sodium restriction results in improved antiproteinuric response to RAS blocking agents. J Am Soc Nephrol 2005;16:474–481.

Franco V, Oparil S. Salt sensitivity, a determinant of blood pressure, cardiovascular disease and survival. J Am Coll Nutr 2006;25: 247S–255S.

He FJ, MacGregor GA. Effect of modest salt reduction on blood pressure: a meta-analysis of randomized trials. Implications for public health. J Hum Hypertens 2002;16:761–770.

Karppanen H, Mervaala E. Sodium intake and hypertension. Prog Cardiovasc Dis 2006;49:59–75.

Kelly RA, Wilcox CS, Mitch WE, et al. Response of the kidney to furosemide: II. Effect of captopril on sodium balance. Kidney Int 1983;24:233–239.

Ritz E. Lowering salt intake–an important strategy in the management of renal disease. Nat Clin Pract Nephrol 2007;3:360–361.

Sacks FM, Svetkey LP, Vollmer WM, et al. Effects on blood pressure of reduced dietary sodium and the Dietary Approaches to Stop Hypertension (DASH) diet. DASH-Sodium Collaborative Research Group. N Engl J Med 2001;344:3–10.

Schmidlin O, Forman A, Sebastian A, et al. What initiates the pressor effect of salt in salt-sensitive humans? Observations in normotensive Blacks. Hypertension 2007;49:1032–1039.

Weinberger MH. Sodium and blood pressure 2003. Curr Opin Cardiol 2004;19:353–356.

16

Obesity in Kidney Disease

Maarit Korkeila, Olof Heimbürger,
Bengt Lindholm, and Peter Stenvinkel

INTRODUCTION

Overweight and obesity, resulting from the imbalance between energy intake and expenditure, is a worldwide epidemic in both affluent as well as in many developing countries. The relationship between obesity and several major public health problems (diabetes mellitus, cardiovascular disease [CVD], cerebrovascular disease, musculoskeletal disorders, and some types of cancer) is well established, with a significantly increased morbidity and mortality as a consequence. Abdominal obesity is, in addition to hypercholesterolemia, hypertension, and insulin resistance or glucose intolerance, one of the CVD precursors included in the metabolic syndrome (MS).

The emerging problem with overweight and obesity is not only associated with diabetes and hypertension but also a higher risk of chronic kidney disease (CKD). Overweight and obesity share several risk factors together with diabetes, CVD, and CKD, and thus may all mutually contribute to the excess morbidity and mortality in patients suffering from these conditions. In patients with CKD, the impact of overweight and obesity on morbidity and mortality differs depending on CKD stage and treatment. Whereas obesity is a negative prognostic factor both for further progression of CKD and for morbidity and mortality during the CKD stages 1–4, recent epidemiologic evidence suggests it becomes a *positive* prognostic factor in patients receiving maintenance hemodialysis (MHD). Whereas this relationship is not as evident in patients receiving peritoneal dialysis (PD), obesity again is a negative factor for the clinical outcome in kidney transplant patients. In this chapter, we present an overview of clinically important aspects of overweight and obesity in CKD.

ENERGY EXPENDITURE AND MEASURES OF OBESITY IN PATIENTS WITH CHRONIC KIDNEY DISEASE

Whereas resting energy expenditure (REE) in patients receiving PD and hemodialysis (HD) is considered to be similar to that of healthy subjects, factors such as inflammation, secondary hyperparathyroidism, and diabetes may contribute to increased REE in patients with CKD. The current definition of overweight and obesity, based on body mass index (BMI) (Table 16-1), assumes that the proportion between different tissues (including fat and lean body mass [LBM]) is similar among individuals. The fact that BMI fails to make a distinction between these compartments is an obvious weakness. Moreover, age, gender, ethnicity, various diseases, nutritional intake, exercise, fluid overload, and many other factors may affect the validity of BMI as a measure of overweight. For example, BMI may relate better to body fat in overweight subjects than in subjects with normal weight. Despite the

Table 16-1.   The international classification of adult underweight, overweight, and obesity by body mass index in Caucasians according to World Health Organization (WHO)*

Category	BMI (kg/m^2)
Underweight	<18.5
Normal weight	18.5–24.9
Overweight	25.0–29.9
Obese	≥30.0
Obese class I	30.0–34.9
Obese class II	35.0–39.9
Obese class III	≥40.0

*Other values apply to the Asian population.
BMI, body mass index.

many limitations of BMI, it has the advantage of always being available, and therefore it has been widely used in numerous population studies as a measure of obesity.

Studies of body weight in patients with CKD is influenced by several confounding factors, like the water balance before and after dialysis and muscle depletion because of protein-energy wasting (PEW). *Obese sarcopenia* is defined as relative PEW and loss of LBM and has been shown to be common among obese patients with stage 5 CKD and associated with inflammation. Most of the studies on obesity in CKD are based on BMI because other, more specific measures of body composition are not ready available (Table 16-2). Many studies have indicated that the assessment of body composition (in particular LBM) is a more important prognostic determinant than BMI.

Recently, waist circumference and the waist-hip ratio (WHR) have emerged as measures that better reflect *abdominal* or *central* obesity. Many studies have concluded that compared with BMI, waist circumference and/or WHR are better predictors of mortality both in the general population and in CKD stages 1–3. Preliminary data show strong correlations between WHR and visceral fat mass assessed by computed tomography. Only a few systematic studies have compared the prognostic value of different measures of weight and body composition among patients with different stages of CKD.

THE PATHOGENESIS OF OBESITY

The increased prevalence of obesity is considered to result not only from increased caloric intake and a more sedentary lifestyle with reduced physical activity but also from genetic factors. Indeed, heritability studies have suggested that genetic effects determine as much as 70% of the variability in body weight in a given population. As the prevalence of obesity differs markedly between regions, nutritional factors are most certainly also of importance. It has been suggested that the markedly increased consumption of fructose in the United States (used as a soft drink sweetener in the United States, in contrast to Europe where

Table 16-2. Different methods for estimating weight and body composition in patients with chronic kidney disease

	BMI	WHR	Skinfold Thickness	Bioimpedance	Dual Energy X-ray Absorptiometry	Computed Tomography
Easy-to-use/cost	+ + +	+ + +	+ +	+ +	+	+
Reproducibility	+ + +	+ + +	+	+ + +	+ +	+ +
Distinction fat mass vs. lean body mass	0	0	+	+ +	+ + +	+ + +

+ + + Excellent
+ + Good
+ Moderate
0 Poor
BMI, body mass index; WHR, waist-hip ratio.

Table 16-3.   List of factors known or believed to be involved in the pathogenesis of obesity

- Increased caloric intake, especially rapid carbohydrates
- High fat intake
- Low physical activity/sedentary lifestyle
- Genetics
- Epigenetics
- Insulin resistance
- Drugs (such as steroids, insulin)
- Comorbidity

mainly saccharine is used for this purpose) may contribute to the increasing prevalence of obesity and cardio-renal disease in the United States. Many patients with CKD have a low physical activity because of decreased physical performance and increased tiredness because of CKD and comorbidity. In patients undergoing HD, the time needed for dialysis treatment and the common tiredness after a HD session may further contribute to physical inactivity. In patients treated with PD, the glucose absorption from the dialysate may represent a significant additional caloric load. Furthermore, many drugs commonly used in patients with CKD may contribute to obesity, such as steroids and insulin (Table 16-3).

OBESITY-RELATED KIDNEY DISEASES

Obesity leads to hyperfiltration, enlarged glomeruli, and pathologic changes resembling diabetic nephropathy. These morphologic changes are called *obesity glomerulopathy* and are defined as the histopathologic changes resembling focal segmental glomerulosclerosis (FSGS). Early changes seen in obesity-related FSGF are segmental or global glomerulosclerosis, glomerular hypertrophy, and minimal podocyte effacement. These changes have been described in subjects with apparently normal kidney function. The degree of glomerulomegaly is reported to correlate with the degree of obesity. Weight loss is shown to decrease proteinuria in overweight patients, but whether the histopathologic changes in obesity glomerulopathy are reversible is unclear. The risk of developing an obesity-related FSGS is considerable, and the glomerular lesions do differ from other types of FSGS. Both failing kidney function and microalbuminuria have lately been recognized as cardiovascular risk factors associated with MS. Although microalbuminuria is considered as a marker for endothelial dysfunction leading to increased CVD morbidity, the exact mechanisms for such a relationship are unknown. Overweight increases the risk for progressive renal disease in IgA nephropathy, mainly through hypertension and increased proteinuria. It is likely that obesity glomerulopathy, hypertension, and proteinuria at obesity are unspecific prognostic factors for developing CKD at several glomerulopathies and after unilateral nephrectomy (Table 16-4).

**Table 16-4.   Chronic kidney diseases in
which overweight and obesity have been
demonstrated to be independent risk factors**

- Proteinuria of other causes
- Diabetic nephropathy/metabolic syndrome
- Ischemic nephropathy/nephrosclerosis
- IgA nephropathy
- Obesity-related focal segmental glomerulosclerosis
- Unilateral nephrectomy
- Chronic allograft nephropathy

DIABETES, METABOLIC SYNDROME, AND INSULIN RESISTANCE

The MS is defined and caused by multiple risk factors correlating with each other. Metabolic syndrome and CKD share many cardiovascular risk factors, such as hypertension, insulin resistance, atherosclerosis, dyslipidemia, inflammation, and abdominal obesity, which predict increased mortality. The association between increased mortality and overweight in patients with MS may be weaker among patients with CKD. Prevention of obesity and overweight has been shown to decrease the development of type-2 diabetes and related complications in subjects without CKD.

Metabolic syndrome increases the incidence of CKD in nondiabetic adults, and the strength of association increases by the number of metabolic traits. Hypertension and obesity as a part of MS increase the risk for proteinuria, a well-known risk factor for CKD. However, similar to obesity, some of the risk factors included in the MS show a paradoxical inverse relation with mortality in CKD stages 4–5. Most studies show a clear survival advantage associated with high serum total cholesterol levels, most likely because they reflect low degree of inflammation and improved nutritional state. Interventions with statins have not been shown to improve survival in diabetic dialysis patients, and there is little evidence that the uremic dyslipoproteinemia is associated with increased mortality. Morbidity and mortality are increased in diabetic obese patients, and BMI is demonstrated to be the most important contributor to insulin resistance in patients with stage 3–4 CKD.

It should be noted that the clinical value of the MS in the general population is questioned. Indeed, a recent study showed that a fasting plasma glucose test is as good as or potentially better than a diagnosis of the MS for predicting diabetes and that diagnosis of the MS has less important association with risk of CVD than expected. Considering the great overlap between manifestations of CKD and the MS, the clinical value of using MS as a prognostic marker in patients with CKD is much debated.

ADIPOKINES

Adipose tissue is a hormonally active organ that releases a large number of bioactive proteins regulating not only body weight and energy homeostasis but also insulin resistance, dyslipidemia, inflammation, fibrinolysis, endothelial function, and coagulation.

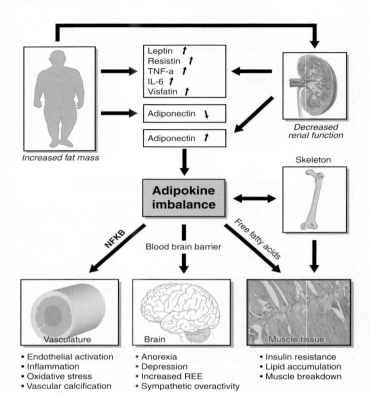

Figure 16-1. Retention of adipokines because of decreased renal function leads to an adipokine imbalance, which may have detrimental effects in the vasculature, brain, and muscle tissue. These local tissue effects may contribute to premature vascular disease, insulin resistance, and protein-energy wasting in chronic kidney disease.

While the pluripotent role of fat is still not completely elucidated, it appears likely that a reduced renal clearance contributes to the accumulation of *adipokines* (such as leptin, adiponectin, and visfatin) originating in part or whole from the adipose tissue, offering novel pathways to explain the marked dysmetabolism, or uremic MS (Fig. 16-1).

Leptin was initially described as a modulator of feeding behavior and thus of fat mass. While leptin signalling is more complex in humans, there is no doubt that loss of kidney function leads to inappropriately elevated serum concentrations of leptin. Serum leptin levels increase with initiation of PD and are related to body fat mass and inflammation. Because most studies have demonstrated an association between inflammatory biomarkers and leptin in CKD, it has been suggested that leptin may play a role in uremic PEW. Indeed, as experimental uremic cachexia can be ameliorated by blockade of leptin signalling through the hypothalamic melanocortin-4 receptor, melanocortin receptor antagonism may provide a novel therapeutic strategy for inflammation-associated wasting. The fact that low leptin levels have been shown to predict poor outcome in dialysis patients probably reflects the detrimental effects of state of energy wasting and loss of fat mass on outcome in this patient group.

Adiponectin is another adipokine that has attracted much interest as it improves insulin sensitivity in the liver and periphery, ameliorates endothelial dysfunction, and counteracts proinflammatory signalling. In contrast to other adipokines, increasing adipose tissue mass is inversely and paradoxically associated with low circulating levels of adiponectin. Low circulating adiponectin is generally found in populations at enhanced risk of CVD. Although plasma adiponectin levels are generally markedly elevated in patients with CKD, it has been reported that patients with CKD with relatively lower adiponectin levels have an increased risk of cardiovascular events. However, studies in larger patient materials have shown that a high, rather than a low, adiponectin level predicts mortality in both CKD and congestive heart failure. Further studies are needed to study if the effects of adiponectin in the brain that decrease body weight can explain the paradoxical relationships between adiponectin and outcome.

Emerging evidence suggests that adipose tissue is also a significant contributor to systemic inflammation. In fact, it has been estimated that adipose tissue (with resident macrophages) may contribute to about 20% to 30% of systemic IL-6 production. Other proinflammatory mediators, such as TNF-α and pentraxin-3, are also expressed in adipose tissue. Visceral adipose tissue releases more cytokines than subcutaneous fat. In accordance, one cross-sectional study of patients with stage 5 CKD showed that whereas a significant association was observed between visceral adipose tissue depots and circulating IL-6 levels, no such association was observed for subcutaneous fat tissue.

EPIDEMIOLOGY OF OBESITY IN CHRONIC KIDNEY DISEASE

Overweight and Risk for Chronic Kidney Disease in Healthy Subjects

It is now generally accepted that obesity is a risk factor for developing CKD and for accelerating the rate of decline of glomerular filtration rate (GFR) in patients with CKD stages 1–2. Thus, a high BMI correlates with higher cystatin C as a marker for kidney function in a healthy population without micro- or macroalbuminuria and estimated GFR >60 mL/minute/1.73 m^2. Several studies have shown that the risk for developing CKD (and eventually terminal CKD) increases linearly by increasing weight when adjusted for several confounders. Although part of this association is possibly mediated by the high prevalence of hypertension among overweight subjects, the association has remained significant fceven after adjustment for blood pressure. Nondiabetic subjects with MS have a 50% higher risk for developing CKD over 9 subsequent years than those without MS. Thus, the likelihood of developing CKD is markedly increased in subjects with known MS. This could be because of several factors; for example, a variety of glomerular abnormalities have recently been described among extremely obese subjects without overt CKD. Moreover, the risk for developing proteinuria and CKD after unilateral nephrectomy is markedly increased in obese subjects. However it is most likely that the most important risk factors linking MS with risk of CKD are hypertension, insulin resistance, and hyperlipidemia.

Overweight and Obesity in Patients Receiving Hemodialysis

Studies in North American patients receiving HD have demonstrated that a high body weight is associated with improved survival. This paradox may not exist in European patients receiving HD because one study showed that mortality patterns were rather similar to those in general populations, i.e., both low and increased body weight is associated with a moderate risk increase during a follow-up period of 7 years. One explanation for the discrepancy of the results might be the much higher prevalence of obesity in the United States compared with Europe. Also, the obesity paradox may be stronger in some ethnic subgroups, such as African Americans. In addition, obese patients starting dialysis in the United States may represent a selected group of survivors because North American patients with CKD are more likely to die than to progress to CKD stage 5. Other possible factors that might explain why obesity could represent a survival advantage are that the uremic toxin load may be less in patients receiving dialysis who have a high BMI because of larger distribution volume, or that these patients receive a larger dialysis dose in proportion to the higher V in the KT/V index, or that the observed protective effect of BMI is due more to a well preserved LBM than fat mass per se. Not unexpectedly, obese and underweight patients receiving dialysis report poorer self-rated health status, and physical function in particular, than normal weight or moderately overweight patients receiving HD. Some additional potential protective factors of increased fat mass in the context of uremia are shown in Figure 16-2.

Overweight and Obesity in Patients Receiving Peritoneal Dialysis

Weight gain and accumulation of fat mass after starting PD is a common problem. Some patients undergoing PD may have excessive weight gain mainly consisting of fat mass, and, in particular, intra-abdominal fat mass. Weight prior to PD, diabetes, female gender, genetics, comorbidity, and being a high transporter are the main determinants of weight gain and accumulation of fat mass during PD. Although the glucose load from PD solutions amounts to 100–200 g/day, most studies have not found any relation between the amount of absorbed glucose and gain in fat mass. However, this factor in combination with obesity-predisposing gene polymorphisms may contribute to the excessive PD-related weight gain in some patients. Long-term body weight on PD treat-

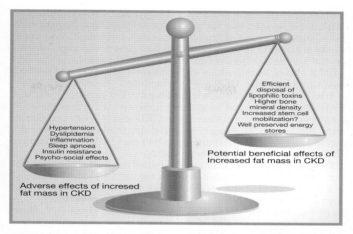

Figure 16-2. Balance between potential beneficial as well as adverse effects of increased body fat mass in the context of advanced chronic kidney disease.

ment seems to be relatively stable, but studies on body composition show a relative increase of fat mass over time. Interestingly, patients receiving PD who do not accumulate fat may risk losing LBM during PD. There is some evidence that patients with low energy stores may benefit from choosing PD as a dialysis modality because of possible weight gain after PD start. High BMI and preserved LBM in particular may be favorable for survival, whereas low body weight is a bad prognostic sign also in patients undergoing PD.

The results on associations between overweight, obesity, and mortality in patients undergoing PD are conflicting. Whereas some studies report that the risk of death for obese patients receiving PD is equal or increased in comparison with patients receiving PD who have normal body weight, others reported a survival benefit for overweight and obese patients who are undergoing PD. Furthermore, overweight and obesity in patients undergoing PD have been reported to be associated with increased incidence of peritonitis, catheter loss, technique failure, and more rapid decline of residual renal function.

WHAT ARE THE PRACTICAL CONSEQUENCES OF OBESITY IN CHRONIC KIDNEY DISEASE?

Several epidemiologic studies have demonstrated a J- or U-shaped relationship between mortality and BMI, and the risks for comorbidities are shown to increase linearly with increasing BMI in healthy populations. Assessing mortality attributed by obesity in population studies is confounded by several risk factors. These associations are even more complex in patients with CKD with high mortality and with several risk factors in common with cardiovascular morbidity and mortality. The significance of intentional weight loss for mortality among obese healthy subjects is controversial. Although unintentional weight loss in patients with CKD is an established bad prognostic sign, studies on the long-term effects of intentional weight loss or increase of LBM with a concomitant loss of fat mass on mortality and morbidity in patients with CKD are still lacking.

BMI is an imperfect metric for obesity. Fat mass (as assessed by BMI or bioelectrical impedance analysis [BIA]) has shown to be a proxy for insulin resistance in CKD stages 3–4. A combined approach, i.e., BMI along with WHR, particularly in physically active patients with CKD aiming to increase LBM, could improve their diagnostic and prognostic utility.

Obesity and overweight are established risk factors for developing CKD in healthy populations. In earlier CKD stages, obesity is a cardiovascular and metabolic risk factor comparable to that seen in the general population. In theory, decreased weight may have beneficial effects on the glomerular hemodynamics. However, the prognostic value of weight loss in patients with CKD is not yet established. In CKD stage 5 no excess risk for mortality because of overweight and obesity has been proven, probably much because of several competing risk factors and the common presence of PEW and/or inflammation in this patient group. LBM and WHR may be more important determinant for survival in CKD stages 3–5 than BMI. Loss of LBM and inflammation occur in CKD stages 3–5 regardless of body weight and are more dominating clinical problems than obesity per se in these patients.

There is no scientific evidence to support a recommendation for decreasing weight in obese patients undergoing dialysis, but increasing LBM is very likely beneficial in all stages of CKD. High physical activity is recommended (see Chapter 17). Energy intake should be scaled to normal BMI and not to actual body weight in all stages of CDK.

Pharmacologic treatment of obesity is not established in patients with CKD, and many of the drugs available are either contraindicated or not tested in patients with CKD. Orlistat can be used, but the clinical effect is very modest in patients with CKD. Anecdotal cases of surgical treatment of obesity in patients with CKD have been reported successful in kidney transplanted patients in particular.

Selected Readings

Allison DB, Kaprio J, Korkeila M, et al. The heritability of body mass index among an international sample of monozygotic twins reared apart. Int J Obes Relat Metab Disord 1996;20:501–506.

Axelsson J, Stenvinkel P. Role of fat mass and adipokines in chronic kidney disease. Curr Opin Nephrol Hypertens 2008;17:25–31.

Axelsson J, Qureshi AR, Suliman ME, et al. Truncal fat mass as a contributor to inflammation in end-stage renal disease. Am J Clin Nutr 2004;80:1222–1229.

Elsayed EF, Tighiouart H, Weiner DE, et al. Waist-to-hip ratio and body mass index as risk factors for cardiovascular events in CKD. Am J Kidney Dis 2008;52:49–57.

Fouque D, Kalantar-Zadeh K, Kopple J, et al. A proposed nomenclature and diagnostic criteria for protein-energy wasting in acute and chronic kidney disease. Kidney Int 2008;73:391–398.

Heimburger O. Obesity on PD patients: causes and management. Contrib Nephrol 2003:140:91–97.

International Obesity Taskforce. Available at: http://www.iotf.org/aboutobesity.asp. Accessed March 28, 2009.

Johnson, RJ, Segal MS, Sautin Y, et al. Potential role of sugar (fructose) in the epidemic of hypertension, obesity and the metabolic syndrome, diabetes, kidney disease, and cardiovascular disease. Am J Clin Nutr 2007;86:899–906.

Liu Y, Coresh J, Eustace JA, et al. Association between cholesterol level and mortality in dialysis patients. Role of inflammation and malnutrition. JAMA 2004;291:451–459.

de Mutsert R, Snijder MB, van der Sman-de Beer F, et al. Association between body mass index and mortality is similar in the hemodialysis population and the general population at high age and equal duration of follow-up. J Am Soc Nephrol 2007;18:967–974.

Sattar N, McConnachie A, Shaper AG, et al. Can metabolic syndrome usefully predict cardiovascular disease and diabetes? Outcome data from two prospective studies. Lancet 2008;371:1927–1935.

Serra, A, Romero R, Lopez D, et al. Renal injury in the extremely obese patients with normal renal function. Kidney Int 2008;73:947–955.

Sorensen TI, Rissanen A, Korkeila M, et al. Intention to lose weight, weight changes, and 18-year mortality in overweight individuals without co-morbidities. PLoS Med 2005;2:e171.

Utaka S, Avesani CM, Draibe SA, et al. Inflammation is associated with increased energy expenditure in patients with chronic kidney disease. Am J Clin Nutr 2005;82:801–805.

Van Gaal LF, Mertens IL, De Block CE. Mechanism linking obesity with cardiovascular disease. Nature 2006;444:875–880.

Verani RR. Obesity-associated focal segmental glomerulosclerosis: pathological features of the lesion and relationship with cardiomegaly and hyperlipidemia. Am J Kidney Dis 1992;20:629–634.

17

Exercise and Physical Function in Kidney Disease

Kirsten L. Johansen

There has been increasing recognition of the inextricable link between nutrition and physical activity over the last decade. This evolution in thinking is evident if one reviews the *Dietary Guidelines for Americans*, a publication that is produced jointly by the U.S. Department of Health and Human Services and the U.S. Department of Agriculture and updated every 5 years to provide science-based advice "to promote health and to reduce the risk for chronic diseases" in the population. Recommendations about physical activity have become increasingly prominent and detailed over successive revisions of this document from 1995 through 2005 because physical activity is a major determinant of energy expenditure, a key component of energy balance. Weight gain and the increase in obesity in the United States is a major public health concern and can be attributed to excessive caloric intake, inadequate energy expenditure in the form of physical activity, or a combination of the two. The *Dietary Guidelines* recommend that individuals consume a wide variety of foods to meet their nutrient needs. However, adequate nutrient intake must be achieved within calorie needs if neutral energy balance is to be maintained and weight gain avoided, and this can be difficult when energy expenditure is low. For these reasons and because of the recognition of the overall health benefits related to physical activity, its prominence has steadily increased to the point that the third of nine key messages conveyed by the *Dietary Guidelines for Americans, 2005 Edition* reads, "be physically active every day," and the dietary pyramid was modified to include physical activity.

EXERCISE AND ITS BENEFITS IN THE GENERAL POPULATION

It is necessary to review some general aspects of the terminology and physiology related to exercise and exercise training in the general population before applying these principles to chronic kidney disease (CKD) populations. Physical activity refers to any movement of the body that results in an increase in energy expenditure and includes activities of daily living as well as home maintenance and occupational activities. In contrast, exercise generally refers to physical activity that is planned, structured, repetitive, and purposive in the sense that improvement or maintenance of one or more components of physical fitness is the objective (Table 17-1). Physical activity is often classified by its intensity, which itself can be characterized on an absolute or a relative scale. The most common way of classifying activity is as a function of energy expenditure, in units of metabolic equivalents (METs), where one MET is the energy expended (or oxygen consumed) at rest. In this classification, light activity constitutes activity that

Table 17-1.   Glossary

Activities of daily living (ADLs)—Personal care activities necessary for everyday living, such as eating, bathing, grooming, dressing, and toileting.

Aerobic training—training that improves the efficiency of the aerobic energy-producing systems and that can improve cardiorespiratory endurance or fitness.

Body composition—A health-related component of physical fitness that relates to the relative amounts of muscle, fat, bone, and other vital parts of the body.

Cardiorespiratory endurance or fitness—A health-related component of physical fitness that relates to the ability of the circulatory and respiratory systems to supply oxygen during sustained physical activity.

Disability—The inability to perform or a limitation in the performance of actions, tasks, and activities usually expected in specific social roles that are customary for the individual or expected for the person's status or role in a specific physical environment.

Endurance training—repetitive, aerobic use of large muscles (e.g., walking, bicycling, swimming).

Exercise—Planned, structured, and repetitive bodily movement done to improve or maintain one or more components of physical fitness.

Flexibility—A health-related component of physical fitness that relates to the range of motion available at a joint.

Functional limitation—A deficit in the ability to perform a discrete task, such as stair climbing.

Instrumental activities of daily living (IADLs)—The more complex skills, such as maintaining a home, performing household chores, shopping, and managing finances, that are important components of independent living.

Maximal heart rate—The highest heart rate value attainable during an all-out effort to the point of exhaustion (often estimated as 220-age).

Maximal oxygen consumption (VO$_2$ max)—The maximal capacity for oxygen consumption by the body during maximal exertion. Also known as aerobic power, maximal oxygen uptake, and cardiorespiratory endurance capacity.

Metabolic equivalent (MET)—A unit used to estimate the metabolic cost (oxygen consumption) of physical activity. One MET equals the resting metabolic rate of approximately 3.5 mL O$_2$/kg/minute.

Moderate physical activity—Activity that causes some increase in breathing or heart rate and is perceived as light to somewhat hard (e.g., brisk walking).

Muscle fatigue—The decline in ability of a muscle to generate force as a result of prolonged or repetitive contraction.

Muscular endurance—The ability of the muscle to continue to perform without fatigue.

Physical activity—Bodily movement that is produced by the contraction of skeletal muscle that increases energy expenditure above basal levels.

(continued)

Table 17-1.   Glossary (*continued*)

Physical fitness—A set of attributes that people have or achieve that relates to the ability to perform physical activity.

Physical function or functioning—A fundamental component of health status describing the state of those sensory and motor skills necessary for usual daily activities.

Physical performance—The execution or accomplishment of specific physical tasks (e.g., walking, stair climbing).

Rating of perceived exertion (RPE)—A person's subjective assessment of how hard he or she is working. The Borg RPE scale® is a numerical scale for rating perceived exertion.

Resistance training—Training designed to increase strength, power, and muscular endurance.

Strength—The ability of the muscle to exert force.

Vigorous physical activity—Activity that causes a large increase in breathing or heart rate and is perceived as hard or very hard.

requires less than 4 METS (or less than 3 for older individuals), moderate activity requires 4 to 6 METs (or 3 to 6 for older individuals), and vigorous activity requires $\geq$6 METs (see Table 17-2 for specific examples of moderate and vigorous activities). Another way to categorize the intensity of physical activity is according to an individual's rating of perceived exertion, or (RPE). Gunnar Borg, a Swedish exercise physiologist, developed the Borg RPE Scale®, which starts at 6, corresponding to no exertion and goes to 20, or maximal exertion. Moderate activities are those for which the perceived exertion is in the range of 11 to 13 or "somewhat hard," and vigorous activities are in the range of 14 and above or "hard" to "very hard." It has been noted that in healthy individuals, heart rate during exertion can be approximated as 10 times the RPE.

Exercise is additionally classified as endurance (or aerobic) exercise or resistance (or strengthening) exercise. Endurance exercise involves repetitive, dynamic, and rhythmic use of large muscles (e.g., walking, running, bicycling) and is the major form of exercise that can improve cardiorespiratory fitness or maximal oxygen consumption (VO_{2max}). Resistance exercise generally involves lifting weights or all or part of one's body weight, or moving the body against an externally imposed resistance (e.g., using a strength training machine or stretching elastic bands). There is overwhelming evidence that both types of exercise have large health benefits in the general population, including prevention of disease and disability as well as improvement in symptoms or management of chronic disease or disability. Higher levels of physical activity have been linked to lower risk of overall and cardiovascular mortality and to reduced risk of outcomes such as cardiovascular events and development of diabetes mellitus, hypertension, colon cancer, and depression. In addition, regular physical activity can improve the control of hypertension and diabetes among those with established disease, increase bone den-

Table 17-2.   Examples of moderate and vigorous physical activities

Setting	Moderate	Vigorous
Exercise and leisure	Walking briskly, dancing, leisurely bicycling, or roller skating, horseback riding, canoeing, yoga	Jogging or running, fast bicycling, aerobic dance, martial arts, jump rope, swimming, step climbing
Sports	Volleyball, golfing, softball, baseball, badminton, doubles tennis, downhill skiing	Soccer, field hockey or ice hockey, lacrosse, singles tennis, racquetball, basketball, cross-country skiing
Home activities	Mowing the lawn with a push power mower, general lawn and garden maintenance, scrubbing floors or washing windows, vacuuming, sweeping	Mowing the lawn with a hand mower, shoveling, carrying and hauling, masonry, carpentry, moving or pushing furniture
Occupational activity	Walking and lifting as part of work, general carpentry	Heavy manual labor (e.g., digging ditches, carrying heavy loads)

sity and improve symptoms of arthritis, and improve physical functioning and psychological well-being among those with limitations. In 1996, the U.S. Surgeon General developed a report on physical activity and health, which concluded that "sedentary living habits clearly constitute a major public health problem." The report summarized the expected benefits of physical activity and included a series of conclusions and recommendations, among which were:

- People of all ages, both male and female, benefit from regular physical activity.
- Significant health benefits can be obtained by including a moderate amount of physical activity (e.g., 30 minutes of brisk walking or raking leaves, 15 minutes of running, or 45 minutes of playing volleyball) on most, if not all, days of the week. Through a modest increase in daily activity, most Americans can improve their health and quality of life.
- Additional health benefits can be gained through greater amounts of physical activity. Physical activity reduces the risk of premature mortality in general and of coronary heart disease, hypertension, colon cancer, and diabetes mellitus in particular. Physical activity also improves mental health and is important for the health of muscles, bones, and joints.
- More than 60% of American adults are not regularly physically active. In fact, 25% of all adults are not active at all.

The report also included some discussion of the dose-response relationship between physical activity and health benefits, but it was noted that the wide variation among studies summarized made it difficult to define an optimal dose that includes duration, intensity, and frequency of activity. Nevertheless, it was noted that there "appears not to be a lower threshold [to the dose-response relationship], thereby indicating that any activity is better than none." However, this finding was not highlighted, nor were specific recommendations given for implementation of increased physical activity among elderly individuals or those with chronic diseases.

In 1998, the American College of Sports Medicine issued a position stand on exercise and physical activity for older adults, which was updated to include individuals with chronic conditions and was endorsed by the American Heart Association as well in 2007. They noted that the goals of exercise appropriate to younger adults, such as prevention of cardiovascular disease, cancer, and diabetes, and increases in life expectancy, should perhaps be replaced in the oldest adults with a new set of goals, which include minimizing biological changes of aging, reversing disuse syndromes, the control of chronic diseases, maximizing psychological health, increasing mobility and function, and assisting with rehabilitation from acute and chronic illnesses. In addition, these guidelines highlighted the importance of defining the intensity of physical activity on a relative rather than an absolute scale. In other words, what would be light activity to a younger, healthier individual might well qualify as moderate intensity activity for an elderly individual or an individual with "clinically significant chronic conditions and/or functional limitations" (such as CKD).

POTENTIAL BENEFITS OF INCREASED PHYSICAL ACTIVITY AMONG PATIENTS WITH CHRONIC KIDNEY DISEASE

As a group, patients with end-stage renal disease (ESRD) on maintenance hemodialysis are extremely inactive, and inactivity is associated with lower survival in this population. In one study of 286 patients on maintenance hemodialysis (MHD), 59% of subjects reported that they were doing no physical activity beyond that needed for activities of daily living, and only 12% reported doing 30 minutes of physical activity on 3 or more days per week (as recommended by the Surgeon General). Another group took a quantitative approach and compared the level of physical activity among a group of 34 patients receiving MHD to that of 80 healthy individuals who were well matched by age and gender and who were chosen because they reported that they did not participate in regular physical activity. Despite the sedentary nature of the control group, the patients receiving MHD were 35% less active on average over a 1-week period.

Not only is physical inactivity prevalent in the ESRD population, but it has also been shown to be associated with loss of muscle mass, reduced physical functioning, and higher 1-year and 4-year mortality among patients beginning maintenance dialysis. Low cardiorespiratory fitness (peak oxygen consumption) is usually associated with inactivity and is typically seen in patients with advanced CKD. Patients undergoing maintenance dialysis have peak oxygen consumption that is usually about 50% to 60% of age-predicted norms, patients with stage 3–4 CKD are similarly low, and transplant patients are about 70% of age-predicted values. Low cardiorespiratory fitness has been shown to be associated with higher mortality among patients with ESRD on MHD as well as in the general population. Several studies have reported that exercise training can improve peak oxygen consumption among patients with advanced CKD as well as ESRD treated both with dialysis and transplantation. It should be noted, however, that with the exception of highly active transplant recipients, patients with CKD do not generally achieve normal levels of exercise capacity even after exercise training, suggesting that inactivity is not the only cause of reduced fitness in this population.

Although peak oxygen consumption is an important physiologic variable directly linked to level of physical activity and relevant to physical functioning and survival, it is problematic in the CKD population. First, many patients are so limited that they cannot perform the maximal treadmill testing or bicycle ergometry needed to measure exercise capacity in this way, limiting participation in studies to those who are healthy and active enough to perform maximal exercise testing. Second, the impact of improvements in peak oxygen consumption on patients' functioning is difficult to quantify. Therefore, it is important to consider other aspects of physical functioning, such as self-reported functioning, physical performance, and physical frailty, which are more closely related to quality of life.

Patients on maintenance dialysis report poor physical functioning when asked about their level of difficulty in performing various tasks, and they perform poorly when asked to do such things as walk a short or longer distance, rise repeatedly from a chair, or climb a flight of stairs. Both self-reported functioning and physical performance are correlated with physical activity as measured by recall questionnaires and by accelerometry. Inactivity-associated muscle atrophy and muscle weakness have also been observed among patients with CKD and contribute to poor physical performance. These aspects of poor physical functioning have been associated with lower health-related quality of life, with higher mortality in the dialysis population, and with worse outcomes following kidney transplantation. Fortunately, several recent studies have shown that both aerobic exercise training and resistance exercise training interventions can improve self-reported physical functioning among patients on dialysis and that resistance exercise training can increase muscle mass and strength.

Recently, the concept of physical frailty has been operationalized to allow its impact to be investigated among elderly community-dwelling individuals, where frailty has been associated with increased risk of disability, hospitalization, institutionalization, and death. Low physical activity is one of five key components of this definition of frailty, and two of the others are related to poor physical performance (weak grip strength and slow gait speed). The final two components are weight loss and exhaustion, with a total of three or more of these marking a person as frail. Both frailty and its components have been associated with kidney function. In the Cardiovascular Health Study, the original cohort used to develop this classification of frailty, patients with CKD, defined as serum creatinine greater than 1.3 mg/dL in women or 1.5 mg/dL in men, were almost 3 times as likely to be frail as individuals with normal kidney function (OR 2.85). After adjusting for demographic characteristics, comorbidity, and laboratory parameters such as hemoglobin and C-reactive protein (CRP), persons with CKD remained 1.5 times more likely to be frail than others. Furthermore, some aspects of the frailty phenotype, in particular tests of physical performance, have been shown to correlate with cystatin C-based estimates of glomerular filtration rate (GFR), even at levels of GFR above 60 mL/minute/1.73 m^2, with worse kidney function associated with worse physical performance. Carrying this into the dialysis arena, 67% of patients recently initiating dialysis were found to be frail by a similar definition, despite the fact that this cohort was not restricted to older individuals. In addition, the links between frailty and hospitalization and mortality were equally strong in this dialysis cohort as within cohorts of healthy elderly individuals.

In addition to the physical sequelae of inactivity, patients on dialysis, as well as those with earlier stages of CKD and kidney transplant recipients, suffer from a great burden of other chronic conditions that are potentially modifiable by exercise participation, including hypertension, dyslipidemia, coronary heart disease, diabetes, and depression. There is little data specific to patients with CKD on whether exercise actually improves most of these conditions. However, there are studies to suggest that blood pressure control and symptoms of depression are improved by

Table 17-3. Kidney disease outcomes quality initiative guidelines about physical activity*

- All dialysis patients should be counseled and regularly encouraged by nephrology and dialysis staff to increase their level of physical activity.
  - Unique challenges to exercise in dialysis patients need to be identified to refer patients appropriately (e.g., to physical therapy or cardiac rehabilitation) and to enable the patients to follow regimens successfully. Such challenges include orthopedic/musculoskeletal limitations, cardiovascular concerns, and motivational issues.
- Measurement of physical functioning:
  - Evaluation of physical functioning and re-evaluation of the physical activity program should be done at least every 6 months.
  - Physical functioning can be measured using physical performance testing or questionnaires (e.g., SF-36).
  - Potential barriers to participation in physical activity should be assessed in every patient.
- Physical activity recommendations:
  - Many dialysis patients are severely deconditioned and therefore may need a referral for physical therapy to increase strength and endurance to the point where they are able to adopt the recommended levels of physical activity.
  - Patients who qualify for cardiac rehabilitation should be referred to a specialist.
  - The goal for activity should be for cardiovascular exercise at a moderate intensity for 30 minutes most, if not all, days per week. Patients who are not currently physically active should start at very low levels and durations and gradually progress to this recommended level.
- Follow-up:
  - Physical functioning assessment and encouragement for participation in physical activity should be part of the routine patient care plan. Regular review should include assessment of changes in activity and physical functioning.

---

*Available at http://www.kidney.org/professionals/kdoqi/guidelines_cvd/guide 14.htm

exercise training among patients on MHD, and the evidence in the general population is quite convincing.

Thus, CKD is associated with a host of conditions that are associated with physical inactivity and potentially modifiable by increasing activity. In some cases, particularly in the arena of exercise capacity and physical functioning, exercise has been shown to result in significant improvement among patients with CKD, but we must extrapolate from studies in healthy individuals when considering such benefits as reduced cardiovascular events and increased survival. Nevertheless, the recent Kidney Disease Outcomes Quality Initiative (K/DOQI) Clinical Practice Guidelines for Cardiovascular Disease in Dialysis Patients included a set of guidelines related to physical activity (Table 17-3). Specifically, guideline 14.2 states that, "All dialysis patients should be encouraged by nephrology and dialysis staff to increase their level of physical activity."

RISK OF PHYSICAL ACTIVITY

It is important to consider the potential risks of increasing physical activity, particularly in the CKD population where physical functioning is generally poor and the risk of cardiovascular events is high relative to the general population. The two types of risks to consider are that of musculoskeletal injury and of cardiovascular events. Regular physical activity is associated with an increased incidence of activity-related injury, particularly in the case of vigorous exercise and sports activities. However, there is some evidence that moderate physical activity may confer some protection against injuries, possibly through gains in neuromuscular control, balance, and muscle strength. A recent study used data from the 2000 to 2002 National Health Interview Survey to examine this question. Respondents were asked about their level of physical activity, which investigators classified as inactive, insufficiently active, or active. They were also asked about any injuries that occurred in the last 3 months and about the setting in which the injuries occurred. Not surprisingly, there was a dose-response relationship between leisure-time physical activity level and increasing incidence of injury episodes related to sports or leisure-time activities. Conversely, they also found that inactive individuals had the greatest incidence of nonsport or nonleisure-time activity injury episodes, and leisure-time physical activity level was not associated with the odds of reporting any injury after adjusting for age, sex, education, and race/ethnicity. The increase in injuries related to leisure-time activity was offset by a reduction in nonleisure-time activity-related injuries.

As with musculoskeletal injuries, the risk of cardiovascular events such as myocardial infarction or cardiac arrest increases during vigorous physical exertion, and this is especially true for persons who are sedentary and who have coronary disease, either documented or undiagnosed. The increased risk of an event occurring during exercise compared with during a period of inactivity is greater with higher intensity exercise and with lower habitual physical activity level. In other words, compared with sedentary people who suddenly begin exercising vigorously, persons who exercise regularly have a lower risk of exercise-related sudden death, although even this group has a transient elevation of risk during and immediately after vigorous exercise. However, it should be noted that physically active or physically fit individuals have a 25% to 50% lower overall risk of developing cardiovascular disease, an important consideration for patients with earlier stages of CKD.

Patients with CKD have the potential to be at higher risk for both of these complications of exercise than the general population. Musculoskeletal risk may be increased as a result of hyperparathyroidism and bone disease, which may place patients at greater risk for fracture and spontaneous tendon ruptures. Overall, the Surgeon General's report states that most musculoskeletal injuries related to physical activity are preventable by gradually working up to a desired level of activity and by avoiding excessive amounts of activity and that the net effect of regular

Table 17-4. **Minimizing risk of exercise participation**

Proper Screening	Rule Out Contraindications
	• Recent myocardial infarction or electro-cardiogram changes consistent with myo-cardial infarction
	• Unstable angina
	• Uncontrolled arrhythmia
	• Third-degree heart block
	• Acute progressive heart failure
	• Elevated blood pressure
	• Any acute condition that would make ex-ercise participation high risk
	• Inability to walk or unstable gait
Proper equipment	Comfortable, stable footwear
	Loose-fitting clothing
Exercise considerations	Begin at low intensity and short duration
	Encourage stretching before and after exer-cise
	Progress gradually according to perceived exertion
	Avoid excessively vigorous activity
	Include 5 minutes of warm-up before and cool-down after any session that is of at least moderate intensity
Evaluate frequently	• Provide encouragement, reinforcement
	• Monitor for problems
	• Reinitiate after intercurrent illnesses

physical activity is a lower risk of mortality from cardiovascular disease. Similarly, it is likely that the risk of cardiac events is higher because of the high prevalence of known cardiac disease and risk factors for cardiac disease. Therefore, it is important to take steps to minimize these risks (Table 17-4). The first step is risk assessment. Individuals should be screened for contraindica-tions to exercise participation, including recent electrocardi-ogram changes suggestive of myocardial infarction or recent myo-cardial infarction, uncontrolled arrhythmia, unstable angina, third-degree heart block, severe symptomatic aortic stenosis, sus-pected or known aortic dissection, or acute progressive heart fail-ure. In addition, uncontrolled hypertension with a systolic blood pressure >200 mm Hg or diastolic blood pressure >120 mm Hg is a relative contraindication to exercise participation. Because adverse effects of exercise are more common with vigorous exer-cise, especially if undertaken by sedentary individuals, the second step is to start exercising at moderate intensity and for short duration.

APPROACH TO PHYSICAL ACTIVITY PROMOTION IN THE CHRONIC KIDNEY DISEASE POPULATION

As a result of the growing body of literature on the benefits of physical activity among members of the general population as well as among persons with CKD, recently published K/DOQI Clinical Practice Guidelines for Cardiovascular Disease in Dialysis Patients included a series of recommendations about physical activity (see Table 17-3). Key elements of these recommendations include a statement that assessment and counseling about physical activity should be done by nephrologists or dialysis unit staff. These guidelines specifically recommend a target of 30 minutes of moderate activity on most days, in accord with the Surgeon General's recommendation and with the American Heart Association/American College of Sports Medicine recommendations for older individuals and persons with chronic conditions and stress that patients should be started at low levels and gradually progressed to recommended levels. Unfortunately, however, a survey of nephrologists showed that most nephrologists are not counseling patients to become more active, and a major reason cited by nephrologists for not counseling was a lack of confidence in their ability to discuss this topic. Although the guidelines provide specific targets, they do not address implementation, something nephrologists urgently need.

Reasons for the lack of focus on the mechanics of exercise prescription include the facts that exercise was only one part of a large set of guidelines on cardiovascular disease and that there are no data specific to CKD populations on how to increase physical activity levels. Therefore, strategies for increasing physical activity among patients with CKD, as for many other aspects of their care, must be extrapolated from information available in persons without kidney disease. Nephrologists have several options available to increase physical activity participation among their patients. These include asking patients about their level of activity, educating them about the benefits of increasing physical activity, providing them with written information about physical activity participation, referring them for physical therapy or cardiac rehabilitation, or, in the case of dialysis patients, providing opportunities to participate in physical activity during dialysis.

First, simply asking patients about their level of physical activity lets them know that this is an important aspect of their medical care. Second, nephrologists can educate patients about the potential benefits of exercise to further reinforce its role in their care. Third, nephrologists can provide written information about exercise and its benefits. A detailed exercise guide specifically designed for patients on dialysis is available at no cost online through Life Options, a program of research-based education and outreach that aims to improve quality of life among patients with kidney disease. This booklet contains information about the benefits of regular exercise as well as specific information about how to get started on an exercise program. Physicians can refer patients to this Web site, or they can download the booklet and provide it to patients directly. In addition, there are a multitude of internet-based sources of exercise information directed at the general public or older individuals provided by such organizations as the Centers for Disease Control and Prevention, the U.S. Department of Agriculture, the American College of Sports Medicine, Harvard School of Public Health, and many others. These resources are valuable for patients who are healthy except for kidney disease, but some patients may need additional help or

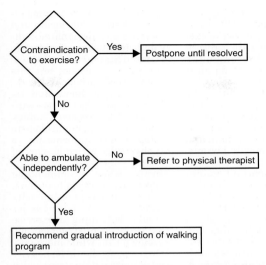

Figure 17-1.   General algorithm for starting aerobic exercise program.

support. Patients who are unable to walk or who have difficulty walking can be referred to physical therapists for evaluation and for recommendations on how to increase strength and physical activity, which should be covered by Medicare. Patients who have known or suspected cardiac disease or congestive heart failure can be referred for cardiac rehabilitation, a large component of which is geared toward beginning an exercise program.

Finally, nephrologists can discuss the specifics of exercise with patients (Fig. 17-1) or can provide opportunities for physical activity participation during dialysis sessions for patients receiving in-center hemodialysis. The latter strategy has been shown to be beneficial and in some cases to improve the efficiency of dialysis and reduce adverse effects such as hypotensive episodes and cramping. Several authors have advocated exercise during dialysis because of better adherence because it does not require additional time commitments from the patients and because it can reverse the forced inactivity of dialysis that does not include exercise. However, although there are many programs in Canada and elsewhere that have successfully incorporated in-center exercise, in the United States, the dialysis provider system does not lend itself easily to incorporating such activity during the dialysis treatment. Dialysis staff are often less than enthusiastic about supporting dialysis-unit based exercise programs, citing concerns about lack of time, patient safety (the difficulty of maneuvering around exercise equipment in the case of a dialysis-related emergency), and staff safety (the possibility of injury when moving bulky exercise equipment to allow patient participation). These barriers are not trivial in any circumstance, but they become effectively insurmountable in the absence of strong physician and unit leadership support of exercise, as well as a designated individual to manage the prescription and monitoring of exercise. Unfortunately, very few units in the United States currently have the resources to provide an on-site exercise program, but this should not preclude encouragement of exercise outside of the dialysis setting. In addition, because patients on home dialysis (peritoneal dialysis or other hemodialysis modality), those with CKD not requiring dialysis, and those who have received kidney transplants are also in need of exercise counseling, nephrologists should develop a mechanism to provide specific information to patients about how to become more physically active as part of their lifestyle.

The most important guiding principle when recommending that patients increase their level of physical activity is to encourage patients to start slowly and gradually increase the intensity and duration of their activity (see Table 17-4). A major barrier to exercise counseling by physicians and to beginning an exercise program for patients is the notion that exercise must be vigorous to be beneficial. Newer research has shown that while more may be better, "even a little is good," and this concept should be heavily emphasized when discussing physical activity with patients with CKD. The idea of "no pain, no gain" should be abandoned, and patients should be advised to start at a level that can be accomplished *without* pain. Although the target is 30 minutes of moderate exercise on most days of the week, it is important to recognize that many patients will need to start with a much shorter duration of activity and that "moderate exercise" should be defined relative to the individual's level of fitness rather than in absolute terms. Thus, rather than advising patients to walk at a certain speed (a difficult recommendation to follow in any case), patients should be advised to walk at a speed that they perceive as "somewhat hard" to "hard" but not "very hard." The example of walking will be used throughout this section, but bicycling or other activity can be prescribed following similar principles. Walking, however, has several advantages: it is generally safe; there is no need for special equipment; it can be done anywhere; intensity can be varied; and it can be tracked by time, distance, or number of steps. In addition, there is specific evidence for the benefit of walking through the Nurses' Health Study, the Harvard Alumni Health Study, and the National Health Interview Survey, and the Women's Health Initiative, among others.

A key component of a successful exercise program is monitoring, and this is where nephrologists or dialysis unit staff could make exercise a part of the patient care plan even without instituting a unit-based program. If patients were routinely asked about the time spent in physical activity and the intensity of the activity, progression to recommended levels could be facilitated. The first goal is usually to increase the duration of exercise to at least 20 minutes per session, and preferably 30 minutes. This can be done gradually, with an increase of 1 to 2 minutes per week as tolerated. Then patients can be encouraged to increase the intensity of the activity. In the case of walking, this can be accomplished by increasing speed, adding uphill segments to the route, or by carrying hand weights and/or wearing ankle weights. Most patients should not be encouraged to increase the velocity to the point of jogging because this may increase the chances of injury. All patients should be advised of the target perceived level of exertion ("somewhat hard" or "hard" but not "very hard") and should be told that exertion should not be so strenuous that they cannot talk during exercise.

In addition to walking or other aerobic activity, physical activity guidelines also state that to promote and maintain health and physical independence, older adults will benefit from performing activities that maintain or increase muscular strength and endurance for a minimum of 2 days each week. These activities include a progressive weight training program, weight bearing calisthenics, and similar resistance exercises that use major muscle groups. The general principle of starting low and increasing gradually applies here as well. The starting weight should be one that can be lifted at least 10 to 15 times for each exercise at a level of exertion that is moderate. However, it may be more difficult for nephrologists to discuss the specifics of resistance training than walking programs, so the option of a physical therapy referral for detailed instructions should be utilized liberally, and physicians can reinforce progress by asking periodically and re-referring as needed for progress assessments and updated recommendations.

Finally, physical activity guidelines for older individuals also state that to maintain the flexibility necessary for regular physical activity and daily life, older adults should perform activities that maintain or increase flexibility on at least 2 days each week for at least 10 minutes each day. To reduce risk of injury from falls, community-dwelling older adults with substantial risk of falls (e.g., with frequent falls or mobility problems) should perform exercises that maintain or improve balance. Physical therapists are well equipped to provide balance and flexibility exercise recommendations to patients with CKD, and these can be incorporated into an overall exercise plan. Stretching exercises should be performed before and after aerobic exercise to warm up and cool down the muscles while also maintaining mobility.

Unfortunately, increasing physical activity and improving fitness are often not one-time endeavors. Patients with CKD suffer from many comorbid conditions and become ill or require hospitalization frequently, which must be taken into account when discussing physical activity with patients. Fitness declines rapidly during periods of bed rest, and it can be discouraging for patients to experience health-related setbacks. Physicians can help by acknowledging that it is not unexpected for there to be losses in ability to exercise associated with these events and by encouraging patients to repeat the process of initiating physical activity during recovery. They should find a new comfortable level, which may well be lower than previously tolerated activity, and should build gradually from there.

In general, it cannot be emphasized enough that physician involvement increases the chances that patients will increase and sustain their level of physical activity. There have been few studies of the experience of patients with CKD with physical activity, but one study of dialysis patients reported that lack of encourage-

ment from their healthcare team was a barrier to exercise participation. Patients often receive subtle or not-so-subtle messages
from their physicians that they are not capable of being active.
Asking about and encouraging physical activity should be part
of our routine care for these patients.

Internet Resources

American College of Sports Medicine: http://www.acsm.org/AM/
Template.cfm?Section = General_Public.

Center for Disease Control and Prevention: http://www.cdc.gov/
nccdphp/dnpa/physical/.

Harvard School of Public Health: http://www.hsph.harvard.edu/
nutritionsource/staying-active/.

Life Options: http://www.lifeoptions.org/catalog/catalog.php?prod-
Cat = booklets: Exercise: A Guide for People on Dialysis.

U.S. Department of Agriculture and U.S. Department of Health and
Human Services: www.mypyramid.gov.

Selected Readings

American College of Sports Medicine Position Stand. Exercise and
physical activity for older adults. Med Sci Sports Exerc 1998;30:
992–1008.

Borg G. An Introduction to Borg's RPE Scale. Ithaca, NY: Movement
Publications; 1985.

Carlson SA, Hootman JM, Powell KE, et al. Self-reported injury and
physical activity levels: United States 2000 to 2002. Ann Epidemiol
2006:16:712–719.

Cheema B, Abas H, Smith B, et al. Progressive exercise for anabolism
in kidney disease (PEAK): a randomized, controlled trial of resistance training during hemodialysis. J Am Soc Nephrol 2007;18:
1594–1601.

Fried LP, Tangen CM, Walston J, et al. for the Cardiovascular Health
Study Collaborative Research Group. Frailty in older adults: evi-
dence for a phenotype. J Gerontol A Biol Sci Med Sci 2001;56A:
M146–M156.

Johansen KL, Painter PL, Sakkas GK, et al. Effects of resistance
exercise training and nandrolone decanoate on body composition
and muscle function among patients who receive hemodialysis: A
randomized, controlled trial. J Am Soc Nephrol 2006;17:2307–2314.

Johansen KL, Sakkas, GK, Doyle J, et al. Exercise counseling practices among nephrologists caring for patients on dialysis. Am J
Kidney Dis 2003;41:171–178.

Kesaniemi YK, Danforth E, Jensen MD, et al. Dose-response issues
concerning physical activity and health: an evidence-based sympo-
sium. Med Sci Sports Exerc 2001;33(Suppl 6):S351–S358.

National Institute on Aging. Exercise: a guide from the National Institute on Aging. U.S Department of Health and Human Services,
Public Health Service, National Institutes of Health, National Institute on Aging. NIH Publication No. 01-4258, April 2008.

National Kidney Foundation. K/DOQI Clinical Practice Guidelines
for Cardiovascular Disease in Dialysis Patients. Am J Kidney Dis
2005;45(Suppl 3):S1–S154.

Nelson ME, Rejeski WJ, Blair SN, et al. Physical activity and public
health in older adults: recommendation from the American College

of Sports Medicine and the American Heart Association. Circulation 2007;116:1094–1105.

Office of the U.S. Surgeon General. Physical activity and health: A report of the Surgeon General. Washington, D.C.: U.S. Department of Health and Human Services, National Center for Chronic Disease Prevention and Health Promotion; 1996.

Painter PL, Hector L, Ray K, Lynes L, et al. A randomized trial of exercise training after renal transplantation. Transplantation 2002;74:42–48.

Shlipak MG, Stehman-Breen C, Fried LF, et al. The presence of frailty in elderly persons with chronic renal insufficiency. Am J Kidney Dis 2004;43:861–867.

U.S. Department of Health and Human Services and U.S. Department of Agriculture. Dietary Guidelines for Americans, 2005. Washington, D.C.: U.S. Department of Health and Human Services and U.S. Department of Agriculture; 2005.

Nutritional Interventions in Chronic Kidney Disease

Lilian Cuppari

NUTRITIONAL INTERVENTION IN CHRONIC KIDNEY DISEASES

In serious chronic diseases such as chronic kidney disease (CKD) the nutritional condition has important impact on many outcomes. Protein-energy wasting (PEW) is highly prevalent in patients with advanced CKD and is strongly associated with morbidity and mortality, particularly in patients undergoing maintenance dialysis therapy. Conversely, overweight and obesity are also common nutritional abnormalities in CKD and may have undesirable effects, especially in earlier stages of CKD and transplant patients. Additionally, the development of several metabolic and hormonal disturbances, the presence of comorbidities, and the effect of renal replacement therapies make the nutritional interventions complex because multiple nutrients must be altered simultaneously. Therefore, a successful intervention depends not only on knowledge on the various nutrition-related aspects of the disease but also on the appropriate approaches to implement dietary plans that can be effectively followed by the patients.

This chapter addresses the main applicable clinical information regarding the nutritional status evaluation, dietary planning, and nutritional intervention for patients with CKD in different stages of the disease.

Assessment and Monitoring Nutritional Status

Assessing and monitoring the nutritional status of patients with CKD during every stage of the disease are critical to prevent, diagnose, and treat nutritional abnormalities. Assessment of nutritional status requires multiple different parameters because there is not a single measurement that provides unequivocal and complete diagnosis of the nutritional condition. Therefore, several methods have been proposed including those that are simple and readily available in the clinical practice and others that are expensive and sophisticated and usually used for research purposes. It is beyond the scope of this chapter to describe in detail each method, but instead this chapter provides a panel of methods that has been considered the most reliable by the majority of published clinical practice guidelines on nutrition in kidney disease. There is a consensus that the panel should include anthropometrics and biochemical measurements, subjective global assessment (SGA), and dietary intake evaluation.

Recently, the International Society of Renal Nutrition and Metabolism (ISRNM) organized an expert panel to re-examine the

Table 18-1.   Readily utilizable criteria for the clinical diagnosis of protein-energy wasting in acute kidney injury and chronic kidney disease

CRITERIA

Serum chemistry
Serum albumin <3.8 g per 100 mL (Bromocresol Green)*
Serum prealbumin (transthyretin) <30 mg per 100 mL (for patients on maintenance dialysis only; levels may vary according to GFR level for patients with CKD stages 2–5)*
Serum cholesterol <100 mg per 100 mL*

Body mass
BMI <23 kg/m^{2†}
Unintentional weight loss over time: 5% over 3 months or 10% over 6 months
Total body fat percentage <10%

Muscle mass
Muscle wasting: reduced muscle mass 5% over 3 months or 10% over 6 months
Reduced mid-arm muscle circumference/area‡ (reduction >10% in relation to 50th percentile of reference population)
Creatinine appearance§

Dietary intake
Unintentional low DPI <0.8 g/kg/day for at least 2 months¶ for dialysis patients or 0.6 g/kg/day for patients with CKD stages 2–5
Unintentional low DEI <25 kcal/kg/day for at least 2 months¶

*Not valid if low concentrations are because of abnormally great urinary or gastrointestinal protein losses, liver disease, or cholesterol-lowering medicines.
†A lower BMI might be desirable for certain Asian populations; weight must be edema-free and stable, for example, postdialysis dry weight.
‡Measurement must be performed by a trained anthropometrist.
§Creatinine appearance is influenced by both muscle and meat intake.
¶Can be assessed by dietary diaries and interviews, or protein intake by calculation of normalized protein equivalent of total nitrogen appearance (nPNA or nPCR) as determined by kinetic measurements.
AKI, acute kidney injury; BMI, body mass index; CKD, chronic kidney disease; DEI, dietary energy intake; DPI, dietary protein intake; GFR, glomerular filtration rate; nPCR, normalized protein catabolic rate; nPNA, normalized protein nitrogen appearance; PEW, protein-energy wasting.
Reprinted from Fouque D, Kalantar-Zadeh K, Kopple J et al. A proposed nomenclature and diagnostic criteria for protein-energy wasting in acute and chronic kidney disease. Kidney Int 2008;73:391–398.

terms and criteria used for the diagnosis of PEW. Table 18-1 shows the expert panel recommendations for four main and established categories to the diagnosis of PEW. At least three out of the four listed categories (and at least one test in each of the selected category) must be satisfied for the diagnosis of kidney disease-related PEW.

Undoubtedly, these proposed criteria have a great applicability in clinical practice not only because the measurements and methods are readily available in the majority of the centers but also because it provides clearly indications on how to use them to reach a diagnosis. However, the validity of this proposal has to

Table 18-2. Main limitations of commonly used parameters for nutritional assessment in chronic kidney disease

Parameter	Limitations
Serum albumin	Large pool size and long half-life. Decreases with fluid overload and inflammation.
Serum prealbumin	Decreases with inflammation and is elevated because of decreased renal catabolism.
Serum cholesterol	Poor sensibility and specificity to nutritional condition.
BMI	Influenced by lean mass and hydration status. Cutoff point may differ according to ethnicity and age.
Body fat	High inter- and intraobserver variability when estimated by skinfold thickness.
Midarm muscle circumference/ area	Indirect estimation of muscle mass, high inter and intraobserver variability.
Creatinine appearance	Depends on the precision of collected urine and dialysate. Is affected by meat ingestion.
Dietary intake Food records	Underreporting of energy intake.
nPNA	Great day-to-day variation in energy intake. In catabolic condition nPNA may exceed protein intake. A single measurement may not reflect the usual protein intake. Errors in urine collection can lead to misleading results.

nPNA, normalized protein nitrogen appearance.

be tested. In addition, despite the recognized association of most of these parameters with poor outcomes in the population of patients with CKD, it is important to be aware of their limitations as markers of PEW to properly interpret the results. Table 18-2 lists the main limitations of the commonly used parameters.

Additionally, the National Kidney Foundation Kidney Disease Outcomes Quality Initiative (NKF-K/DOQI) Clinical Practice Guidelines for Nutrition in CKD as well as the European Best Practice Guideline on Nutrition have recommended the use of 7-point Subjective Global Assessment because low SGA values are associated with high rates of morbidity and mortality in patients undergoing maintenance dialysis. Many other potential indicators of PEW such as appetite assessment questionnaires, composite nutrition score systems, handgrip strength, and inflammatory markers have been proposed and could also be included in the panel of nutritional assessment parameters.

Monitoring the nutritional status on a regular basis is the key to early detect nutritional disturbances, to evaluate the response of nutritional interventions, and to motivate and improve patient's compliance to the dietary therapy. There is no definitive protocol for routine follow-up, but in general body weight, body mass index (BMI) and normalized protein equivalent of nitrogen appearance (nPNA) should be measured monthly for patients undergoing dialysis therapy and every 1 to 3 months for CKD stages 4 and 5. Serum albumin, prealbumin, and cholesterol should be determined every 3 months in clinically stable patients. Other anthropometric measurements, dietary interviews, and SGA should be obtained every 6 months or more often in those patients at risk of developing PEW or with established PEW.

Diet Therapy for Adult Patients with Chronic Kidney Disease

For assessing and prescribing energy and most nutrient intake for patients with CKD, actual edema-free body weight (BW_{ef}) should be used if BW is between 95% and 115% of the median standard body weight (SBW). Adjusted edema-free body weight (aBW_{ef}) should be calculated when patient's weight is lower than 95% or higher than 115% according to the following equation:

$$aBW_{ef} = BW_{ef} + [(SBW - BW_{ef}) \times 0.25]$$

Energy

Chronic Kidney Disease Stages 2 to 5 Not on Maintenance Dialysis

There is compelling evidence suggesting that the energy expenditure of clinically stable patients with CKD not on dialysis treatment is similar or even lower than that of healthy subjects. For this reason, the energy recommendation ranges between 30 and 35 kcal/kg/day, which are values close to those recommended for healthy individuals. Ideally, for estimating the energy requirement of a patient with CKD, factors such as age, gender, physical activity level, nutritional status, and the presence of metabolic disturbances and comorbidities should be considered. However, the contribution of these factors for the daily energy expenditure for this particular group of patients is unknown. Therefore, predictive equations and physical activity factors developed for other populations have been used as an alternative for patients with CKD. Harris and Benedict's equation and Schofield's equation are among the most used in clinical practice to estimate resting energy expenditure or basal metabolic rate. However, there are concerns regarding the validity of these equations for patients with CKD. Physical activity is another important component for the estimation of energy requirement. Although some studies indicate that most patients with CKD have low physical activity level (PAL), it is not known whether the PAL factor of these patients is similar to the ones proposed for healthy subjects. For these reasons, estimation of energy requirement by using either the energy recommended by guidelines or estimated by equations can be very helpful only as an initial guide for planning the diet.

The best way to evaluate whether the estimated energy requirement is adequate in a patient with CKD is by monitoring the
patient's nutritional status and making appropriate adjustments
as needed.

Most patients with CKD stage 2–5 who are not on maintenance
dialysis are potentially on a low-protein diet, and thus it is important to provide an amount of energy sufficient to guarantee at
least a neutral nitrogen balance. Therefore, diets containing less
than 25 kcal/kg/day should be avoided even for patients who need
to lose weight.

Chronic Kidney Disease Stage 5 on Maintenance Dialysis

It is well demonstrated that hemodialysis is a catabolic event
leading to increased energy and protein catabolism, not only during the dialysis session but also over 2 hours following the completion of hemodialysis. However, several lines of evidence indicate
that this effect can be reverted by intradialytic nutritional supplementation. Therefore, it seems advisable to provide, whenever
possible, oral supplements or even a well-designed meal/snack
for patients during hemodialysis. To avoid vomiting, it is recommended to provide the supplement/food during the initial hours of
the dialysis session or potentially within 1 hour prior to initiating
hemodialysis.

Metabolic derangements such as hyperparathyroidism and acidosis as well as inflammation may become more severe in patients
with CKD undergoing maintenance dialysis and can result in
increased energy expenditure. However, except if persistent and
severe, the impact of these abnormalities on the energy requirement may be small. Indeed, the daily energy expenditure of patients on dialysis seems to be comparable to that of subjects with
normal renal function as demonstrated by several studies. The
NKF-K/DOQI Clinical Practice Guidelines for Nutrition in
Chronic Renal Failure recommends a daily energy intake of 35
kcal/kg/day for patients who are less than 60 years of age and
30–35 kcal/kg/day for those older than 60 years. The recent published European Best Practice Guideline on Nutrition recommends 30–40 kcal/kg/day adjusted for age, gender, and to the best
estimation of physical activity level.

For patients receiving peritoneal dialysis therapy, the energy
provided by the absorbed glucose has to be considered in the estimation of energy requirement, particularly in those patients with
overweight or obesity. Although the extra source of energy could
be helpful for planning a high-energy diet for patients with PEW,
the constant glucose absorption may have a negative effect on
appetite.

Episodes of low energy intake because of decreased appetite are
not uncommon in patients undergoing dialysis treatment. This
condition is often challenging for the dialysis care team, and efforts should be made to identify the underlying causes of anorexia
while intensive dietary counseling should be provided. The first
step is to analyze the actual food intake through a 24-hour recall
or 3-day food record to identify potential modifications on
amounts or food choices to improve energy intake. Prescribing a
less restrictive diet and taking into considerations the patient's
food preferences can also be helpful to improve overall intake.

Additionally, lists containing high-energy density conventional foods and recipes should be provided. If no satisfactory response is achieved within a short period, renal-specific oral supplements or even tube feeding should be considered.

Protein

Chronic Kidney Disease Stages 2 to 5 Not on Maintenance Dialysis

Despite the controversies regarding the role of protein restriction in slowing progression of CKD, the benefits of such dietary manipulation in preventing or ameliorating the accumulation of nitrogen waste products, metabolic and hormonal disorders (acidosis, glucose intolerance, and hyperparathyroidism), and proteinuria are unquestionable. In addition, there is evidence that well-designed diets, planned by skilled dietitians, and followed by motivated and compliant patients are effective and do not have harmful effects on the nutritional condition.

In general, it is recommended a protein intake ranging from 0.6 g/kg/day to a maximum of 0.8 g/kg/day providing at least 50% to 60% of high-biologic-value proteins to ensure a sufficient amount of essential amino acids. For patients with CKD and diabetes, a diet with 0.8 g/kg/day has been recommended. Because typical Western diets contain larger amounts of proteins, usually between 1.0 and 1.5 g/kg/day, the initial adherence to low-protein diets is somewhat difficult. For this reason, the dietary plan should be individualized taking into account the patient food habits and preferences. Food choices lists according to the protein content are important tools to allow greater variability in the diet along with enhanced palatability. Moreover, it has been shown that compliance increases when interventions involve patient self-management, with ongoing feedback, regular monitoring, and support.

A very-low–protein diet (VLPD) supplemented with essential amino acids and keto analogues can be another dietary option, especially for patients with more advanced CKD (glomerular filtration rate [GFR] <25 mL/minute). The dietary prescription consists of a 0.3 g/kg/day of unrestricted quality protein, mainly protein from vegetable source, supplemented with a similar amount of a mixture of amino acids and keto analogues. There are several studies showing the benefits of such dietary regimens when properly conducted. Besides the expected improvement on uremic symptoms, mineral metabolism, glucose tolerance, and metabolic acidosis, a recently published study demonstrated that this dietary approach as compared with either standard low-protein diet or unrestricted diet, allowed a marked and sustained improvement of blood pressure control that was associated with a significant decrement in the extent of proteinuria. It is clear that this dietary regimen represents an important change in patient's lifestyle and is accepted by only a minority of patients even when they are greatly motivated. However, once accepted, compliance with the diet has been shown to be quite high.

Skilled dietitians are essential for planning and implement a VLPD considering the limitation of food choices, the need to achieve energy and nutrient requirements, as well as the need

Table 18-3.   Estimating protein intake by calculating protein equivalent of nitrogen appearance before and after dietary counseling

Example

Well-nourished clinically stable male patient with body weight
= 75 kg.
Prescribed conventional low-protein diet of 0.6 g/kg/day.

Equation*

PNA (g of protein/day) = (UUN [g/day] + 0.031 g N/kg/day)
× 6.25

Measurements	Before	After
UUN (g/day)	12.4	6.1
PNA (g/kg/day)	91.8	52.5
nPNA (g/kg/day)	1.22	0.7

nPNA, normalized protein nitrogen appearance; PNA, protein nitrogen appearance; UUN, 24-hour urinary urea nitrogen.
From Maroni B, Steinman TI, Mitch WA. A method for estimating nitrogen intake of patients with chronic renal failure. Kidney Int 1985;27:58–65.

to adequately control other common complications in this stage of the disease such as hyperkalemia. Thus, besides an individualized dietary plan it is important to provide the patient special recipes, menu samples, as well as food choice lists. Vitamin and iron supplements are often necessary. Additionally, constant monitoring and reinforcement by the health care team are essential to achieve compliance with low impact in the patient's quality of life.

The adherence with the dietary protein restriction can be easily monitored by calculating the nPNA when a neutral nitrogen balance is assumed. In clinical practice a neutral nitrogen balance is considered when the patient's nutritional parameters are maintained and no catabolic conditions (infection, inflammation, persistently poor glycemic control, catabolic medications) are present. Table 18-3 shows an example of calculated PNA of a patient before and after dietary counseling. As can be seen, although the prescribed amount was not fully achieved, a significant reduction in protein intake was obtained and the protein intake was no greater than 20% over the prescribed what can be considered a good compliance.

Chronic Kidney Disease Stage 5 on Maintenance Dialysis

Clinical practice guidelines recommend a dietary protein intake in the range of 1.1 to 1.2 g/kg/day in patients on maintenance dialysis. More recently, some researchers have claimed that a high protein intake may be not necessary for maintaining good nutritional status of patients on dialysis. Indeed, several studies have shown that a level of protein intake higher than 1.1 g/kg/day seems to have no further nutritional benefits. However, epidemiologic studies have suggested a survival advantage of a protein intake slightly higher. Hence, until stronger evidence is provided, the recommended values should be used as an initial guide for planning the dietary therapy. Regular clinical and nutritional monitoring allows determining with more confidence the patient's actual protein requirement. The challenge for dietitians is to keep the patient's protein intake within a range that is nutritionally safe while controlling for common metabolic disorders, in particular hyperphosphatemia, because foods with high protein content have large amounts of phosphorus as well. The approaches to deal with this particular dietary aspect are discussed below.

Low protein intake, as a result of decreased appetite or of aversion to high protein foods is usually observed in patients on hemodialysis, and for unknown reasons, it seems to be more common in patients on peritoneal dialysis. In this situation the patient should be assisted in choosing foods that have high protein content in small portions such as cheese, eggs, and lean meats. Protein bars and oral modular protein supplements can be good choices to improve protein intake. Patients should be encouraged to consume these products between meals and not as a substitute of conventional foods. To maximize the beneficial effect of a diet with higher protein content, an adequate energy intake should also be provided.

Sodium and Fluids

Chronic Kidney Disease Stages 2 to 5 Not on Maintenance Dialysis

Although the kidney's ability to excrete sodium is usually maintained intact until the GFR falls to less than 15 mL/minute, moderate sodium restriction is beneficial to control hypertension and to avoid fluid overload, particularly in patients with nephrotic syndrome, congestive heart failure, and ascites. A sodium intake below 2000 mg/day has been recommended. This amount of sodium corresponds to approximately 5 to 6 g of salt (NaCl). In patients on sodium balance, sodium intake can be estimated from the sodium excretion from a 24-hour urine collection.

To achieve a satisfactory sodium intake control, patients should be instructed to reduce at a minimum the intake of processed, canned, frozen, and fast foods. To enhance the flavor of foods cooked without salt, herbs such as parsley, chives, basil, oregano, curry, ginger, garlic, and pepper are good options. Salt substitutes should be avoided, especially in patients with stage 5 CKD because they consist mostly of potassium chloride (KCL). Fluid control is usually not necessary for patients with CKD because the thirst mechanism regulates water balance when sodium balance is well controlled. A more detailed review of this subject can be found in Chapter 15.

Chronic Kidney Disease Stage 5 on Maintenance Dialysis

Sodium and fluid restrictions are essential to control blood pressure, extracellular volume, and to avoid excessive interdialytic body weight gain in oliguric and anuric patients on maintenance dialysis. Clinical practice guidelines recommend a sodium intake of below 2000 mg/day ($\sim$5 g of NaCl). For patients on maintenance

**Table 18-4.   Selected fruits and
vegetables with high and low potassium content**

High-potassium (>200 mg per serving)
Avocado, banana, orange, papaya, melon, guava, kiwi, figs, dried
fruits, coconut water, carrots raw, tomatoes, spinach, beans, potatoes, nuts, cocoa.

Low-potassium (<200 mg per serving)
Apple, pineapple, watermelon, plums, grapes, strawberries, water-
cress, lettuce, cucumber, okra, cabbage.

hemodialysis (MHD), a low sodium intake facilitates the fluid
control by reducing thirst. Although there is a general recommendation for daily fluid intake of no more than 1000 mL plus urine
output, the interdialytic weight gain is likely to be the best way
to assess whether fluid and sodium intake are under control. A
weight gain of no more than 3.0% to 4.0% of "dry" body weight
has been recommended for patients on MHD.

Fluid restriction is one of the most demanding and difficult
components of the diet therapy for most patients on MHD. In
clinical practice some approaches such as chewing gum, eating
hard mint candies, brushing teeth often, using a few drops of
lemon in drinking water, chewing on one or two ice cubes, and
avoiding foods with great sugar and salt content can help to control thirst. Patients on peritoneal dialysis typically have fewer
problems with fluid retention. However, when it is necessary to
restrict the use of hypertonic dialysate bags, sodium and fluid
intake should be controlled to avoid fluid retention.

Potassium
Normal serum potassium is maintained during progression of
CKD as a result of increased tubular secretion of potassium and
by enhancing potassium excretion through the feces. Thus, hyperkalemia is more commonly found in patients with CKD in stages
4 or 5 when dietary potassium restriction is often necessary. Predialysis patients with normal serum potassium but with GFR
below 20 mL/min should also be instructed to avoid foods with
high potassium content (Table 18-4). A diet providing approximately 50 to 75 mmol/day of potassium should be prescribed to
patients undergoing dialysis. It is of note that several factors can
contribute to elevated serum potassium level in addition to the
dietary potassium intake and should be treated to allow a less
restrictive diet (Table 18-5).

**Table 18-5.   Factors Contributing to
Hyperkalemia in Chronic Kidney Disease**

- Constipation
- Hypercatabolism
- Angiotensin-converting enzyme inhibitor and angiotensin
  receptor 2 blocker therapies
- Beta blocker therapy
- Acidemia and hypoaldosteronism
- Hypoinsulinemia

The main sources of dietary potassium are fruits and vegetables. Significant amounts (~60%) of potassium from vegetables can be extracted by cooking processes such as soaking and boiling. Therefore, using these techniques on foods with high potassium content allows inclusion of low-potassium fresh (raw) fruits and vegetables in the dietary plan, which may guarantee a reasonable amount of essential nutrients and bioactive compounds such as vitamin C, folic acid, fiber, carotenoids, and flavonoids.

Phosphorus

Phosphate retention and/or elevated serum phosphorus are among the factors that contribute to secondary hyperparathyroidism. More importantly, elevated serum phosphorus is a risk factor for vascular calcification, all-cause and cardiovascular hospitalization, and all-cause and cardiovascular mortality. Although several factors can contribute to serum phosphorus increase, dietary phosphorus plays an important role in controlling and treating hyperphosphatemia.

Chronic Kidney Disease Stages 2 to 5 Not on Maintenance Dialysis

As kidney function declines, the ability to maintain phosphorus homeostasis is compromised. The initial compensatory mechanism to maintain phosphorus levels is a decrease in the rate of renal tubular reabsorption of phosphorus, which is partially mediated by parathyroid hormone (PTH). This usually allows the maintenance of serum phosphorus within the normal range until GFR falls below 20–25 mL/minute. At this point, the phosphorus excretion cannot compensate the phosphorus intake, and serum phosphorus increases. According to the K/DOQI Guidelines for Bone Metabolism and Disease in CKD, dietary phosphorus should be maintained between 800 and 1000 mg/day when serum phosphorus is higher than 4.6 mg/dL at stages 3 and 4 or when plasma levels of PTH are elevated above the target range. If these approaches do not result in controlling serum phosphorus, phosphate binders should be prescribed.

Phosphorus is present in a significant amount in a large number of foods, mainly in protein sources. The intestinal absorption of phosphorus derived from animal sources such as meats, eggs, and dairy products is in general quite efficient ranging from 70% to 90%. In food from vegetable sources, a significant amount of phosphorus is in the form of fitate, a nondigestible compound, resulting in low phosphorus absorption. More recently, food containing phosphate additives has been identified as another important source of phosphorus. It is estimated that the contribution of phosphorus additives for total phosphorus intake may be up to 1000 mg/day in the United States. Phosphorus additives are used by food manufacturers to ensure foods quality, flavor, and longer shelf life. The so-called convenience foods such as restructured meats, processed and spreadable cheeses, instant and refrigerated bakery products, and beverages have been pointed out as important contributors to phosphorus additives in the diet. To provide renal dietitians information regarding the phosphorus content in popular manufactured foods, a series of reports named

"Hidden Phosphorus" have been published elsewhere (see Selected Readings).

For patients with CKD stages 3 and 4 the recommended amount of phosphorus is relatively easy to achieve if the patient complies with a normal/low-protein diet. Obviously, nonprotein sources with high phosphorus content should be strongly avoided.

Chronic Kidney Disease Stage 5 on Maintenance Dialysis

The efficiency of phosphorus removal by standard dialysis schedule is quite limited. It is estimated that 800 to 1000 mg of phosphorus are eliminated in each hemodialysis session, which represents an excretion of 350 to 450 mg of phosphorus if extrapolated to 24 hours in patients with minimal residual renal function. A similar amount of phosphorus is removed daily in peritoneal dialysis. Considering intestinal phosphorus absorption of 60%, approximately 600 mg of phosphorus would be the maximum intake to balance with phosphorus removal by the dialysis. Such low phosphorus intake is incompatible with the protein requirement for most patients on dialysis therapy. Therefore, a combination of a well-planned diet with phosphate binder therapy is often necessary for maintaining serum phosphorus within acceptable values for the majority of the patients. According to the K/DOQI Guidelines for Bone Metabolism and Disease in CKD, serum phosphorus should be maintained between 3.5 and 5.5 mg/dL, and the phosphorus intake should be restricted to 800 to 1000 mg/day.

The dietary counseling should include a detailed evaluation the patient's phosphorus intake. A semiquantitative dietary frequency questionnaire focused on foods with high phosphorus content can be a useful tool to evaluate not only the phosphorus intake but also food habits and practices in a representative period of time. Together with phosphorus intake, it is important to analyze the use of phosphate binders, vitamin D, the dialysis adequacy, and the bone remodeling conditions because these factors are also determinants of serum phosphorus.

To avoid compromising protein intake at the expense of phosphorus restriction, the first step in dietary planning is to estimate the patient's protein requirement considering a minimum of 50% of high-biologic value proteins, and then to make adjustments by choosing foods with the lowest phosphorus/protein ratio (Table 18-6). It has been shown that the cooking process of boiling allows a significant reduction of the phosphorus content while preserving the protein content of beef and poultry.

The second step is to adjust the phosphate binder dose according to the amount of phosphorus in each meal and snacks. Several different types of phosphate binders are available, including calcium-based ones (calcium carbonate and calcium acetate) and noncalcium-based binders (sevelamer hydrochloride and lanthanum carbonate). Practice guidelines recommend that calcium-containing binders should be avoided if corrected serum calcium is higher than 10.2 mg/dL for patients with severe vascular and/or other soft-tissue calcification or if the total intake of calcium (binder plus diet) exceeds 2000 mg of elemental calcium. A combination of phosphate binder types is also possible whenever necessary.

**Table 18-6.   Phosphorus
content of protein-containing foods**

Food	Common Measure	Phosphorus (mg)	Protein (g)	mg P/g Protein
Beans, Legumes, Tofu				
Beans, kidney	1 cup	251	15	16.7
Beans, lima	1 cup	209	15	13.9
Beans, navy	1 cup	286	16	17.9
Beans, black	1 cup	241	15	16.1
Beans, refried	1 cup	217	14	15.5
Soybeans, boiled	1 cup	421	29	14.5
Soybeans, roasted	1 cup	624	61	10.2
Sunflower seeds	1 oz	322	6	53.7
Tofu, firm	100 g	76	6	12.7
Tofu, soft	100 g	52	4	13.0
Tofu, lite	100 g	68	5	13.6
Cheese/Cheese Products				
Cheese, cheddar	1 oz.	145	7	20.7
Cheese, Swiss	1 oz.	171	8	21.4
Cottage cheese, reg.	1 cup	297	28	10.6
Cottage cheese, 1%	1 cup	151	14	10.8
Cottage cheese, 2%	1 cup	340	31	11.0
Cottage cheese, nonfat	1 cup	151	25	6.0
Cheese, cream	2 Tb	30	2	15.0
Combination Foods				
Bean/Cheese burrito, FF	2 small	180	15	12.0
Breakfast biscuit, FF	1 egg/cheese/ bacon	459	16.3	28.2
Cheeseburger, FF	Single with condiments	310	28.2	11.0
Chicken sandwich, FF	1 sandwich	405	29.4	13.8
Fried shrimp, FF	6 to 8 small	344	18.9	18.2
Hot fudge sundae	1 small	227	5.6	40.5
Morningstar breakfast patty	1 patty	106	9.9	10.7
Pepperoni pizza, 1 slice	Frozen pepperoni	222	16	13.9
Roast beef sandwich	1 sandwich	239	21.5	11.1
Sub sandwich, FF	1 cold cuts	287	21.8	13.2
Taco, FF	Large	313	31	10.1
Dairy and Milk				
Buttermilk	1 cup	219	8	27.4
Cream, light	1 cup	192	7	27.4
Cream, sour	1 Tb	32	1.2	26.7
Cream, half and half	1 cup	230	7	32.9
Cream, heavy	1 cup	149	5	29.8
Milk, 2%	1 cup	232	8	29.0
Milk, low sodium	1 cup	209	8	26.1
Milk, nonfat	1 cup	247	8	30.9
Milk, whole	1 cup	227	8	28.4

(continued)

Table 18-6. (*continued*)

Food	Common Measure	Phosphorus (mg)	Protein (g)	mg P/g Protein
Yogurt, low fat	4 oz.	162	6	27.0
Yogurt, nonfat	4 oz.	177	6	29.5
Yogurt, reg	4 oz.	107	4	26.8
Fish and Seafood				
Crab, blue	3 oz.	175	17	10.3
Crab, Dungeness	3 oz.	149	19	7.8
Halibut	3 oz.	214	23	9.3
Oysters, fried	3 oz.	196	13	15.1
Salmon	3 oz.	282	21	13.4
Shrimp	3 oz.	116	18	6.4
Meats/Poultry/Egg				
Beef liver	3 oz.	392	23	17.0
Beef, top sirloin	3 oz.	203	25	8.1
Chicken, breast	3 oz.	196	27	7.3
Chicken, thigh	3 oz	148	22	6.7
Egg, large	1 large	86	6	14.3
Ham	3 oz.	239	19	12.6
Lamb sirloin chop	3 oz.	190	22	8.6
Pork loin	3 oz.	146	22	6.6
Turkey	3 oz.	210	28	7.5
Veal loin	3 oz.	189	22	8.6
Nuts/ Nut Butter				
Almonds	1 oz.	139	6	23.2
Macadamia	1 oz.	56	2	28.0
Peanut butter, chunky	2 Tb	101	8	12.6
Peanut butter, smooth	2 Tb	118	8	14.8
Peanuts, roasted	1 oz.	147	8	18.4
Walnuts	1 oz.	98	4	24.5
Other Sources of Phosphorus				
Beer	12 oz.	43	1	43.0
Chocolate, milk	1 miniature	95	3	31.7
Chocolate, semisweet	1 oz.	37	1	37.0
Coffee, brewed	1 cup	2.3	0	
Coffee, instant	1 tsp.	4.5	0	
Cola	12 oz.	44	0	
Lemon lime	12 oz.	0	0	
Lemonade	1 cup	5	0.3	16.7
Root beer	12 oz.	0	0	
Tea, brewed	1 cup	2.4	0	

FF, fast food; oz, ounce; Tb, tablespoon.
From NKF-K/DOQI Clinical practice guidelines for bone metabolism and disease in chronic kidney disease. Am J Kidney Dis 2003;42(Suppl 3):S1–S200, with permission.

Despite the expanding knowledge, the development of relatively efficient tools and the continued efforts of the multidisciplinary team members, the management of hyperphosphatemia is still a challenge. Although hyperphosphatemia is multifactorial, the dietary noncompliance is one of the major reasons responsible for high serum phosphorus in patients on maintenance dialysis. Studies show that several barriers are implicated in the lack of patient's dietary adherence. They include inadequate understanding of importance of strict phosphorus control, failure to understand how phosphate binders act, ignorance of the difference among food constituents, functional inability to prepare meals, and socioeconomic constrains. Therefore, intensive and focused individualized dietary counseling that includes the patients and their family in a decision-making process combined with continuing educational programs are shown to result in increased motivation and awareness with positive impact on compliance and phosphorus control.

CONCLUSION

It is clear that the nutritional management of patients with CKD is complex and demanding. The success of the dietary intervention depends on the patient's adherence, which can only be achieved by using effective tools. Despite the extensive and continually expanding scientific literature on nutrition therapy for patients with chronic kidney disease, there is still a need of well-designed, randomized, and controlled studies to identify suitable nutritional intervention approaches for implementation of the overall nutritional care.

Selected Readings

Adamasco C, D'Alessandro C, Baldi R, et al. Dietary habits and counseling focused on phosphate intake in hemodialysis patients with hyperphosphatemia. J Ren Nutr 2004;14:220–225.

Bellizzi V, Di Iorio BR, De Nicola L, et al. Very low protein diet supplemented with ketoanalogs improves blood pressure control in chronic kidney disease. Kidney Int 2007;71:245–251.

Byham-Gray LD. Weighing the evidence: energy determinations across the spectrum of kidney disease. J Ren Nutr 2006;16:17–26.

Campbell KL, Ash S, Davies PSW, et al. Randomized controlled trial of nutritional counseling on body composition and dietary intake in severe CKD. Am J Kidney Dis 2008;51:748–758.

Cuppari L, Avesani CM. Energy requirements in patients with chronic kidney disease. J Ren Nutr 2004;14:121–126.

De Brito I, Dobbie H. A randomized controlled trial of an educational intervention to improve phosphate levels in hemodialysis patients. J Ren Nutr 2003;13:267–274.

Drueke TB, Moe SM, Langman CB. Treatment approaches in CKD. In: Olgaard K, ed. Clinical Guide to Bone and Mineral Metabolism in CKD. New York: National Kidney Foundation; 2006:111–131.

Fouque D, Aparicio M. Eleven reasons to control protein intake of patients with chronic kidney disease. Nat Clin Pract Nephrol 2007; 3:383–392.

Fouque D, Kalantar-Zadeh K, Kopple J, et al. A proposed nomenclature and diagnostic criteria for protein-energy wasting in acute and chronic kidney disease. Kidney Int 2008;73:391–398.

Fouque D, Vennegoor M, Wee PT, et al. EBPG guideline on nutrition. Nephrol Dial Transplant 2007;22(Suppl 2):ii45–ii87.

Ikizler TA. Protein and energy intake in advanced chronic kidney disease: how much is too much? Semin Dial 2007;20:5–11.

Kamimura MA, Majchrzak K, Cuppari L, et al. Protein energy depletion in chronic hemodialysis patients: clinical applicability of diagnostic tools. Nutr Clin Pract 2005;20:162–175.

Mitch WE, Remuzzi G. Diets for patients with chronic kidney disease, still worth prescribing. J Am Soc Nephrol 2004;15:234–237.

Murphy-Gutekunst L. Hidden phosphorus at breakfast: Part 2. J Ren Nutr 2005;15:e1–e6.

Murphy-Gutekunst L. Hidden phosphorus-enhanced meats: Part 3. J Ren Nutr 2005;15:e1–e4.

Murphy-Gutekunst L. Hidden phosphorus in popular beverages: Part 1. J Ren Nutr 2005;15: e1–e6.

NKF-K/DOQI Clinical practice guidelines for bone metabolism and disease in chronic kidney disease. Am J Kidney Dis 2003;42 (Suppl 3):S1–S200.

NKF-K/DOQI Clinical practice guidelines for nutrition in chronic renal failure. Am J Kidney Dis 2000;35(Suppl 2):S1–S140.

Sanches FMR, Avesani CM, Kamimura MA, et al. Waist circumference and visceral fat in CKD: A cross-sectional study. Am J Kidney Dis 2008;52:66–75.

Sample Menus for Chronic Kidney Disease Patients

Jane H. Greene

MEAL PLANNING

No matter what stage of kidney disease, planning meals to meet nutritional requirements, prevent malnutrition, and maintain acceptable blood chemistries, blood pressure, and fluid status is a daunting task for any patient.

Most renal dietitians use the *average* calorie, protein, sodium, potassium, and phosphorus content for the food groups lists developed by the Renal Dietitians dietetic practice group of the American Dietetic Association when calculating a meal plan for a patient with chronic kidney disease (CKD). Steps involved to calculate a meal plan for any patient are as follows:

- Determine the nutrition prescription.
- Determine amount of high biological value (HBV) protein needed.
- Determine the number of meat and milk choices needed to supply the HBV protein.
- Distribute the remainder of protein between starch, milk substitute, fruit, and vegetable choices.
- Provide for the remainder of caloric requirements with fat and high calorie choices (foods high in carbohydrates that contain only a trace of protein and minimal electrolytes).
- Total each nutrient and adjust the diet to meet the previously established nutrition prescription.

The following sample menus and meal planning suggestions are a starting point for the health care team to assist patients and their caregivers. Each example will be based on the nutritional requirements of a 70-kg patient, using the Kidney Disease Outcomes Quality Initiative (K/DOQI) guidelines for the nutrition prescription.

CHRONIC KIDNEY DISEASE STAGES 3 AND 4

Nutrition Prescription: 0.6 g protein/kg body weight (42 g) and 30 calories/kg (2100 calories) <2400 mg sodium, 800 mg phosphorus, <2400 mg potassium.

Goals/Outcomes: prevent malnutrition, slow progression of kidney disease, decrease nitrogenous waste products, and prevent symptoms of uremia.

Meal Plan: 4 oz meat or meat substitute, 1 milk substitute, 5 starches, 3 vegetables, 1 fruit, 15 fats, and 4 high-calorie choices.

Day 1:

Breakfast: ½ cup liquid nondairy creamer, 1 cup Fruit Loops cereal, 1 medium powdered sugar donut, 1 cup Tang Breakfast drink,1 cup coffee with cream and sugar

Lunch:	Chicken salad on croissant (2 oz cooked chicken, 1 Tb mayonnaise, ¼ tsp dried tarragon, 2 Tb chopped celery), wedge of iceberg lettuce with 1 Tb Catalina dressing, poached pear with 1 Tb brown sugar, 1/4 tsp nutmeg, 12 oz lemon-lime soda
Dinner:	2 oz fish and 2 hushpuppies fried in ¼ cup olive oil, ½ cup green beans seasoned with onion, ½ cup coleslaw with 1 Tb mayonnaise, 12 oz lemonade
Snacks:	Fruit-flavored Popsicle and 8 oz cranberry juice cocktail

Nutritional Analysis: 2140 calories, 42.5 g protein, 1979 mg sodium, 803 mg phosphorus, and 1535 mg potassium.

Day 2:

Breakfast:	½ cup liquid nondairy creamer, ½ cup cream of wheat cereal, 1 Tb granulated sugar, 1 Tb unsalted tub margarine, 1 tsp cinnamon, 1 slice white bread, toasted and buttered, ½ cup red raspberries, 8 oz hot tea with 1 Tb honey
Lunch:	Chef's salad (approximately 2 cups): 1 cup red leaf lettuce, 2 Tb chopped red and yellow pepper, 2 Tb grated carrot, 2 Tb diced celery, ¼ cup cucumber slices, 4 cherry tomatoes, 1 boiled egg, diced, 3 Tb ranch dressing; 8 club crackers, 12 oz orange-flavored drink mix with sugar, ½ cup canned peaches
Dinner:	3 oz grilled pork tenderloin with rosemary and thyme, 1 cup fresh lemon rice, 6 small asparagus spears sautéed in 1 Tb olive oil, 12 oz sugar sweetened iced tea, 1 cup fruit sorbet
Snacks:	2 oz package Skittles, 1 Fruit Roll-Ups

Nutritional Analysis: 2122 calories, 41.8 gm protein, 1855 mg sodium, 1909 mg potassium, and 784 mg phosphorus.

- Patients should be warned that many "fresh" pork and chicken cuts are actually "processed" to improve moisture and flavor when cooked. Patients should avoid any cuts of meat with the following claim: "Enhanced up to 10% with solution containing water, salt, and sodium phosphate."
- **Dietary Reference Intake:** The diet for CKD contains less than the Dietary Reference Intake (DRI) for several water-soluble vitamins because of the restriction of high protein and high potassium foods.

Chronic Kidney Disease Stage 5—Hemodialysis

Nutrition Prescription: 1.2 g protein/kg body weight (84 g protein) and 35 calories/kg (2450 calories) <2400 mg sodium, <1200 mg phosphorus, and <2400 mg potassium with 1000 mL fluid restriction.

Goals/Outcomes: adequate protein and calorie intake to maintain nutritional status, interdialytic fluid weight gains within acceptable range, laboratory values within acceptable range, blood pressure within appropriate limits, and level of functional ability maintained.

Meal Plan: 8 oz meat or meat substitute, 1 milk, 9 starches, 4 vegetables, 4 fruits, 6 fats, and 4 high-calorie choices.

Day 1 (nondialysis day):

Breakfast:	½ cup fresh blueberries, 1 cup frosted corn flakes, 4 oz 2% milk, 1 scrambled egg, 1 toaster muffin, 6 oz brewed coffee with nondairy creamer and sugar
Lunch:	2 slices white bread, ½ cup low sodium, water-packed tuna, 1 Tb mayonnaise with 2 tsp sweet pickle relish and ¼ tsp celery seed and lettuce leaf, ½ cup carrot sticks, ½ cup sweetened applesauce, 10 vanilla wafers, 8 oz lemon-flavored drink mix with sugar
Dinner:	4 oz braised chuck roast, ½ cup parsley buttered noodles, ½ cup frozen French-style green beans, 1½–2 cups tossed salad: Bibb lettuce, red and yellow bell pepper strips, sliced cucumbers, 2 Tb Catalina dressing, dinner roll with 2 Tb unsalted tub margarine, ½ cup fruit sorbet, 8 oz iced tea with sugar
Snack:	2 Fruit Roll-Ups

Nutritional Analysis: 900 mL fluid, 2327 calories, 81.5 gm protein, 2519 mg sodium, 1120 mg phosphorus, and 2267 mg potassium.

Day 2 (dialysis day)

Breakfast:	4 oz grape juice, 2 scrambled eggs, 2 slices lower sodium bacon, 2 slices white bread, toasted, 2 Tb unsalted tub margarine, 2 Tb blackberry jam, 8 oz brewed coffee with sugar and creamer
After dialysis: Meal:	Frozen microwave meal with at least 18–20 g protein and <600 mg sodium, 8 oz cranberry juice cocktail, 1 pouch chewy fruit snacks
Third meal:	½ cup chicken salad with mayonnaise, tarragon, and chopped celery in medium pita bread, fresh pear, 10 vanilla wafers, 8 oz can of renal nutritional supplement (NovaSource Renal, Nutren Renal, or Nepro)

Nutritional Analysis: 840 mL fluid, ~2450 calories, ~85 g protein, ~2200 mg sodium, <2000 mg potassium, and <1200 mg phosphorus.

- Dialysis patients may be tired and not interested in cooking on the days they receive their hemodialysis treatment. Offering ideas for quick meals at home and nutritional supplements could prevent a trip to the drive-thru window for a high-sodium fast-food meal on the way home.
- **Dietary Reference Intake:** The diet for hemodialysis patients contains less than the daily recommended intake for several water-soluble vitamins because of the restriction of

Table 19-1. Nutrition recommendations for the immediate posttransplant recovery phase

Goals	1. Promote wound healing 2. Promote anabolism 3. Prevent infection 4. Minimize side effects of medications
Nutrient requirements	**Recommendations**
Calories	• 1.3–1.5 (BEE or 30–35 kcal/kg dry wt or wt, adjusted for obesity)
Protein	• 1.3–2.0 g/kg dry wt or wt, adjusted for obesity
Carbohydrate	• 50%–70% nonprotein kcal; diabetic diet as appropriate
Fat	• 30%–50% nonprotein kcal
Fluid	• Ad lib or 1.0 mL/kg dry wt; increase intake to equal output unless diuresis is goal
Vitamins	• RDA; supplementation usually not necessary
Minerals	• Sodium: 4.0 g/day or no added salt; unrestricted if HTN/edema absent • Potassium: unrestricted unless necessary • Calcium: 1000–1500 mg/day; supplement if necessary • Phosphorus: supplementation may be necessary • Magnesium: supplementation may be necessary

BEE, basal energy expenditure; HTN, hypertension; RDA, recommended dietary allowance.

foods high in potassium and phosphorus, dialysate losses, and decreased intestinal absorption.

Kidney Transplant (Table 19-1)

Kidney Transplant—Maintenance Needs

Nutrition Prescription: 1 g protein/kg body weight (70 g protein) and 25 to 30 cal/kg body weight (1750–2100 calories or adequate to maintain desirable weight), fat <30% total calories (70 g total fat for 2100 calories) with <300 mg cholesterol/day. Vitamins and minerals, restrict or supplement as needed to meet recommended daily intake.

Goals/Outcomes: achieve or maintain desirable weight, maintain acceptable blood glucose levels, maintain serum cholesterol levels <200 mg/dL, maintain normal blood pressure, maintain optimal bone density, minimize side effects of medications, and maintain healthy lifestyle.

Meal Plan: 6 oz lean meat or meat substitute, 1 cup skim or 1% milk, 8 starches, 3 vegetables, 4 fruits, 5 servings of mono- or polyunsaturated oils, minimal sweets.

Day 1:

Breakfast: ¾ cup oatmeal, ½ cup blueberries, 8 oz skim milk, 1 slice whole grain toast, 2 tsp tub margarine, 2 tsp jelly, 4 oz orange juice, coffee or tea

Lunch: 3 oz turkey breast, 2 slices whole grain bread, lettuce, tomato, mustard, 1 cup carrot sticks, ½ cup apple, celery and walnut salad, iced tea

Dinner: 3 oz flank steak, steamed broccoli with lemon, small baked potato, 2 tsp tub margarine, 1 slice Italian bread, ½ cup sliced strawberries, 1 slice angel food cake, iced tea

Nutritional Analysis: 1776 calories, 74 g protein, 39 g fat.

Subject Index

Page numbers followed by *f* or *t* indicate material in figures or tables, respectively.